SHORT-TERM COUPLE THERAPY

THE GUILFORD FAMILY THERAPY SERIES
Michael P. Nichols, Series Editor

Recent Volumes

Short-Term Couple Therapy

Edited by

JAMES M. DONOVAN

THE GUILFORD PRESS
New York   London

© 1999 The Guilford Press
A Division of Guilford Publications, Inc.
72 Spring Street, New York, NY 10012
http://www.guilford.com

Printed in the United States of America

This book is printed on acid-free paper.

Last digit is print number: 9 8 7 6 5

Library of Congress Cataloging-in-Publication Data

Short-term couple therapy / edited by James M. Donovan.
        p.   cm.—(The Guilford family therapy series)
    Includes bibliographic references and index.
    ISBN 1-57230-431-6 (hc.)   ISBN 1-57230-833-8 (pbk.)
    1. Marital psychotherapy. 2. Brief psychotherapy.
    I. Donovan, James M.   II. Series.
RC488.5.S497 1999
616.89′156—dc21   98-32163
                                                          CIP

To Connie, Liz, Abbie, Brian—
Thank you for teaching me long-term
family therapy at its best . . .

ABOUT THE EDITOR

James M. Donovan, PhD, received his undergraduate education at Stanford University and his doctorate from the University of Michigan. A veteran of HMO mental health work, he has served as staff psychologist at Harvard Community Health Plan, now Harvard Vanguard Medical Associates, for 25 years. Dr. Donovan founded and has codirected the Mental Health Fellowship at Harvard Pilgrim Health Care for 15 years and is Assistant Professor of Psychiatry in Psychology at Harvard Medical School.

CONTRIBUTORS

Simon Budman, PhD, Innovative Training Systems, Inc., Newton, Massachusetts

Andrew Christensen, PhD, Psychology Department, University of California, Los Angeles, Los Angeles, California

Phyllis M. Cohen, PhD, New Hope Guild Center, Brooklyn, New York; Department of Applied Psychology, New York University, New York

Victoria C. Dickerson, Bay Area Family Therapy Training Associates, Cupertino, California

Kathleen Eldridge, MA, Psychology Department, University of California, Los Angeles, Los Angeles, California

Joseph B. Eron, PsyD, Catskill Family Institute, Kingston, New York

Leo F. Fay, PhD, Department of Sociology and Anthropology, Fairfield University, Fairfield, Connecticut

Thomas F. Fogarty, MD, Center for Family Learning, Rye Brook, New York

Steven Friedman, PhD, Beacon Health Strategies, Boston, Massachusetts; Lesley College Graduate School, Cambridge, Massachusetts

Philip J. Guerin, Jr., MD, Center for Family Learning, Rye Brook, New York

Neil S. Jacobson, PhD, Department of Psychology, University of Washington, Seattle, Washington

Susan M. Johnson, EdD, Department of Psychology, University of Ottawa, Ottawa, Ontario, Canada

Judith G. Kautto, ACSW, Center for Family Learning, Rye Brook, New York

James Keim, MSW, LCSW, Department of Social Work, Colorado State University, Fort Collins, Colorado

Erika Lawrence, MA, Psychology Department, University of California, Los Angeles, Los Angeles, California

Eve Lipchik, MSW, ICF Consultants, Inc., Milwaukee, Wisconsin

Thomas W. Lund, PsyD, Catskill Family Institute, Kingston, New York

Salvador Minuchin, MD, Family Studies, Inc., Boston, Massachusetts

John H. Neal, PhD, Mental Research Institute, Palo Alto, California; Department of Psychiatry and Behavioral Sciences, Stanford Medical School, Stanford, California

Michael P. Nichols, PhD, Department of Psychology, College of William & Mary, Williamsburg, Virginia

Richard Vogel, PhD, San Francisco Psychotherapy Research Group, San Francisco, California

Daniel B. Wile, PhD, private practice, Oakland, California

Jeffrey L. Zimmerman, Bay Area Family Therapy Training Associates, Cupertino, California

PREFACE

When an angry couple walks through your door, it is important to know where to turn for guidance about what to do. Should you draw from your training as a family therapist, or should you draw from what you have learned doing individual therapy? What should you tackle first, especially if there will be only a few sessions and a lot of work to do? The picture gets complex quickly. We hope this book will help guide you to choose the intervention that best suits the situation and your own theoretical background.

Couple therapy is a kind of stepchild treatment. It mixes both family therapy and individual therapy. It has traditionally been time-limited, yet the principles of short-term couple therapy have never been closely defined. In this book I have brought together some of the key people whose work with couples distinguishes them. They describe various approaches and show how these can be conducted in an effective, time-managed way. Perhaps the book will point toward a clearer understanding of what works and what doesn't—doing brief therapy with couples—and will help bring couple therapy more in the main body of therapeutic practice.

As therapists, we all want to add new approaches and techniques to our repertoire. But for me, as an avid reader of psychotherapy books, though I have often been intrigued by a new approach, I have been frustrated because the writer has not told me what he or she actually does with clients. I say to myself, "This sounds interesting and creative, but how should I change what I say to my patient?" Perhaps you've had the same experience? Understanding theory is not enough. We need to see the sequential stages of the treatment and see examples of specific interventions in which the approach is applied to the type of case we might encounter tomorrow in the office. I wanted this volume to be a guidebook to therapeutic models, something any therapist could consult for real direction about what to say and when to say it.

To this end I have shamelessly nagged my authors to be more specific, to label the stages of change illustrated by each intervention, and to explain why they chose the tact they did and why it carried the power it did. Brief therapy only works when there is a clear plan of action. It is not the same old long-term therapy tape played at fast forward. The authors in this book needed to explain how to find the focus quickly, how to stick to it, how to quickly form a therapeutic alliance and plan treatment, how to introduce reframing of events, how to be active without being overly intrusive, and how to deal with strong affect but not be submerged by it. I am grateful that the authors agreed with my plan to explicate brief couple therapy more specifically and then patiently crafted their chapters with this objective in mind. They took time from other projects and heard perhaps more about sentence structure, punctuation, and clarity than they may have, at first, felt they were signing up for. I appreciate their hard work and perseverance and hope they are as proud of the outcome as I am.

I am grateful also to Kitty Moore, my editor at The Guilford Press, for her patience as submission of the final manuscript was delayed again and again. Kitty understood that a good book about brief therapy cannot necessarily be completed briefly.

Most of all I am indebted to Michael P. Nichols, editor of The Guilford Family Therapy Series, for his X-ray editorial vision. Mike looks at a paragraph, a sentence, or even a word, sees to its core, and judges whether it captures the meaning the writer intended. Without him, this book would definitely have suffered in quality.

I am grateful, too, to the Harvard Pilgrim Health Care Foundation for giving me continued intellectual and clerical support through its Teaching Center. Lynda Pozerski did a great deal of typing and suffered evening emergency calls with characteristic good nature.

Our patients also deserve great thanks. Nothing cuts so deeply into people's self-esteem and ego-ideal than the fear that they might not be as good a parent or marital partner as they thought. It takes courage to lay themselves bare in front of a stranger and admit shortcomings in these, the two most important roles in life. Couple treatment, challenging for the therapist, is even more demanding for the patient, who must be an observer, a learner, and a completely personally involved participant, all simultaneously. Without our courageous patients, there would be no time-effective couple therapy for us to explore and write about.

JAMES M. DONOVAN
Chestnut Hill, MA

CONTENTS

1

—◄o►—

SHORT-TERM COUPLE THERAPY AND THE PRINCIPLES OF BRIEF TREATMENT

JAMES M. DONOVAN

Forty percent of mental health referrals involve marital conflict (Budman & Gurman, 1988). Some 120 million patients receive their mental health coverage through one or another managed care arrangement (Shore, 1996). If we ever needed workable models of time-effective couple therapy, we need them now.

In the preface, I emphasized the need for a practical, specific guide to what actually works and doesn't work in brief treatment with couples, but there are other reasons I edited this volume. Effective time-managed therapy for couples clearly represents a key goal for mental health practitioners, but couple therapy has an identity problem, which we address in this book. No one seems sure whether couple treatment is individual therapy in double focus, a subspecialty of family work, or some unique enterprise (Gerson, 1996). Marital counseling, in various formats, has been with us for decades (Nichols & Schwartz, 1998), but couple therapy as a definitive treatment form has only come into its own in the last decade (Jacobson & Gurman, 1995). Couple therapy is, thus, a less mature field than its close cousins on either side—short-term individual therapy (see Gustafson, 1986, and Budman & Gurman, 1988) and family therapy (see Nichols & Schwartz, 1998). As recently as

1

1991, Susan Johnson noted that we still lack a comprehensive theory of couple intimacy and therefore of marital dysfunction on which to base our work (Johnson, 1991).

We constructed this book to assemble examples of the major schools of short-term couple therapy in one place. An examination of the similarities and differences between these approaches represents the only reliable method to ascertain the present conceptual and technical state of the field. Our hope is that the book will then propel couple therapy toward a consolidation phase, one reached by short-term individual therapy and family therapy in recent years. These two other fields of psychotherapy boast many well-defined schools of approach, multiple treatment manuals, substantial outcome statistics covering many methods, and their own journals. By illustrating where we are now in the field, perhaps we can take stock and outline where we need to go next.

"Couple therapy" is part of our title, and an additional reason for writing the book can be found in the title as well. Couple treatment is the only form of psychotherapy that began as *brief therapy* (Budman & Gurman, 1988). (Freud originally conceived of psychoanalysis as a short treatment, but as we see today, it became the longest of all therapies.) Two-thirds of couple treatment still comprises fewer than 20 sessions (Budman & Gurman, 1988), so when we refer to couple treatment, we are inevitably speaking of a brief modality.

With the advent, some would say the outbreak, of managed care, practicing brief therapy has become singularly important. Brief treatment is not just rapid long-term therapy, it carries specific principles of its own that we will learn much more about as we study each chapter. The book, then, is about *couple therapy* but also about how to do time-effective treatment. The balance of this chapter outlines the important principles about brief therapy.

In this volume we encounter a spectrum of approaches: dynamic–gestalt (Johnson), structural (Nichols and Minuchin), narrative (Neal, Zimmerman, and Dickerson), solution-focused (Friedman and Lipchik), and on and on. Neither research evidence (Johnson, 1991), nor clinical experience, nor common sense, can persuade us that one model here is superior to others. Couple therapy will never have a world series or choose a most valuable player. Rather than competitively contrasting our models, it seems more rewarding to trace the common struggles of our authors and to search for parallel elements in the models that they have constructed to help couples toward effective change within the brief therapy format.

Reading through the chapters, we discover that all the authors, sometimes explicitly, sometimes not, grasp and then integrate within their systems at least six principles of brief therapy. These represent the same action premises that organized the work of the brief individual treatment pioneers 20 years earlier (Donovan, 1998). We will encounter these six guidelines frequently, so let's name them now:

1. Find the focus.
2. Maintain flexibility.
3. Build affective intensity.
4. Encourage the alliance.
5. Arrange an emotionally affirming experience.
6. Plan the treatment.

The differences among the models emerge from the alternate positions that our writers assume on each of these principles, but if the treatment promises efficacy and brevity, each of these six sign posts that mark the trail must be carefully observed and heeded.

PRINCIPLE 1: FIND THE FOCUS

If the three most important attributes of real estate are location, location, location, then the three most important features of time-effective therapy are *focus, focus,* and *focus.* Our practitioners ask themselves again and again what emotional conflict, blurred boundary, behavioral snare, or misplaced view of self lies at the core of this couple's dilemma? How will I clarify, deepen, or reframe that focus to bring it to the center of the treatment?

Susan Johnson searches for the point of "emotional softening." Does fear of abandonment underlie the angry wife's tirade as she lashes out at her withdrawn husband? Steven Friedman and Eve Lipchik hunt for positive interactions between the couple and use these as an antidote to the problem-laden story. Richard Vogel looks for the pathogenic belief in one partner that will explain his or her proclivity to respond in some unhelpful way: to withdraw, explode, or provoke.

The landscape becomes more cluttered, though, the further we study the focus. The authors choose their focus based on a conceptual framework, which underlies their approach. Johnson relies on Bowlby's attachment theory to help her understand the largely unconscious affects surrounding loss of connection. These she will map as she pursues an intervention that will help the couple share an empathic experience. One partner must "soften" in his or her affective response to the other. Michael Nichols and Salvador Minuchin keep a structural framework as they search for enmeshed boundaries in the family seated before them, the nexus of the couple or family conflict. To develop an understanding of each author's approach, examine first his or her *theoretical base.*

Understanding the different approaches becomes still more complex, since each author has developed *core technical maneuvers* that will allow him or her access to the focus he or she seeks. Joseph Eron and Thomas Lund know a great deal about enlarging upon preferred views of self. Susan Johnson has become expert at integrating into the couple's relationship the repressed affect behind their paralyzed stance. I comb the past of the patient and bring it into the present at the right moment: "Your mother was hypochondriacal. You learned to ignore her, but what will you do now with your wife's current complaints?" Study the core techniques that emerge from each theory that the authors use to work their focus.

PRINCIPLE 2: MAINTAIN FLEXIBILITY

However artfully framed the focus, and well-honed the core techniques, brief therapy provides little time to convince the patient of your point of view. Therapists practicing brief couple therapy have learned to flexibly engage patients no matter what their thoughts and feelings when they first come for treatment. Alexander and French (1946), the grandfathers of today's brief treatment, articulated the principle of flexibility early and often in their remarkably modern 1946 book describing short-term dynamic therapy. In one celebrated case, Alexander tolerated rebelliousness at the hands of the glass manufacturer's son because this was exactly the relationship offer that the patient's father could not abide. Eron and Lund and Friedman and Lipchik place flexibility at the center of their approaches and encourage us to understand and work with the patient's world view and preferred view of self from the very first phone call. Different authors promote flexibility in different ways, again consistent with their theoretical outlook. Flexibility, however, remains at the center of time-managed couple therapy.

Flexibility does not imply a free-for-all treatment in which anything goes. Each writer grapples with the question of *patient selection*. Not every set of clients is encouraged to continue with couple therapy after the assessment period. Again proceeding from their theory and their core techniques, Johnson and Erika Lawrence, Kathleen Eldridge, Andrew Christensen, and Neil Jacobson designate the first three or four sessions as evaluative. I organize a pregroup workshop before offering couples group therapy. Daniel Wile, though, is less concerned with exclusionary criteria and is more likely to start right out in helping his couple partners construct a shared platform from which to view their relationship.

All our authors engage a wide variety of patients in their treatment, espousing as they do the principle of flexibility, but most exclude psychotic, actively addicted, or assaultive individuals. Trace how these writers confront and work with the patient selection issue.

PRINCIPLE 3: MANAGE THE EMOTIONAL INTENSITY—TO STOKE THE FIRE OR COOL THE JETS?

Brief, dynamic, individual therapists assumed that change could only come through stirring emotional intensity. Malan (1963), Davanloo (1980), and Gustafson (1986), as a central technique of their therapies, attempted to put the patient in touch with as much of his or her true feelings as he or she could tolerate at any given moment. Johnson and I stand as the couple therapy heirs to Malan, Davanloo, and Gustafson. Johnson's therapy turns on the breakthrough of "hard" feelings into the "soft" emotions beneath. Anger covers fear of abandonment. Silent withdrawal masks confusion and guilt. I, too, search for the affect. I push my patients to connect the bitter disappointments of the past with the present marital conflict.

Wile takes a midway position on emotional expression. He coaches his couples to feel entitled to their affective storms and to incorporate these reactions into the relationship conversation. However, he is not primarily interested in fanning the coals to create greater heat. Friedman and Lipchik and Eron and Lund attempt to circumnavigate the tornado of feeling by emphasizing present positive experiences and resurrecting the preferred views of self within the relationship. We know all too vividly that couples present with plenty of emotional intensity. All our authors assume a definitive position toward that intensity dictated by their conceptual stance and enacted through their core clinical techniques. The fascination comes in the different paths that therapists take as they confront the affective storm.

PRINCIPLE 4: BUILD THE ALLIANCE

Brief therapists have learned that the satisfactory engagement of Principles 1–3 helps foster the therapeutic alliance. Gustafson (1995) repeats the one common finding across all psychotherapy research: Positive therapeutic alliance abets positive outcome, and negative alliance, negative outcome. The couple must feel that the therapist has grasped their most important issue (the focus), that he or she can tolerate their most disturbing feelings (emotional intensity), and that the clinician accepts them in the distressed condition in which they arrive (flexibility).

Once again our authors build the alliance according to their own theories and move toward it with their own techniques. The Lawrence, Eldridge, Christensen, and Jacobson camp work hard to reduce the couple's polarization by increasing emotional acceptance. Then the partners will be sufficiently allied with each other and with the therapist to enter fully into the behavioral exchange and communication problem training, the second half of the treatment, which will increase their intimacy and satisfaction. Johnson's empathy with the hidden affective dilemma of each member of her couples helps each individual feel understood and attached, so they can reattach with each other in Steps 6 and 7 of her model. Johnson reports that her research on emotionally focused therapy suggests that therapeutic alliance, once again, is the most important predictor of positive outcome.

Whatever their approach to alliance building, it remains a high priority for our therapists, and they are willing to work for it, each in his or her own way.

PRINCIPLE 5: ARRANGE AN AFFIRMING EMOTIONAL EXPERIENCE

Every couple's treatment begins with more of the same. The members of the couple share their fight with their therapist by reenacting it for him or her. Each partner first enters the office feeling confused, blamed, frightened, angry, bitter, and most of all, powerless to alter the destructive downward plunge of this important relationship. Demoralization is the order of the day. To address this despair, any brief treatment, and particularly couple treatment, must offer an affirming emotional experience—"a new ending to an old beginning" (Alexander & French, 1946). Or, as Budman, Hoyt, and Friedman (1992) tell us, the time-effective therapist must rapidly introduce novelty into this complex situation to shed light on the first steps out. Implicitly or explicitly, our therapists guide their patients toward experiences and actions that lead to empowering capabilities, the only real antidote to their desperation.

The novelty introduced, of course, differs from therapist to therapist and reflects their core techniques. Wile teaches his couples to discuss the fight openly and to include it in their relationship. When they do this, they have a plan and a methodology to use that renders them less powerless and returns them to the status of communicative adults, actively working toward shared goals. Friedman and Lipchik immediately start their couples in search of overlooked positive experiences in their relationship. Eron and Lund, from the first minute, work to help the partners reconnect with their preferred view of self through which they can activate solutions to their dilemma.

I help my couples to see that their fighting makes psychological sense, given their past family experiences, and then guide them in developing "tools" to understand and redirect the "fight." Eschewing subtlety, as is my wont, I exhort my patients to apply the just-learned techniques.

> "Paul, you've gained a new tool here. If you act condescendingly when Mary complains, you can always arrange a fight, but when you ask sincerely, 'Okay, tell me all your feelings about this; I'll help if I can,' then you've learned you simply aren't going to have a fight, and you'll gain some new knowledge in the process."

Note the number of optimistic, action words I have unconsciously piled into my coaching, "gained," "new tool," "learned," "gain" (again), "new knowledge." To avoid the trap of the fight, the patient must act in his or her own constructive fashion, the efficacy of which he or she already has proof.

We now have a hint about the secret of the emotionally affirming experience. The new skills need to be nurtured *less* with the therapist and *more* with the couple. The affirming emotional experience works outside the office as well—the true novelty. When members of the couple can practice and gain confidence in their "new tools," they no longer must travel to see their therapist. The treatment becomes both brief and effective.

PRINCIPLE 6: PLAN THE TREATMENT

"If you want therapy to be brief, plan it as brief" (S. Budman, personal communication, February 15, 1997). Malan (1963) and Mann (1973) demonstrated that treatment could be effectively planned within a preset number of sessions. My couples group always lasts 15 sessions, never more, never less. But Eron and Lund spy the possible pitfall here—the therapist can become procrustean and attempt to constrain therapy within too rigid a time limit. Both practitioner and patient might then lose confidence if positive change does not quickly appear. Better to keep the focus, nurture the alliance, search for the new perspective, and let these forces control the time limit. Budman, Eron and Lund, and Phyllis Cohen space sessions more widely later on as couples practice their new skills. Therapy can be brief in number of sessions but long in elapsed

time. All our authors agree, however, that termination must be anticipated and planned for rather than allowed to arrive willy-nilly.

Another planning dimension seems more subtle but carries equal
importance. The therapy needs to unfold in a series of *general phases* so
that therapists can gauge the couple's journey within the treatment plan
as it develops. Johnson knows that if "softenings" seem few and hard to
find by Session 7 or 8, her therapy is in trouble. I stay alert for couples
who have yet to begin to process the fight psychologically by session 6
of my group or who have fashioned few tools by Session 12. Therapists
need not view such aberrant courses with undue alarm, but they need to
actively intervene to nudge their couples back on track. The lack of a
therapy template introduces a virus into the system by exposing the
treatment to the potential of uneven progress or the unfortunate surprise
of a patient dropout: no therapy template, no safeguard for self-
correction.

Not all of our authors describe definite phases of treatment. The
postmodernists—for example, John Neal, Jeffrey Zimmerman, and Victoria Dickerson, and Friedman and Lipchik—stand resolutely as "anti-
pattern and anti-normative structures" (S. Friedman, personal communication, March 20, 1997). They attempt to "co-create" a new language
and a new conversation with each new client. However, a general outline of what to expect remains necessary for the working therapist and
for us, the students. How to begin most treatments seems plain. How to
end also clear, particularly if the outcome is a happy one, but the curative action tends to take place in the middle acts of the play. The therapist and the student must approach these middle sections alertly, learn
how to recognize each, and how to predict which stage comes next.

Obviously no practitioner can or should plan a therapy in minute
detail; this would violate the principle of flexibility. Therapists do need a
good guidebook for the journey, though, and should be able to chart their
location landmark by landmark. If they can't, they need to ask why.

CONCLUSION

Our introduction is becoming a place in which several truths about
short-term couple treatment are revealed ahead of time. The last of these
is that no one principle of time-effective therapy assumes more importance than another. The pioneers of brief individual treatment Malan,
Mann, and Gustafson learned that the most important principle was to
practice with all the principles in mind. Leave out any at your peril. Our
authors heed the same warning; we find most of our six principles fully
on display in chapter after chapter.

Our writers have allowed us the privilege of entering their minds and their offices as they take on the exciting challenge of explaining and illustrating the brief couple therapy models they've worked so hard to develop. The education in this book can be found in the details. It's important to study exactly how our experts apply their trade. With which conceptual framework do the writers venture forth? What are their core techniques? How do our authors achieve focus, promote flexibility, build the alliance, and regulate emotional intensity? How do they use treatment planning to augment the strength of their interventions?

No book can substitute for actual clinical experience. However, our writers have given us a file of road maps. We must choose a few and start on the trip on our own, but we can refer back to this volume when we begin to lose our way.

REFERENCES

Alexander, F., & French, T. M. (1946). *Psychoanalytic therapy: Principles and applications.* New York: Ronald Press.

Budman, S. H., & Gurman, A. S. (1988). *Theory and practice of brief therapy.* New York: Guilford Press.

Budman, S. H., Hoyt, M. F., & Friedman, S. (1992). *The first session in brief therapy.* New York: Guilford Press.

Davanloo, H. (Ed.). (1980). *Short term dynamic psychotherapy.* New York: Jason Aronson.

Donovan, J. M. (1998). Brief couples therapy: Lessons from the history of brief individual treatment. *Psychotherapy, 35,* 116–129.

Gerson, M. J. (1996). *The embedded self.* Hillsdale, NJ: Analytic Press.

Gustafson, J. P. (1986). *The complex secret of brief psychotherapy.* New York: Norton.

Gustafson, J. P. (1995). *Brief versus long psychotherapy.* Northvale, NJ: Jason Aronson.

Jacobson, N. S., & Gurman, A. S. (Eds.). (1995). *Clinical handbook of couple therapy.* New York: Guilford Press.

Johnson, S. M. (1991). Marital therapy: Issues and challenges. *Journal of Psychiatric Neuroscience, 16,* 176–181.

Malan, D. H. (1963). *A study of brief psychotherapy.* New York: Plenum Press.

Mann, J. (1973). *Time limited psychotherapy.* Cambridge, MA: Harvard University Press.

Nichols, M. P., & Schwartz, R. C. (1998). *Family therapy: Concepts and methods* (4th ed.). Boston: Allyn & Bacon.

Shore, M. F. (1996). An overview of managed behavioral health care. In M. F. Shore (Ed.), *Managed care, the private sector and Medicaid: Mental health and substance abuse services.* San Francisco: Jossey-Bass.

PART I

◄○►

PSYCHODYNAMIC
METHODS

Spread across my living room floor are the 15 chapters that comprise the body of this book. I ponder the order of presentation—which should come first and which chapters should be grouped together? The pieces describe a wide spectrum of approaches indeed. It's tempting, but a disservice to our understanding, to round off the corners and present different approaches as if they were more similar than they really are. However some models do, in fact, hold more in common with others. Eron and Lund, and Friedman and Lipchik offer quite similar approaches to each other and quite different ones from Johnson's or my own, for example.

I've decided to begin with psychodynamic methods—partly because these are close to traditional, psychoanalytically oriented therapy and therefore perhaps more familiar to a general readership. I then move to systemic models, then advance toward collaborative approaches, and close with representatives of the postmodern school. In a very rough way, this arrangement reflects the historical evolution of the field. Psychodynamic writings preceded systemic work, which, in turn, preceded collaborative models. The postmodern approaches appeared last chronologically.

My chapter, as well as the ones by Johnson and Vogel, are psychodynamically oriented, since they help patients to bring their unconscious or unacknowledged feelings to the surface of their awareness. Johnson supports partners of her couples to feel the "softer" affects beneath their angry recriminations. Mutual experience of these affects then allows the partners of the couple to bond more closely. In my couples group, interestingly the only group model in the book, I help my patients bear their anxiety and suspend their defenses to feel their fears and their anger. These affects acknowledged, the members of the couples can move, less defensively, to develop their own particular strategies to help them find their way through their fight. Vogel supports one or both partners to discover unconscious survivor or separation guilt, which explains their need to explode, withdraw, or provoke.

As well as introducing a panoply of important, specific techniques for couple intervention, these chapters illustrate one common crucial assumption. For the pair to change, there must be a breakthrough into previously unconscious or preconscious feelings and insights. The remaining models in the book do not, for the most part, share this assumption, which poses a fascinating controversy in the field, for us, the students, to wrestle with as we read on.

JAMES M. DONOVAN

2

◄◦►

EMOTIONALLY FOCUSED
COUPLE THERAPY

Straight to the Heart

SUSAN M. JOHNSON

Emotionally focused couple therapy (EFT; Johnson, 1996; Greenberg &
Johnson, 1988) is an effective short-term approach to modifying distressed couples' constricted interaction patterns and emotional responses
and fostering the development of a secure emotional bond. Such bonds
are powerfully associated with physical and emotional health and well-
being, with resilience in the face of stress and trauma, with optimal personality development, and with adaptation to the environment (Willis,
1991; House, Landis, & Umberson, 1988; Feeney & Ryan, 1994;
Burman & Margolin, 1992; Mikulincer, Florian, & Weller, 1993). Perhaps because of this focus on the creation of secure bonds, over the last
decade, EFT has also been used to successfully address marital distress
complicated by other problems such as depression, posttraumatic stress
disorder (PTSD), and chronic physical illness (Johnson & Williams
Keeler, 1998). EFT is now one of the best empirically validated
approaches to changing distressed relationships (Baucom, Shoham,
Mueser, Daiuto, & Stickle, 1998; Alexander, Holtzworth-Munroe, &
Jameson, 1994; Dunn & Schwebel, 1995). Research has clarified how
the process of change occurs (Johnson & Greenberg, 1988) and who is
best suited to this kind of intervention (Johnson & Talitman, 1997). A
version of EFT is also used with families (Johnson, 1996, 1998). EFT

also compares well with other approaches in terms of treatment effect sizes (Johnson, Hunsley, Greenberg, & Schindler, 1999), rates of recovery and improvement, and evidence of long-term effectiveness (Gordon Walker, Manion, & Cloutier, 1998) after relatively short treatment (10 sessions; Gordon Walker, Johnson, Manion, & Cloutier, 1996).

To create lasting change in a brief and efficient manner, a treatment approach should optimally have certain characteristics. It should be founded on a clear, empirically validated theory of dysfunction and health, that is, the target of interventions and the goals of the change process should be as specific as possible. Interventions should be clearly specified. The therapist must know not only *what* to do and *how* to do it but *when* particular interventions are required. The change process in therapy should be specified so that the therapist knows when he or she is on track, and there should be some evidence as to how to match client to treatment. The treatment model should also be able to deal with the fact that marital distress often occurs in tandem with other problems and symptoms. The literature on EFT addresses the issues outlined above (Johnson, 1996). EFT is able to create change efficiently, perhaps because this approach integrates the intrapsychic and the interpersonal, using the compelling power of emotion to restructure the drama of distressed relationships and choreographing powerful bonding events that redefine the attachment bond between partners.

THE EFT PERSPECTIVE ON MARITAL DISTRESS AND ADULT INTIMACY: THE THEORETICAL MODEL

EFT assumes that the key factors in marital distress are the ongoing construction of absorbing states of distressed affect and the constrained, destructive interactional patterns that arise from, reflect, and then in turn prime this affect. This assumption combines an experiential intrapsychic focus on inner experience, particularly affect, with a systemic focus on cyclical self-reinforcing interactional responses. This focus on affect and interaction, and how they create and reflect each other, echoes the empirical work of John Gottman (1991). Gottman emphasizes the power of negative affect, as expressed in facial expression, to predict long-term stability and satisfaction in relationships and the destructive impact of repeated cycles of interaction, such as criticize and defend or complain and stonewall. The inability of distressed couples to sustain emotional engagement is also noted in this research (Gottman & Levenson, 1986) and appears more central in maintaining distress than the number of disagreements or whether disagreements can be resolved. Gottman notes that there appear to be differences in affect regulation between men and women. Women seem to be more able to regulate their affect in interpersonal conflict and therefore more often seem to take the complaining position, whereas their male partners withdraw to contain their affect. Gottman's thorough and empirically validated description of marital distress and his ability to predict marital outcomes suggest that emotional responses and particular self-reinforcing interaction patterns are the most appropriate targets of intervention in marital therapy (Gottman, 1994).

To understand why affect and the interactional patterns outlined above are so central to marital distress, we need to place these empirical findings in the context of a theory of relationship. Marital therapy has, in general, lacked a clear theory of adult intimacy and therefore a clear sense of the primary goals and targets for the change process and of what constitutes health in relationships (Manus, 1966; Segraves, 1990; Roberts, 1992). If a therapy is to be brief, it's crucial to define what specific changes are necessary to create recovery from distress and promote long-term health and resilience. We must define what difference will really make a difference.

One theory that has come to the fore to provide a rich theoretical context for understanding adult intimacy is attachment theory (Bowlby, 1969; Hazan & Shaver, 1987). This theory was first elaborated in the context of parent–child relationships and has now been applied to adult bonds. From an attachment perspective, the description of marital distress outlined above is best understood in terms of separation distress and an insecure bond. A bond here refers to an emotional tie, a set of attachment behaviors to create and manage proximity to the attachment figure and a set of working models, or what are usually termed "schemas." These schemas are concerned with the dependability of others and the worth or lovableness of self.

Attachment theory states that compelling fear, anger, and sadness will automatically arise when an attachment figure is perceived as inaccessible or unresponsive. These emotions have what Tronick (1989) terms control precedence; they override other cues. Seeking and maintaining contact with others are viewed as the primary motivating principles in human beings and an innate survival mechanism, providing us with a safe haven and a secure base in a potentially dangerous world (Bowlby, 1988). When attachment security is threatened, affect organizes attachment responses into predictable sequences. Bowlby suggests that, typically, protest and anger will be the first response to such a threat, followed by some form of clinging and seeking, which then gives way to depression and despair. Finally, if the attachment figure doesn't respond, detachment and separation will occur. The potential loss of an attachment figure, or even an ongoing inability to define the relationship as generally secure, is significant enough to prime automatic fight, flight, or freeze responses that limit information processing and constrict interactional responses (Johnson, 1996). So a husband corners his wife and yells "kiss me" in enraged protest at his wife's unresponsiveness, and so he ensures that she will completely shut him out. Fear narrows options.

Much of the research on adult attachment has concerned attachment styles. These styles can be seen in terms of the answer to the crucial question, "Can I count on this person to be there for me if I need him or her?" (Hazan & Shaver, 1994). There are a limited number of answers to this question and limited ways of dealing with these answers. Attachment styles, expectations, and responses formulated in past relationships help to create present interactions, and, in turn, present interactions tend to mitigate or intensify a person's habitual style. Many partners basically believe that significant others will be there if they need them and are able to trust their partners; they have a secure attachment style. They tend to see others as reliable and themselves as lovable and worthy of care. They are able to process attachment information, give clear emotional signals when their attachment needs arise, and they tend to feel confident enough to assert themselves in the face of the differences that inevitably arise in any long-term relationship. If and when a bond is threatened, they can then respond with resourceful flexibility. If, however, the answer to the question above is a tentative "maybe," and the attachment is thus defined as anxiously insecure, partners tend either to cling to attachment figures or aggressively demand reassurance, often fearing that they are somehow deficient or unlovable. If the answer to the above question is "no," partners tend to avoid closeness with others, exhibiting an avoidant, fearful style, or they tend to deny their need for attachment and frame others as untrustworthy, displaying an avoidant, dismissing attachment style (Bartholomew & Horowitz, 1991).

Insecure attachment styles, then, predispose people to certain predictable emotional responses and behavior and ways of experiencing self and other that make the repair of distressed relationships more difficult and help maintain marital distress. For example, avoidantly attached partners tend to particularly restrict contact when they or their partners are most anxious and in need of comfort (Simpson, Rholes, & Nelligan, 1992). A husband says, "It's not that I don't care. I get overwhelmed. I'm not sure how to comfort you. I'm scared that I won't do it right. So I freeze and withdraw. I guess this happens just when you need me the most."

Attachment theory provides a map for adult intimate relationships.

It outlines attachment needs for contact, comfort, security, and closeness as the features that define this landscape. These needs are viewed as adaptive and inherently human, rather than in any way a reflection of immaturity or pathology (Bowlby, 1988). This perspective is consonant with new directions in feminist thought (Jordan, Kaplan, Miller, Stiver, & Surrey, 1991) that stress the definition of self in relation to others, rather than in terms of self-sufficiency and separateness. It's not attachment needs themselves that are problematic in distressed relationships. It is, rather, how partners process and enact such needs in a context of perceived danger and insecurity that primes this distress (Johnson, 1996).

Attachment theory has room for the consideration of both self and system, inner experience and organized interaction with others. It takes into account both the past, reflected in habitual attachment styles, and the present ongoing interactions, which may modify such styles. Attachment theory is, then, nonpathologizing and interactional and now has a considerable research base as a theory of adult love and relatedness (Bartholomew & Perlman, 1994; Shaver & Hazan, 1993).

An attachment perspective focuses the couple therapist on attachment insecurities, longings, and needs. It stresses the significance of experiences of deprivation and loss of trust and connection. It directs the process of therapy toward the creation of the accessibility and responsiveness that foster safe emotional engagement. Such engagement encourages partners to express their attachment needs. This perspective also gives us a potent and useful way of reframing typical problematic behaviors to make them accessible to reorganization. For example, angry blaming is viewed most often as an attempt to modify the partner's inaccessibility and a protest response to abandonment. Distancing is often framed as a way of regulating fears of loss or avoiding anticipated feedback about the self's unworthiness. This perspective also allows us to reframe each partner's responses in a manner that fosters compassion and contact. For example, an anxious partner's critical pursuit of the other may be framed as a fear of loss and a compelling desire for reassurance rather than as a desire for control or as hostility. These kinds of reframes then help the other partner to respond more positively. In general, placing distressed responses in an attachment context allows spouses to see and relate to their partner's pain. Partners talk in life and death terms about key interactions in attachment relationships. This is because they are facing basic concerns about security and contact and how they are defined by the person they depend on the most: So a wife says to her spouse, "You watch me drown. You don't respond. You throw me away like I am nothing."

In terms of the process of change, attachment theory directs the therapist's attention to the accessing and reprocessing of attachment-related affect, the modifying of interactions that block contact, and the creation of bonding interactions. It also stresses the need for exploring and sometimes modifying the working models of self and other that underlie negative attribution patterns and so help to maintain marital distress.

This theory also complements Gottman's research on the importance of affect in the definition of close relationships. In attachment theory, emotion may be seen as alerting partners to the significance and nature of key relational experiences, evoking working models in a state-dependent fashion (when I'm anxious, I easily formulate all my fears about myself) and, most importantly for the couple therapist, priming attachment behaviors. In constructivist terms, emotion is seen as an organizing force in the processing of attachment information and the definition of the nature of the bond between partners. Emotion is the music of the attachment dance (Johnson, 1996). In marital distress, this interactional dance and each partner's experience of the relationship are constricted by compelling attachment fears and insecurities. The role of affect in close relationships and the change process in therapy are addressed further in the intervention section of this chapter.

The goals of EFT, which arise out of this attachment perspective and the view of marital distress summarized above, are: first, to expand attachment-related affect and so expand interactional positions, so when I experience and express my fear rather than my anger, I take a less dominating and more contactful stance with my partner; second, to do this in a manner that fosters emotional engagement, the expression of bonding needs and the attainment of comfort and security. EFT is conducted in 8 to 20 sessions in which the therapist uses both experiential techniques to explore and reconstruct the key emotional responses that arise in the session and directive, systemic techniques to shape new interactions. Change strategies occur in the context of a positive therapeutic alliance that provides a secure base (Bowlby, 1988) for the therapy process. The role of the therapist is that of a process consultant, working with partners to construct new experiences and new interactions that redefine their relationship.

KEY PHASES IN TREATMENT

The process of change in EFT has been delineated in nine treatment steps. The first four steps involve assessment and the deescalation of problematic interactional cycles. The middle steps (5–7) emphasize the creation of specific change events where interactional positions shift, and new bonding experiences occur. The last two steps of therapy (8–9) address the consolidation of change and the integration of these changes into the everyday life of the couple. These steps are described in linear form. In fact, the therapist circles through them in spiral fashion as one step incorporates and leads into another. In a mildly distressed, securely attached couple, the partners generally work quickly through the steps at a parallel rate. In more distressed couples, the more passive or withdrawn partner is usually invited to go through the steps slightly ahead of the other. The increased emotional engagement of this partner then helps the other more active, critical partner shift to a more trusting stance.

The nine steps of EFT are as follows:

Cycle deescalation

Step 1 Assessment. Creating an alliance and explicating the core issues in the marital conflict using an attachment perspective.

Step 2 Identifying the problem interactional cycle that maintains attachment insecurity and marital distress.

Step 3 Accessing the unacknowledged emotions underlying interactional positions.

Step 4 Reframing the problem in terms of the cycle, the underlying emotions, and attachment needs.

Changing interactional positions

Step 5 Promoting identification with disowned needs and aspects of self and integrating these into relationship interactions.

Step 6 Promoting acceptance of the partner's new construction of experience in the relationship and new interactional behavior.

Step 7 Facilitating the expression of specific needs and wants and creating emotional engagement. Key change events, withdrawer reengagement and blamer softening, evolve here. The events are completed in Step 7. When both partners complete Step 7, a prototypical bonding event usually occurs, either in the session or at home.

Consolidation/integration

Step 8 Facilitating the emergence of new solutions to old problematic relationship issues.

Step 9 Consolidating new positions and new cycles of attachment behavior.

In all of these steps, the therapist moves between: first, helping partners to crystallize their emotional experience in the present, tracking, reflecting, and then expanding this experience; and second, setting interactional tasks that add new elements to and reorganize the interactional cycle. The therapist might, then, first help a withdrawn, guarded spouse formulate his sense of paralyzed helplessness that primes his withdrawal, then help the partner to hear his experience, and finally move to structure an interaction around this helplessness: as in, "So can you turn your chair, please, and can you tell her, 'I feel so helplessness and defeated. I just want to get away and hide.'" This kind of statement, in and of itself, represents a move away from passive withdrawal and the beginning of active emotional engagement. The steps of EFT are described in greater detail elsewhere (Johnson, 1996, 1998).

Stages of Therapy

In terms of the change process, it is especially helpful to the therapist who is committed to brief structured interventions to delineate key change events in the therapy, so that the process stays focused and on course. In EFT, the first shift, which usually occurs at the end of Step 4, is a deescalation of the negative cycle. This is a first-order change (Watzlawick, Weakland, & Fisch, 1974). The way interactions are organized hasn't changed, but the nature of the elements has. Reactive emotional responses are less intense; negative attributions about the partner are less rigidly held, and responses toward the spouse are generally less extreme. Partners are more hopeful and experience the therapy sessions as a safe place to learn about their relationship. The couple begins to risk more engagement and to view the cycle as the enemy, rather than the other spouse. If the partners have very different agendas for therapy, for example, if one has already emotionally divorced the other, this may be the end of the therapy process. The therapist is able at this point to clarify the nature of the present relationship and the choices open to the couple. In most couples, however, this shift sets the stage for the work of second-order change, reorganizing the interactional dance in the direction of safe attachment. At this point, a partner might say, "Well, things are better. We're fighting less, and I see him a little differently, but it's a truce. He still runs and hides, and I still go for him. We're still not dancing in the dark together."

In the middle stage of therapy (Steps 5–7) there are two change events that are crucial turning points in EFT. The first is withdrawer reengagement where this partner changes his or her interactional position and becomes more active in defining the relationship and more accessible to his or her partner. So, for example, a silent and always distant partner might become angry and assert her need for respect and support in the relationship in a way that gives her mate a chance to respond to that need.

The second change event, a softening, occurs when a previously critical, active spouse is able to risk expressing needs and vulnerabilities and to begin to trustingly engage with his or her partner. Research on the process of change has found that this event predicts recovery from marital distress in EFT (Johnson & Greenberg, 1988). If there is only partial engagement in these change events, or if the couple reach an impasse here, the relationship may still improve, but the impact of therapy will be less potent. For example, problem cycles will have diminished, but the trust in the relationship is often limited, since positions are essentially unchanged. Bonding is then also circumscribed, and the couple are more susceptible to relapse. Transcripts and detailed descriptions of a softening can be found elsewhere (Johnson & Greenberg, 1995; Johnson & Williams-Keeler, 1998).

This softening event is a shift in the critical partner's position, both in terms of affiliation and control, that then restructures the cycle of interactions. In its final stages, it is also a prototypical bonding event where two now accessible partners initiate a new cycle characterized by engagement and responsiveness. This kind of bonding event (occurring when the second partner completes Step 7) has the ability, because of its emotional salience in terms of basic attachment needs, to heal past injuries and wounds in the relationship and to redefine the nature of the bond. So a critical, often accusing partner is able to share his deep fears of loss and abandonment and let himself be comforted and reassured by the partner. He then experiences a shift from isolation to connectedness and from frustration in the face of the problem cycle to a sense of efficacy in the creation of a new kind of relationship. Once this kind of change event has occurred, the couple naturally moves into consolidating this new positive cycle and begin effectively problem solving conflictual, pragmatic issues.

ASSESSMENT AND THE SELECTION OF CLIENTS

In brief therapy, it's particularly important to have some way of matching client to treatment. Addressing this issue, first, EFT is not used for couples where abuse is an ongoing part of the relationship and is used only in an abbreviated form (as referred to above) for couples who are separating. Abusive partners are referred to group or individual therapy to help them deal with their anger and abusive behavior. They are offered EFT only after this therapy is completed and their partners no longer feel at risk. It is important that the latter is used as a criterion for readiness for marital therapy rather than the abusive partner's assessment that his or her behavior is now under control. The goal of treatment, after the assessment, is then to encourage the abusive spouse to enter treatment and the victimized partner to seek supportive counseling or individual therapy.

Research on success in EFT (Johnson & Talitman, 1997) allows us to make some specific predictions as to who will benefit from EFT. First, the quality of the alliance with the therapist predicts success in EFT. This is to be expected; it is a general finding in research on all forms of psychotherapy that a positive alliance is associated with success, However, to be more specific, the quality of the alliance in EFT seems to be a much more powerful and general predictor of treatment success than initial distress level. In our study, initial distress level was not an important predictor of success 3 months after therapy. This is an unusual finding because initial distress level is usually by far the best predictor of long-term success in marital therapy (Whisman & Jacobson, 1990).

In addition, our research indicated that the perceived relevance of the tasks of therapy seems to be the most important aspect of the alliance. Perceived task relevance was more central than a positive bond with the therapist or a sense of shared goals. The couple's ability to join with the therapist in a collaborative alliance and to view the tasks of EFT, tasks that focus on issues such as safety, trust, and control, as personally relevant seem to be crucial. This may, of course, also be a reflection of the therapist's skill in presenting these tasks and in creating an alliance. Generally, this research suggests that EFT works best for couples who still have an emotional investment in their relationship and therefore some willingness to genuinely engage in the therapy process and who are able to see their problems in terms of insecure attachment and conflicts around closeness and distance. These results suggest that the first concern of the EFT therapist must be to form and maintain a strong supportive alliance with each of the partners. EFT interventions are only as potent as the alliance.

A lack of expressiveness or of emotional awareness has not been found to hamper the EFT change process. In fact, EFT seems to be particularly powerful in helping male partners who are described by their partners as inexpressive. This may be because when such partners are able to discover and express their experience, the results are often compelling, both for them and for their partners. Traditional relationships, where the man is oriented to independence and is often unexpressive while the woman is oriented to affiliation, were found to be responsive to EFT interventions. EFT was also more effective with older men (over 35), who may be more responsive to a focus on intimacy and attachment.

The female partner's initial level of trust, specifically her faith that her partner still cared for her, was a very strong predictor of treatment success. In a culture in which women have traditionally taken most of the responsibility for maintaining close bonds in families, if the female partner no longer has this faith that her partner cares for her, this may define the bond as nonviable and may stifle the emotional investment necessary for change. Accumulating evidence suggests that emotional disengagement, rather than factors such as the inability to resolve disagreements, is predictive of long-term marital unhappiness and instability (Gottman, 1994) and of lack of success in marital therapy in general (Jacobson & Addis, 1993). Low levels of this element of trust may then be a bad prognostic indicator for couples engaging in any form of marital therapy. In these particular situations, the EFT therapist might then help a couple to clarify their goals and the limits of their engagement. For example, in a small number of cases, the couple may curtail the cycle of distress by choosing to redefine their relationship as a parallel friendship, without expectations of romance or closeness.

Unfortunately marital distress often occurs hand in hand with other symptoms and problems, particularly clinical depression. The brief therapist then has to find a way to address these issues in an integrated fashion, that is to address how these individual symptoms and the distressed marital interactions prime and maintain each other. If not addressed, these individual problems tend to undermine progress in redefining the relationship. Conversely, if they are successfully addressed, the therapist is often able to "kill two birds with one stone." There is empirical evidence that EFT is effective with depressed partners (Dessaulles, 1991; Gordon Walker, 1991). Marital discord is the most common life stressor that precedes the onset of depression, and 25-fold increased risk rate for depression has been reported for those who are unhappily married (Weissman, 1987). Research also demonstrates that EFT works well with couples experiencing chronic family stress and grief, for example families with chronically ill children (Gordon Walker et al., 1996). EFT has also been used for couples where one partner is suffering from PTSD resulting from physical illness, violent crime, or childhood sexual abuse (Johnson & Williams-Keeler, 1998). These clients have typically received some individual therapy before requesting marital therapy and may be referred by their individual therapist, who recognizes the need to address marital issues. Trauma increases the need for protective attachments and, at the same time, undermines the ability to trust and therefore to build such attachments. If the marital therapist can foster the development of a secure bond between the partners, this not only improves the marital relationship but also helps partners to deal with the trauma and mitigate its long-term effects. So a spouse might say to his partner, "I want you to be able to feel safe in my arms and to rest in that safe place when the ghosts come for you. I can help you fight them off."

PLANNING TREATMENT AND
BUILDING AN ALLIANCE

In the initial sessions of EFT, we assess the nature of the problem and the strengths of the relationship by listening to the couple's history of their relationship and their current difficulties, eliciting specific descriptions of problematic responses and incidents, for example, the most recent fight, and inviting the couple to interact in the session. We also probe for instances when the couple partners have experienced their relationship as satisfying and supportive and their understanding of the shift into the problem cycle. We also elicit a very brief personal history from each person. This focuses upon their attachment history, including questions such as "Who were you close to growing up?" "Who held and comforted you?" It's pertinent for the EFT therapist to know if partners have experienced safe attachment with this partner, any partner, or any attachment figure, and if partners have been traumatized in close relationships. We track and reflect sequences of interaction and begin to formulate and reflect each partner's habitual position in the relationship. Consonant with the nonpathologizing stance of EFT, we validate each partner's construction of his or her emotional experience and place this experience in the context of the pattern of interactions. This reflection and validation not only focuses assessment on affect and interaction and encourages disclosure, but it also immediately begins to forge a strong alliance. A focus on the problem interactions or cycles allows us to frame both partners as victims, to assign responsibility without blame, and to begin to link the couple against these cycles. The cycles then become their common enemy.

Assessment and the formation of an alliance are not separate from treatment in EFT; they are an integral part of active treatment. By the end of the first or second session, we usually have a clear sense of the typical problem interactions (e.g., "I feel alone and frustrated, so I pick at you. You feel lost and confused and become intellectual and distant. I then intensify my barbs. You shut down and avoid me for 2 or 3 days."). At this point, we can also assess the strengths of the relationship and form hypotheses as to key underlying emotions and definitions of self and other that operate at an implicit level in the couple's interactions. We actively intervene with the couple and assess how open the partners are and how easy they will be to engage in therapy. From the beginning, the EFT therapist is active and directs the partners' disclosures toward attachment-salient interactions, attributions, and emotional responses. We check with the couple as to their specific treatment goals and formulate a therapy contract briefly describing the process of treatment, setting an expectation that treatment will be concluded in approximately 8 to 15 sessions. We encourage couples to view us as consultants, who can be corrected and who will need their active participation to redefine their relationship. We then can admit mistakes and allow clients to teach us about their unique experience and their relationship.

The creation of the alliance in EFT is based on the techniques of experiential therapy (Rogers, 1951; Greenberg, Rice, & Elliott, 1993). The EFT therapist focuses upon empathic attunement, acceptance, and genuineness. We assume that the alliance must always be monitored and any potential break in this alliance must be attended to and repaired before therapy can continue. The alliance is viewed in attachment terms as a secure base that allows for the exploration and reformulation of emotional experience and engagement in potentially threatening interactions. We begin by taking people as they are (Johnson, 1996). We then try, by the leap of imagination that is empathy (Guerney, 1994), to understand the valid and legitimate reasons for their manner of relating to each other and exactly how this maintains their marital distress. The therapist must be able to validate each partner's experience of the relationship without blaming or invalidating the other. We acknowledge that partners will perceive the relationship differently and are doing their best to protect themselves and the relationship within the present narrow cycles of interaction.

CORE INTERVENTIONS

There are two basic therapeutic tasks in EFT, the exploration and reformulation of emotional experience and the restructuring of interactions. Before describing the interventions associated with these tasks, it is pertinent to discuss briefly the role and significance of emotion as it is conceptualized in this approach.

Emotion, here, refers to a small number of basic universal affects: anger, fear, surprise, hurt/distress, shame, sadness/despair, and joy (Plutchik, 1980). An emotional response integrates physiological arousal, meaning schemes, and action tendencies. For example, I see a movement; I feel hot; I decide it's a tiger, and I run. Emotion gives us compelling feedback as to how our environment is affecting us, organizing and priming us to respond to this impact. It often takes control precedence and overrides other cues, especially in attachment relationships. Specifically, in such relationships, emotion is first a major organizer of responses to our partner and second, emotional expression is a regulator of key dimensions of social interaction, such as closeness/distance and control/submission.

In terms of organizing our experience of and response to significant others, emotion is designed to rapidly reorganize behavior in the interests of security and the fulfillment of basic needs. In intimate relationships, emotion orients us to our own needs as well as colors environmental cues and meanings. So when I'm angry, I focus on my injury and the need implicit in that injury. In a state-dependent fashion, I also recall all the other times when this need has been frustrated, and I move rapidly to address the situation, perhaps by protesting and demanding a response from my partner. Emotion particularly primes attachment behaviors (when I'm afraid, I move closer to you and seek out comfort). It also activates associated core definitions of self and other. For example, my hurt at your criticism touches all my doubts about my own adequacy and worth.

In terms of regulating social interaction, emotional expression, especially tone of voice and facial expression, communicates to others in a manner that defines the nature of a particular relationship and pulls for particular responses. For example, the expression of vulnerability tends to disarm and invite approach. The power of emotion is such that, if unaddressed, it can also easily undermine or block shifts in cognition and behavior by igniting fight or flight responses. If used in the process of change, emotion also has the power to elicit key responses that cannot be elicited by any other means, such as affection and compassionate comforting that can rapidly redefine the attachment relationship and prime new positive behaviors.

The EFT therapist begins by reflecting and validating the secondary reactive responses (see Johnson & Greenberg, 1994, for a discussion of different kinds of affect) that the couple displays, such as anger. The therapist then expands these responses into the primary underlying emotions that are often unattended to, undifferentiated or disowned, and so remain unexpressed in the relationship, such as the hurt underlying rage. Emotion in EFT isn't simply discussed from a distance or relabeled. It is evoked and developed by helping clients to focus on the leading edge of experience and to differentiate new elements in that experience. For example, numbness, when explored, might first become hopelessness and then defiance. A partner might say, "I give up. I can't do it. Then I say to myself, 'I'm not even going to try.'" This defiance may then be used by the therapist to create new kinds of interactions; it could, for example, be used to prime engaged assertiveness.

How does the therapist know which emotion to focus on? The therapist focuses on (1) the most present poignant emotions that arise in the therapy process, the nonverbal gesture, or the "hot" image; (2) the emotion that's most salient in terms of attachment needs and fears; and (3) the emotion that seems to organize problem interactions or has the potential to organize positive ones. For example, the therapist might highlight the look of relief on a husband's face when his partner says that she "interrogates" him out of fear, not out of hostility or contempt. Fear is addressed extensively in EFT, primarily because fear especially constricts and constrains both information processing and interactional responses.

Exploring and Reformulating Emotion

The following interventions are used in EFT to address this task.

Tracking and Reflecting Emotional Experience

Example: "Could you help me to understand? I think you're saying that you are so caught up with your own feelings and how to deal with them that you find it hard to even make sense of his response; everything seems confusing and overwhelming, is that it?"

Main functions: Focusing the therapy process; building and maintaining the alliance; clarifying emotional responses underlying interactional positions.

Validation

Example: "You feel so alarmed that you can't even focus. When we're that afraid, we can't even concentrate, is that it?"

Main functions: Legitimizing responses and supporting clients to continue to explore how they construct their experience and their interactions; building the alliance.

Evocative Responding: Expanding by Open Questions the Stimulus, Bodily Response, Associated Desires, and Meanings or Action Tendency

Examples: "What's happening right now, as you say that?" "What's that like for you?" "So when this occurs, some part of you just wants to run, run and hide?"

Main functions: Expanding elements of experience to facilitate the reorganization of that experience; formulating unclear elements of experience and encouraging exploration and engagement.

Heightening: Using Repetition, Images, Metaphors, or Enactments

Examples: "So could you say that again, directly to her, that you do shut her out?" "It seems like this is so difficult for you, like climbing a cliff, so scary." "Can you turn to him and tell him, 'It's too hard to ask. It's too hard to ask you to take my hand'? "

Main functions: Highlighting key experiences that organize responses to the partner and new formulations of experience that will reorganize the interaction.

Empathic Conjecture or Interpretation

Example: "You don't believe it's possible that anyone could see this part of you and still accept you, is that right? So you have no choice but to hide?"

Main functions: Clarifying and formulating new meanings, especially regarding interactional positions and definitions of self.

These interventions are discussed in more detail elsewhere, together with markers or cues as to when specific interventions are used and descriptions of the process partners engage in as a result of each intervention (Johnson, 1996).

Restructuring Interventions

The following interventions are used in EFT to address this task.

Tracking, Reflecting, and Replaying Interactions

Examples: "So what just happened here? It seemed like you turned from your anger for a moment and appealed to him. Is that okay? But Jim, you were paying attention to the anger and stayed behind your barricade, yes?"

Main functions: Slows down and clarifies steps in the interactional dance; replays key interactional sequences.

Reframing in the Context of the Cycle and Attachment Processes

Example: "You freeze because you feel like you're right on the edge of losing her, yes?" "You freeze because she matters so much to you, not because you don't care."

Main functions: Shifts the meaning of specific responses and fosters more positive perceptions of the partner.

Restructuring and Shaping Interactions: Enacting Present Positions, Enacting New Behaviors Based upon New Emotional Responses, and Choreographing Specific Change Events

Examples: "Can you tell him, 'I'm going to shut you out. You don't get to devastate me again'? " "This is the first time you've ever mentioned being ashamed. Could you tell him about that shame?" "Can you ask him, please?" "Can you ask him for what you need?"

Main functions: Clarifies and expands negative interaction patterns, creates new kinds of dialogue and new interactional steps/positions, leading to positive cycles of accessibility and responsiveness.

TERMINATION

In this phase of treatment, the therapist is less directive, and the couple themselves begin the process of consolidating their new interactional positions and finding new solutions to problematic issues in a collaborative way. We emphasize each partner's shifts in position. For example, we frame a more passive and withdrawn husband as now powerful and able to help his spouse deal with her attachment fears, while this spouse is framed as needing his support. We support constructive patterns of interaction and help the couple put together a narrative that captures the change that has occurred in therapy and the nature of the new relationship. We stress the ways the couple have found to exit from the problem cycle and create closeness and safety. Any relapses are also discussed and normalized. If these interactions occur, they are shorter, less alarming, and are processed differently, so they have less impact on the definition of the relationship. The couple's goals for their future together are also discussed, as are any fears around terminating the sessions. At this point, the couple express more confidence in their relationship and are ready to leave therapy. We offer couples the possibility of future booster sessions, but this is placed in the context of future crises triggered from outside the relationship, rather than any expectation that they will need such sessions to deal with marital problems per se. For example, a couple returned for three sessions of therapy after their son had been killed in an accident.

CASE DESCRIPTION AND TRANSCRIPT

As they walked into my office, I had the image of an annoyed Doris Day marching ahead of a laconic John Wayne. Clara was a pretty lady in her 60s, and she had been married to Len, her tall gangly partner, for 40 years. He grinned at me and lounged in the chair, apparently very relaxed, and he spoke in a slow drawl. She, on the other hand, sat on the edge of her chair, alert and tight-lipped. They immediately told me with pride that they had three children, all of whom had left home, and two grandchildren. Len was a high-profile politician going through the process of retiring as therapy started. They were referred by Len's individual therapist who was treating him for a recent depression. This depression had developed after Len decided to retire because of his arthritis. Clara had undergone treatment for lung cancer the year before. She told me in a steady voice that she felt that she had beaten the disease. However she understood that there was a high risk of recurrence. Clara described the problem between them as "constant bickering" and said that unless something changed she was going to leave Len and "find some peace." Clara referred to a particular past episode again and again. In this episode, Len had become very stressed and overwhelmed in his job and had pressured Clara to help run his office. Clara said passionately, "I hated this job. I told him again and again that I had to stop. I told him the job was killing me." She described how he had minimized her distress at the time, and he continued to do so in the session. He laconically told her that she was exaggerating, turning to me and telling me that "she really didn't mind that much." As he smiled at me and informed me that his wife would "calm down in a minute," she spat out angrily that he had pressured her to keep on running the office for a year until she had been diagnosed with cancer. His unwillingness to listen to her was then associated with the occurrence of a life-threatening illness.

Len and Clara played out the dominant cycle in their relationship while discussing this incident. She attacked him, saying "You discounted me and only took care of yourself, and I hate you for this." He dismissed her statement, responding with, "It wasn't that bad, and you don't hate me, and I took care of you when you were ill." As Len defended himself in a calm reasoning manner, Clara became more and more enraged. "I'm tired of being told how I feel and who I am," she said. "This has gone on for 15 years, and now I'm on the point of leaving." Len's manner immediately changed when she said this. He went still and silent. He then turned to me and began to tell me a rambling detailed story designed to prove his point that Clara hadn't been that upset about working in his office. Clara looked like she was going to explode and then sighed and told me in a quiet hopeless tone, "He buries me in words." She commented that this kind of interaction occurred frequently at home and that this kind of stress "was going to make me sick again." As she said this, he furrowed his brow and looked really upset for the first time in the session.

In the EFT model, the episode that Clara described might be labeled as an attachment "crime" or "injury." Clara had expressed her exhaustion and distress and Len had not responded. He had discounted her pain and remained inaccessible, both in the past and in the current dialogue. Underlying many such attachment injuries, that continue to define the relationship, is a potent experience of danger or physical threat in which the partner was perceived as failing to provide caring and protection.

Clara and Len presented with a classic complain/attack versus stonewall/defend cycle. In this case, Len was withdrawn and also clinically depressed. He was also facing a significant life transition that he experienced as an enormous loss. In the past Clara had usually initiated closeness, but she had now put up a "wall." Len commented that he would try to cuddle her in the mornings in bed, but he often felt "pushed away." Again and again he would comment to me, "She exaggerates; she gets wild-eyed over nothing." Clara acknowledged that Len had taken care of her when she was ill with cancer, but then she wagged her finger at him, saying, "Mostly though, through the years, you've taught me to be alone and put your career first." Illness was very present in this relationship. Clara's sister had recently died of cancer, her daughter was ill, and the specter of a possible remission of Clara's cancer was always present. She said with tears in her eyes, "If I have a shortened life to live, I'm determined not to live it in a box, with him sitting on the lid. I'm tired of trying to get through to him."

After the initial sessions and the building of an alliance, we articulated the interactional cycle described above, putting each person's responses in the context of the other's behavior (Step 2). The couple were framed as victims of this cycle of angry complaint and rational defense. This cycle had robbed them of the comfort and closeness they had experienced at previous times in their relationship. They told their story of the evolution of the relationship. Clara stated that for many years she "had allowed him to define reality," and Len admitted that he had been "rather authoritarian." She felt "bullied by his impenetrable rationalizing." He spoke of the need to convince her to "dampen down her feelings about a few isolated negative incidents." Past events in Len and Clara's personal histories and in the history of the relationship were only pursued if they were directly relevant to present attachment issues and problematic interactions. For example, Len pointed out that, in his career, there were many times when it was very important for him to stay calm and rationalize people's complaints. I used this to validate his style, and we were then able to talk about how, here, it simply seemed to make his wife more angry and desperate.

I then helped the couple to move into Step 3 of therapy, exploring the emotions underlying their interactional positions. Len began to talk about his hurt at being "shut out" by Clara and by her threats to leave him. I focused on his voice and facial expression rather than his words and helped him formulate that he was "sad" and "in shock." I helped him talk about his fear of losing Clara, either through her angry distancing, her leaving the relationship, and/or through a recurrence of her illness. We began to talk about how this fear paralyzed him. Clara spoke of her sense of having no impact on Len, no way of getting him to acknowledge her hurt and desperateness, and so alternating between rage and helplessness. I helped Len to articulate that the loss of his career, where he felt affirmed and valued, had left him feeling vulnerable and sensitive to Clara's criticism. She was able to talk of how she felt abandoned and disqualified by his "denials and discounts" and now by his withdrawal into depression. I framed both of them as isolated and vulnerable and as having lost a sense of control over their lives and their relationship.

The experience and expression of the emotions implicit in the interactional cycle began to expand the dialogue, and moments of engagement began to occur. For example, when Clara talked openly of her cancer, Len was able to directly express his fear of losing her. She was touched by this. She commented to him, "I never knew you were that worried. Maybe you're just trying to calm yourself down with all that rationalizing. I thought you were just trying to bully me." Then she reached over and laid her hand on his arm.

I set interactional tasks based on these emotional responses that promoted the deescalation of the problem cycle and the beginnings of emotional engagement. For example, I asked Len to talk to Clara about how he had lost his sense of power and competence when he retired. Together we articulated that his "job" now was to take care of her and he "didn't know how to do it." "In fact," he said "I'm blowing it. I'm failing." His response to this sense of failure was then to feel hopeless and to withdraw. She began to view his withdrawal in terms of how much impact she had, rather than how little. He became less distant and self-protective, and she became less angry and blaming. At this point, (Step 4), they talked about the cycle and their "sensitivities" as the problem. They were kinder to each other. The cycle had deescalated, and we were through Stage 1.

In Steps 5 and 6 of EFT, first one partner and then the other formulates and expresses attachment-related affect in a way that fosters acceptance from the other and rapidly reorganizes attachment behaviors. In Session 6, Len began to express with much weeping how terrified he was of her anger and of hearing her say that he'd failed her. Her illness, his retirement, and his own depression had all intensified his awareness of how much he needed her. As we explored what happened to him when he got the message that he was disappointing her, he was able to describe the "panic" that preceded his attempts to "cool down" her anger. He was then able to move to Step 7 (creating emotional engagement) and ask her to stop threatening to leave and to control her rage, so that he could, as he put it, "learn to take care of her and become good at this new job." His reengagement then allowed her to move into formulating her sense of helplessness when he did not recognize her experience and her need for his validation and comfort. She moved in terms of her interactional position from a blaming stance to expressing her fear of having her pain denied and therefore being abandoned. She said to him, "It's too scary to count on you when you don't even seem to see or hear me." Both partners were now much more available and responsive to each other and were able to comfort each other.

A new cycle of closeness and comfort began, and this couple was able to create pragmatic solutions to old issues (Step 8), such as his occasional inebriation and the effect this had on her. She was able to share with him that she needed him to "be with" her, rather than against her or distant from her. At the end of therapy, the couple's interactional patterns had changed. They were able to curtail the problem cycle when it occurred and to respond to each other in a manner that initiated new cycles of closeness and confiding (Step 9). Their attributions about their relationship and the other partner had changed. She saw him as overwhelmed and afraid, rather than as a bully. He saw her as desperate for his validation and caring, rather than as hysterical and hostile. The relationship was now defined as a "safe haven" (Bowlby, 1988) where their attachment needs could be articulated and met. Each partner's sense of self had also expanded. For example, Len was able to accept his vulnerability and feel a sense of competence in dealing with his affect and responding to his wife's needs. As a result he became less depressed. By the end of therapy, their emotional experience was formulated differently. They both were able to accept their own emotions and express them in a way that pulled their partner closer to them. They were now also able to use the relationship to regulate distress, such as the fear of illness. Len and Clara completed 12 sessions of therapy.

The following exchange occurred during Session II in the context of a threatened relapse at the end of treatment where Len began to withdraw and is therefore a replay of Steps 5 and 7 for him. Here, he owns vulnerabilities and needs and expresses them in an engaged manner to his partner.

LEN: The relationship is better. I don't spend near as much energy dodging her rage. She's less angry. (*He smiles at her.*)

CLARA: (*She smiles back at him.*) Well, you hear me more, and you're less depressed and withdrawn, so it's less lonely for me. But (*She turns to me and her voice becomes higher and more clipped.*) I have to be sure that he really gets this, that he can keep on doing this.

LEN: (*He studies the nails on his right hand and says slowly:*) I'm not stupid. I understand more than you give me credit for. (*He looks out the window.*)

CLARA: (*Her voice now goes up a decibel, and she moves to the edge of her seat.*) Well, when you have more than one drink you get really pushy and loud. Then on Saturday you got all mopey and distant.

LEN: (*very slowly, still looking out the window*) I got a little pushy, and I got a little down (*long pause*), but I wasn't that bad. (*He tears and looks away.*)

SUSAN: What's happening for you now, Len? (*He mutters that he's fine. I see him as in obvious pain.*) What's it like for you when Clara says she sees you as being easier for her to get close to, to contact, and then she adds a "but"?

LEN: I don't like it. It's hard. (*He looks directly at her, but she stares at her hand.*)

SUSAN: Ah-ha. It's hard. And some part of you even feels like weeping, is that right?

LEN: (*Pause; he focuses on me and rubs his eyes.*) No, it's just my eyes watering. Well, okay, it's like she's accusing me again, and that's scary.

SUSAN: Right. And that's part of the cycle you guys get trapped in.

LEN: Right. (*long silence and then a deep sigh*) Maybe I can't make it.

CLARA: (*She looks up at him. Her voice is soft, and she sits back in her chair.*) I'm trying to give you a chance. We've had some really good days. (*Now her lips tighten again. She smooths her skirt with her hand, and her voice is clipped.*) But then, I gave you the recipe, I suggested no alcohol and . . .

SUSAN: (*I decide to stay with Len and help him stay engaged. I use a soft voice.*) You're disappointed—that she is doubting you?

LEN: Yeah. She starts to accuse me. (*He turns to Clara.*) I can read recipes, but . . . (*He tears and wrings his hands.*)

SUSAN: What happened on Saturday afternoon, Len, before you had a few drinks?

LEN: I got into a . . . (*He is searching for the right words. He then speaks empathically and deliberately.*) a massive internal flap.

SUSAN: A massive internal flap. Can you help me understand? A flap is, like, frantic?

LEN: Yeah. She was talking about the drinking, and I was already uneasy, but then, but then (*His voice cracks, and he squirms in his chair.*) she went in the study and read the medical books my brother gave me.

CLARA: (*She turns to me and speaks in a very calm tone.*) I went and read about my kind of cancer, and it wasn't good. It said that basically recurrence is just a matter of time.

LEN: And she still has that pain. (*He puts his hands over his eyes.*)

CLARA: (*She leans toward him and says very calmly:*) But we knew that, really.

SUSAN: You were able to read the book and look at that with some calmness, Clara? (*She nods.*) But for you, Len, anticipating that Clara is about to be disappointed with you or angry at you was difficult, that's still difficult, but then knowing that she had read that book, the book you had already read, yes? (*He nods and his eyes widen, telling me I am on track here.*) That brought on a massive internal flap, a panic, for you, yes?

LEN: Yes. (*He weeps.*) I want to make her happy. I try. Her anger scares me. She talks of leaving, and we've got better at handling that, but then, then she talked about this recurrence thing. (*His voice trails off.*)

SUSAN: And you start to feel helpless (*He nods.*), like you can't make her happy, at least that's what came up on Saturday afternoon, and the fear that you might loose her, she might leave, by getting mad enough at you, or by getting sick again. Is that it? [We are recycling through Step 5 here. I am reflecting and heightening his panic and his fear of loss.]

LEN: Yes. (*He weeps.*) She used to say the fights we had were killing her. Things have improved a lot, but . . . Saturday . . .

CLARA: (*She now looks concerned and leans toward him. She sees his distress. She is much more empathic than she was the first time we went through this process of him expressing and owning his hurts and fears.*) I know I have said that you're not listening and discounting me kills me, but . . .

SUSAN: (*to Len*) On Saturday afternoon, all your fears of not being able to hold on to Clara, of not being able to keep her, keep her happy and with you, of losing her, came up again, yes? (*He nods emphatically.*) You even heard her say that the relationship was hurting her, making her sick, and you got frantic.

LEN: That's it. (*He weeps and wipes the tears away with his enormous hands.*) It's terrifying. I get totally paralyzed. I do.

SUSAN: And that's the massive internal flap that has you minimizing and trying to persuade Clara that she doesn't hurt, that everything is fine. Finally when that doesn't work, you feel beaten, and you withdraw into your despair; that's what it's all about? [I summarize the inner panic that primes his despair and his withdrawal.]

LEN: Right, I get all scared. I hover around, trying to be optimistic, and she feels discounted.

CLARA: (*looking surprised*) But you were always so separate, so into your work. I never felt you even needed me.

SUSAN: It's a little strange for you to hear his fear, to see how much he needs you, how afraid he is of hurting or disappointing you?

CLARA: (*Long pause; she stares at Len.*) I guess so . . . so, so, you're afraid. (*He nods and tears.*)

SUSAN: Maybe he's even more afraid of fighting the cancer again than you are, maybe?

CLARA: (*again in a surprised tone*) Oh, . . . Oh, well, I guess so . . . yes, maybe he is.

SUSAN: His massive internal flap pulls him into trying to make everything smooth, better. He tries to make your hurts smaller, but then you get even more hurt and angry, and he gets defeated and depressed. You're so precious to him, is that okay, Len? (*He nods.*) He goes into a panic. [His minimizing and discounting are framed in an attachment context. All these formulations of underlying feelings and interpretations have been used before. They are now applied specifically in the context of her possible relapse and his fear of that.]

CLARA: Oh, . . . (*She turns to Len.*) is that it?

LEN: (*in a much more relaxed tone*) That's about it. When you get in a hissy fit and say you're leaving, I just can't handle that. And then you tell me that the way I am with you will bring back the cancer ... I just freeze up.

CLARA: (*She puts her hands up to her face.*) Oh dear, maybe I shouldn't do that.

LEN: (*He leans toward her.*) It doesn't help. I'm trying. I think I'm doing better. I wasn't good at listening in the past. I can't handle being afraid of losing you and then hearing that I'm making you sick. I want to be with you, not hurt you.

SUSAN: (*softly*) What happens for you as you see his fear, Clara?

CLARA: Well, I guess ... it all seems different. It puts things in a different light.

SUSAN: Ah-ha. Maybe it's his fear that he is trying to control when he plays down your feelings and withdraws.

CLARA: Right, and I always saw it as him trying to control me!

LEN: (*He smiles at her and then at me. He's John Wayne again.*) I wouldn't dare. (*He laughs.*)

SUSAN: Len, can you help her see more? Can you help her understand how much you want to protect and hold her, how afraid you are when the shadow of her leaving, through anger or getting ill, looms?

I then drew the session to a close on the theme of how fear isolated them from each other. All of these themes had been touched on before, and Clara and Len had already changed their problem cycle and initiated a more positive bond. However, here the themes all came together and could be addressed in an integrated fashion that prevented relapse, consolidated his engagement and her softening, and explicitly brought the issue of cancer into the interaction. The next session was the last. The couple came in and reported that they had talked for hours together about her need to be seen by him and to depend on his responsiveness and about his fears of failing her and losing her. This process was a repeat and elaboration of the initial process of Len's reengagement that had occurred in earlier sessions. She was able to respond here because she had already expressed her needs in a previous session and experienced his comfort and caring.

They had also talked openly after this session of the possibility of her death and experienced being much closer to each other through the week. She stated that she realized that because they were closer she felt, "no panic" about the idea of recurrence. She said to me in a quiet voice, "If it happens, we will face it together." They had also been able to talk together and formulate pragmatic plans and coping strategies to deal with such a recurrence. The couple here were able to use their relationship as a safe haven and a secure base in dealing constructively with the trauma of cancer.

Many things happened in this session on the level of individual partners, relationship definition, and existential realities. Specifically, this session touched on Len's depression and adjustment to retirement, the nature of Len and Clara's attachment and marital satisfaction, and their ability to cope with the possibility of a recurrence of her illness and possible death.

To further clarify the process of change in EFT, it may be useful to look at key moments in Clara's softening, which occurred in Sessions 8 and 9, and how these moments redefined the relationship:

- In Step 3 of therapy, Clara formulated the emotions underlying her critical angry stance in terms of helplessness. She said, "I can't get through to him. I hurl myself at this mountain. He just defines me away. He tells me I don't hurt."
- In the softening process, in Step 5, she was able to tell him, "I get desperate when you discount me. It's like I don't exist. It's like when I said I felt ill before the cancer diagnosis, you said I was fine, but I was dying (*she wept*). I can't reach you."
- In Step 7, this process evolved into Clara stating with quiet intensity her fear of abandonment and her need for comfort. She said, "I'm afraid of the cancer coming back, but I'm more afraid of being alone. I need you to see me and hold me. Hold me so I'm not so afraid. Please don't leave me all alone." She got up and held onto him.

When these moments occur:

1. Clara focuses on and expresses vulnerability rather than anger. She is then able to formulate her needs. She is also able to express them in a way that makes it easier for Len to respond. It is when we are experiencing intense emotion that we find it easiest to formulate our most pressing needs and concerns. Emotion carries with it a clear message about what matters most to us.

2. Clara's expression of vulnerability constitutes a less dominant, more affiliative stance toward Len. Emotion is an action tendency; as Clara experiences her fear and longing, she reaches for Len and asks for comfort. In doing so, she changes her interactional position. She is no longer simply the critical accuser.

3. As Clara expresses her fears and hurts, Len sees her differently. She is less dangerous. She is therefore easier for him to respond to. The expression of "new" emotion pulls for a "new" response from the

spouse and so reorganizes the interaction, creating a shift from the problem cycle.

4. As interactions expand, so does each partner's sense of self. Both partners see themselves as more able to control their relationship and deal with their emotions. Intense emotions are also a direct route into our core cognitions about who we are. Len is able to touch his sense of failure in this process and have it evolve into a new sense of how essential and irreplaceable he is to his wife.

5. New emotions structure new steps in Len and Clara's dance. A new cycle of confiding and responsiveness begins. This new cycle of trust and confiding creates a more positive relationship and tends to be self-reinforcing.

6. This new cycle is not just a new set of behaviors replacing the destructive cycle. It is a cycle that addresses inherent attachment needs. It redefines the relationship as a place of safety and comfort. This then influences both partners' resilience in the crises and challenges of life.

Perhaps one of the most creative ways to view the whole issue of brief therapy is to view it in terms of efficiency rather than simply in terms of time; that is, rather than thinking in terms of having to create limited change in a very small number of sessions, focusing on making specific changes that have an immediate, lasting, and significant impact on people's lives. Perhaps, of all modalities, marital therapy has the most potential to create multiple impacts (Lewis, Beaver, Gossett, & Phillips, 1979), potentially affecting individual, couple and family functioning. EFT attempts to tap the power of compelling emotional responses and of basic attachment needs and processes to create a difference that really makes a difference in a brief format.

REFERENCES

Alexander, J. F., Holtzworth-Munroe, A., & Jameson, P. (1994). The process and outcome of marital and family therapy: Research review and evaluation. In A. Bergin & S. Garfield (Eds.), Handbook of psychotherapy and behavior change (pp. 595–607). New York: Wiley.

Bartholomew, K., & Horowitz, L. (1991). Attachment styles among young adults. Journal of Personality and Social Psychology, 61, 226–244.

Bartholomew, K., & Perlman, D. (1994). Attachment processes in adulthood: Advances in personal relationships, Vol. 5. London: Penn/Jessica Kingsley.

Baucom, D., Shoham, V., Mueser, K., Daiuto, A., & Stickle, T. (1998). Empirically supported couple and family interventions for marital distress and adult mental health problems. Journal of Consulting and Clinical Psychology, 66, 53–88.

Bowlby, J. (1969). *Attachment and loss: Vol. 1. Attachment.* New York: Basic Books.

Bowlby, J. (1988). *A secure base.* New York: Basic Books.

Burman, B., & Margolin, G. (1992). Analysis of the association between marital relationships and health problems: An interactional perspective. *Psychological Bulletin, 112,* 39–63.

Dessaulles, A. (1991). *The treatment of clinical depression in the context of marital distress.* Unpublished doctoral dissertation, University of Ottawa, Ottawa, Canada.

Dunn, R. L., & Schwebel, A. I. (1995). Meta-analytic review of marital therapy outcome research. *Journal of Family Psychology, 9,* 58–68.

Feeney, J., & Ryan, S. (1994). Attachment style and affect regulation: Relationships with health behavior and family experiences of illness in a student sample. *Health Psychology, 13,* 334–345.

Gordon Walker, J. (1991). *Marital intervention for couples with chronically ill children.* Unpublished doctoral dissertation, University of Ottawa, Ottawa, Canada.

Gordon Walker, J., Johnson, S., Manion, I., & Cloutier, P. (1996). Emotionally focused marital interventions for couples with chronically ill children. *Journal of Consulting and Clinical Psychology, 64,* 1029–1036.

Gordon Walker, J., Manion, I., & Cloutier, P. (1998). *Emotionally focused marital therapy for the parents of chronically ill children: A two year follow-up study.* Manuscript submitted for publication.

Gottman, J. (1991). Predicting the longitudinal course of marriages. *Journal of Marital and Family Therapy, 17,* 3–7.

Gottman, J. (1994). An agenda for marital therapy. In S. M. Johnson & L. S. Greenberg (Eds.), *The heart of the matter: Perspectives on emotion in marital therapy* (pp. 256–296). New York: Brunner/Mazel (now Taylor & Francis).

Gottman, J., & Levenson, R. W. (1986). Assessing the role of emotion in marriage. *Behavioral Assessment, 8,* 31–48.

Greenberg, L. S., & Johnson, S. M. (1988). *Emotionally focused therapy for couples.* New York: Guilford Press.

Greenberg, L. S., Rice, L. N., & Elliott, R. (1993). *Facilitating emotional change: The moment-by-moment process.* New York: Guilford Press.

Guerney, B. G. (1994). The role of emotion in relationship enhancement marital/family therapy. In S. M. Johnson & L. S. Greenberg (Eds.), *The heart of the matter: Perspectives on emotion in marital therapy* (pp. 124–150). New York: Brunner/Mazel (now Taylor & Francis).

Hazan, C., & Shaver, P. (1987). Conceptualizing romantic love as an attachment process. *Journal of Personality and Social Psychology, 52,* 511–524.

Hazan, C., & Shaver, P. (1994). Attachment in an organizational framework for research on close relationships: Target article. *Psychological Inquiry, 5,* 1–22.

House, J. S., Landis, K. R., & Umber Son, D. (1988). Social relationships and health. *Science, 241,* 540–545.

Jacobson, N. S., & Addis, M. E. (1993). Research on couples and couples therapy: What do we know? Where are we going? *Journal of Consulting and Clinical Psychology, 61,* 85–93.

Johnson, S. M. (1996). *The practice of emotionally focused marital therapy: Creating connection.* New York: Brunner/Mazel (now Taylor & Francis).

Johnson, S. M. (1998). Emotionally focused couple therapy. In F. M. Dattilio (Ed.), *Case studies in couple and family therapy* (pp. 450–472). New York: Guilford Press.

Johnson, S. M., & Greenberg, L. S. (1988). Relating process to outcome in marital therapy. *Journal of Marital and Family Therapy, 14,* 175–183.

Johnson, S. M., & Greenberg, L. S. (Eds.). (1994). *The heart of the matter: Perspectives on emotion in marital therapy.* New York: Brunner/Mazel (now Taylor & Francis).

Johnson, S. M., & Greenberg, L. S. (1995). The emotionally focused approach to problems in adult attachment. In N. S. Jacobson & A. S. Gurman (Eds.), *Clinical handbook of couple therapy* (pp. 121–141). New York: Guilford Press.

Johnson, S. M., Hunsley, J., Greenberg, L. S., & Schlindler, D. (1999). The effects of emotionally focused marital therapy: A meta-analysis. *Clinical Psychology: Science and Practice, 6,* 67–79.

Johnson, S. M., Maddeaux, C., & Blouin. (1998). Emotionally focused family therapy or bulimia: Changing attachment patterns. *Psychotherapy: Theory, Research and Practice, 35,* 238–247.

Johnson, S. M., & Talitman, E. (1997). Predictors of success in emotionally focused marital therapy. *Journal of Marital and Family Therapy, 23,* 135–152.

Johnson, S. M., & Williams-Keeler, L. (1998). Creating healing relationships for couples dealing with trauma : The use of emotionally focused couples therapy. *Journal of Marital and Family Therapy, 24,* 25–40.

Jordan, J. V., Kaplan, A. G., Miller, J. B., Stiver, I. P., & Surrey, J. L. (1991). *Women's growth in connection: Writings from the Stone Center.* New York: Guilford Press.

Lewis, J. M., Beaver, W. R., Gossett, J. T., & Phillips, V. A. (1976). *No single thread: Psychological health in family systems.* New York: Brunner/Mazel (now Taylor & Francis).

Manus, G. L. (1966). Marriage counselling: A technique in search of a theory. *Journal of Marriage and the Family, 28,* 449–453.

Mikulincer, M., Florian, V., & Weller, A. (1993). Attachment styles: Coping strategies and posttraumatic psychological distress: The impact of the gulf war in Israel. *Journal of Personality and Social Psychology, 64,* 817–826.

Plutchik, R. (1980). *Emotion: A psycho-evolutionary synthesis.* New York: Harper & Row.

Roberts, T. W. (1992). Sexual attraction and romantic love: Forgotten variables in marital therapy. *Journal of Marital and Family Therapy, 18,* 357–364.

Rogers, C. (1951). *Client-centered therapy.* Boston: Houghton Mifflin.

Segraves, R. J. (1990). Theoretical orientations in the treatment of marital discord. In F. D. Fincham & T. N. Bradbury (Eds.), *The psychology of marriage* (pp. 281–298). New York: Guilford Press.

Shaver, P., & Hazan, C. (1993). Adult romantic attachment: Theory and evidence. In D. Perlman & W. Jones (Eds.), *Advances in personal relationships* (Vol. 4, pp. 29–70). London: Penn/Jessica Kingsley.

Simpson, J. A., Rholes, W. S., & Nelligan, J. S. (1992). Support giving and support seeking within couples in anxiety provoking situations: The role of attachment styles. *Journal of Personality and Social Psychology, 62,* 434–446.

Tronick, E. Z. (1989). Emotions and emotional communication in infants. *American Psychologist, 44,* 112–119.

Watzlawick, P., Weakland, J. H., & Fisch, R. (1974). *Change: Principles of problem formation and problem resolution.* New York: Norton.

Weissman, M. M. (1987). Advances in psychiatric epidemiology: Rates and risks for major depression. *American Journal of Public Health, 77,* 445–451.

Whisman, M. A., & Jacobson, N. S. (1990). Power, marital satisfaction and response to marital therapy. *Journal of Family Psychology, 4,* 202–212.

Willis, T. A. (1991). Social support and interpersonal relationships. In M. S. Clark (Ed.), *Prosocial behavior* (pp. 265–289). Newbury Park, CA: Sage.

3

—◀O▶—

SHORT-TERM COUPLES GROUP PSYCHOTHERAPY

A Tale of Four Fights

JAMES M. DONOVAN

> Eureka! I saw that I carried this black cloud around. It's
> not Eileen. It's me, and it's from my father. He was always
> angry and negative. I don't need to blame Eileen. I felt
> much calmer in the last few days.
>
> —PAUL (46-year-old teacher; Group Session 15)

Paul's realization captures the dilemma of every married person. Is it *her* or is it *me,* and how will I ever know? This chapter describes a 15-session psychotherapy group which consists of four couples all of whom struggle to help Paul with his question.

BACKGROUND

There are very few references to short-term couples group psychotherapy in the literature. A monograph by Judith and Erich Coché, (1990) has been the most helpful single citation. The Cochés contribute a clear description of how cotherapists can organize and conduct a 1 year couples group. The authors' observations concerning patient selection,

43

pregroup preparation, core couples group issues, therapist interventions, and the sequence of group process ring as true for short-term couples group as for long-term. After the Cochés work, we are forced to scour ideas from a wide range of sources to support our model.

Generic short-term group therapy has valuable general lessons for short-term couples group treatment. MacKenzie (1990), Budman and Gurman (1988, Chap. 10), and Budman, Simeone, Reilly, and Demby (1994) provide particularly helpful introductions to short-term group therapy. They emphasize the need to develop with each patient a working interpersonal focus for the group and the need to promote group cohesion as rapidly as possible.

MacKenzie and the Budman camp present research-based summaries of the phases through which each short-term group progresses, models to which we will return. Hoyt (1993) writing specifically about short-term group therapy within the HMO setting, recommends an approach similar to that described by Budman and Gurman. Hoyt also underscores the need for interpersonal focus, rapid group cohesion, homogeneous patient selection, and high therapist activity. But exactly how to develop this focus, select workable patients, and conduct the group actively?

CONCEPTUAL AND TECHNICAL THEORY
OF SHORT-TERM COUPLES GROUPS

Any theory of short-term treatment has to begin with an understanding of the focused presenting complaint. We have found that couples usually play out one recurrent "fight" in which the major unconscious conflicts in the relationship come to a head. They may have only one fight, but they have it hundreds of times.

Scene 3

WILLIAM (40-year-old consultant): I'm a consultant and try to deal with disagreements rationally, but she becomes irrational and blows up at me.

BARBARA (37-year-old social worker): He treats me like a little child. I get furious. There's no point in talking to someone so disrespectful.

Because the concept of the fight represents a very familiar and a very pressing issue for couples, we often begin an evaluation simply with "Okay, what's the fight?" Most couples readily respond with a specific, poignant description. They can describe the fight in detail but, of course, encounter great difficulty altering it, laden as it is with anxiety and defense.

If the group is a "tale of four fights," we must begin with a conceptual grasp of the couple's fight. Enter the mechanism of "projective identification," the concept originally explored by Melanie Klein. Rutan and Smith (1985) have applied projective identification to couples. According to this principle, partners are attracted to one another, in part, because each is the willing recipient for unconscious projections from the other. For example, the motherless boy raised by a taciturn father, though capable intellectually, grows up awkward and bashful, carrying his father's convictions of shame and inferiority. Protecting himself against these painful affects, the boy grows cautious and, like his father, caustic toward the performance of others, particularly those upon whom he is dependent. He marries a bright, timid woman, continually criticized by her mother for failing to reach her sister's level of achievement. Soon the husband can't help noticing and remarking on his wife's incompetent performance. She's inefficient in the kitchen, a poor limit setter with the children, and so on.

This wife readily receives and accepts these attributions. She's used to them. She projects onto her husband the object image of her unsatisfiable mother, which his unconscious rapidly incorporates. Note that the couple shares the same conflict, here over competence, but they appear to embody opposite ends of the issue. She is apparently bumbling and inept, he rational and skilled.

The fight occurs when the husband, stressed from work, denies his dependency still further by accelerating his projections of incompetence onto his wife. She, now feeling utterly devalued as she did as a child, can stand it no more, and lashes back at her husband/mother. The fight then, represents an attempt by the partners no longer to identify with but to repulse the projections of the other and to establish a more realistic identity in the relationship.

Unfortunately the partners' projections activate long-held negative views of self, "pathogenic beliefs." These are central to psychopathology and are often the focus of short- or long-term individual therapy (Weiss, 1993; Donovan, 1987). Therefore, each participant in his or her unconscious is part-way convinced of the shameful validity of the pathogenic belief and thus of the partner's accusations. In the fight, they flail against the projections of the partner in an attempt to disconfirm the pathogenic belief. They're striving toward health but aren't sure of the right direction or proper mode of travel (R. Reilly, personal communication, April 1, 1996).

Of course, the couples barely sense these tenacious unconscious roots of their conflict, all they know is that they are frightened and bewildered.

Their attempts to win the fight, prove themselves innocent of the partner's accusations or resolve the issues through common sense measures always fall frustratingly short. Each partner withdraws, angry, guilty, helpless, and confused. As the pattern recurs, rage and despondence set in.

How can we help these foundering couples? If this complex fight is the problem, the therapeutic work of the group must proceed in two stages:

1. The partners must grasp the connection between present and past (in the example above, the timid wife must allow herself to feel the parallel between critical husband and critical mother).
2. Each member of the pair will need to uncover and bear the unconscious conflicted affects remaining from unresolved problems in the family of origin now wrapped within the marital relationship.

Our husband must begin to feel his dependency and his fear of incompetence. He can't tuck these conflicts into his wife's knapsack for her to carry forever. If the parallel between past and present can be meaningfully established, and if the shards of repressed affects from both time zones can be pulled into consciousness, then each individual will need to project less and comply less with the projections of the partner. The participants will have found the only reliable path out of the thicket. A clear game plan, but what is the opening gambit?

We know from our previous literature discussion that quickly finding a focus is the crucial first move. The fight will be the focus of treatment but how to understand this focus more deeply? Drawing from short-term individual and group treatment respectively, Malan (1979), Malan and Osimo (1992), and MacKenzie (1990) offer theories that focus on a "triangle of person" that targets (1) current relationships, (2) past relationships, and (3) transference feelings. We have instead chosen to work a "triangle of focus." Our "triangle of focus" draws parallels among the action at three critical points: (1) the fight, (2) unresolved problems in the family of origin, and (3) long-term, individual, character conflicts including past and current persons. We have selected these three foci because, in group after group, the most fruitful exchanges center on these concerns.

The discussion of the triangle of focus occupies the first five or six group sessions, but there is more to come. Now we use an affective breakthrough method, akin to the individual couple approach described by Susan Johnson in Chapter 2 of this volume. Step 1 of the process, the triangle of focus, is to relate the present to the past and to individual character issues, but Step 2 is to achieve emotional breakthrough in each of these important areas. Malan's instructions are the most helpful for this work. We apply his triangle of conflict (Malan, 1979; Milan & Osimo, 1992) directly to our triangle of focus in order to investigate conflict (or displaced affect) at each apex within the triangle of focus (see Figure 3.1) and particularly to help us conceptualize the fight.

The triangle of conflict explains that couples become stuck when important feelings are repressed due to *anxiety* (often over anger), and the couple moves toward a *defensive*, dead-end solution such as mutual projective identification to stabilize the turbulent inner life and outer relationship. The therapist needs to chip away at the foreclosed solution, with empathy and support, to help the patients identify and bear their anxiety, so that they can give up defensive solutions and can grasp, experience, and fully acknowledge the *hidden feelings* locked under the anxiety–defense conflict (McCullough, 1993, 1994). For couples, these hidden feelings usually turn out to be desperate wishes for acceptance and mutual cooperation for which neither person can dare to hope.

Although the group members haven't read Malan's and McCullough's texts, they can pursue this strategy for themselves in homespun terms and help other couples with the project. Thus, in our opening example, Paul realizes his blame toward Eileen represents defensive behavior on his part and not her real shortcomings. Below, we learn that wrestling with the triangle of conflict represents the work of the second half of the group. We can see that each fight in each relationship can be conceptualized by the two triangles on their side intersecting at the "defensive solution" pole (see Figure 3.2). We need to unravel this, help

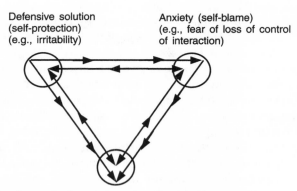

FIGURE 3.1. The triangle of conflict in couple therapy.

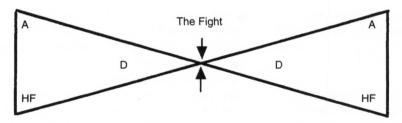

FIGURE 3.2. The fight: Interlocking defensive solutions. A, anxiety; HF, hidden feeling; D, defensive solution.

to mitigate the anxiety, and bring forth the hidden feelings beneath. For me, this is the essence of couples therapy.

PHASES OF TREATMENT

The key steps in short-term couples group psychotherapy are as follows:

1. *Help each couple to describe their fight.* Each partner outlines his or her role, and the therapists and group members explore for more interactional details.
2. *Introduce the triangle of focus.* Support each group member to connect his or her fight to family-of-origin issues and to his or her own long-term, character problems; for example, is William condescending toward his wife in the way that his father is toward William's mother?
3. *Aid the couples in understanding the fight as an interlocking defensive solution to the family-of-origin and character conflicts described in Step 2.*
4. *Outline the triangle of conflict for each couple.* Search for specific anxieties and defensive solutions, many of which will be inherited from unresolved family issues, for example, William is condescending (defense) because he fears being controlled by his wife (anxiety).
5. *Strive for affective breakthrough.* With each member of each couple, first interpret the defensive solutions, then probe the anxiety responsible for these solutions, and finally uncover the hidden feelings beneath.
6. *Support the group in using group cohesion and the insights of all the couples* in the exploration of Steps 1 through 5 for each couple.

7. *For each couple, consolidate partners' breakthroughs and rein-force their identification of tools* to grapple with present and future conflict, using examples from all the couples present.

For reasons that I will explain subsequently, it turns out that the uncovering work with the triangles of focus and conflict proceeds partic-ularly productively within a group context. We can now turn to a description of the group dynamics through which this work unfolds.

GROUP ORGANIZATION
AND PATIENT SELECTION

The Setting

My colleagues and I have led some 20 15-session couples groups over the past 10 years. Nearly all of these groups included four couples, though occasionally two, three, or five. I treated the groups conjointly with a series of postdoctoral fellows, PhDs, and MDs participating in the Harvard Community Health Plan Mental Health Fellowship (Dono-van, Steinberg, & Sabin, 1991, 1994). Each group met in the evening for 90 minutes over 15 consecutive weeks, sometimes interrupted by holidays. The treatment took place at a large, northeastern HMO and was offered within the annual mental health benefit of 20 low-cost psy-chotherapy sessions.

Patient Selection: A Key to Successful
Short-Term Couples Group Therapy

We require a small, stable group that will be able to work with emotion-ally distressing communication issues. Therefore we rule out couples unlikely to be able to participate in such an experience.

We exclude suicidal or violent, unstable individuals, those who are abusing substances, or suffering from major mental illness. Likewise, we exclude couples on the brink of divorce. These common sense selection criteria are similar to those used by the Cochés (1990, p.7) and by many other short-term group therapists (Budman & Gurman, 1988, Chap. 10; MacKenzie, 1990). Patient selection is crucial because the short-term group offers little opportunity to absorb couples rashly included.

Motivation for change is another crucial selection criterion, but it is one usually harder to assess than the degree of psychiatric or marital dis-turbance. To start, we require that prospective group members *have a previous track record of marital commitment* and of attempts to resolve their difficulties. We ask that they have been married for at least 3 years and have engaged in some previous treatment if only a few evaluation sessions with the referring therapist. The partners need a little pregroup time to ventilate their hurt and to demonstrate that they can grapple with the problem without regressing into the never-ending story of blame and mistrust.

Couples rarely admit to ambivalent motivation, since they are attempting to gain entrance to the group, but certain tell-tale presentations alert the vigilant clinician. Some couples *minimize the seriousness of their difficulties.* After describing great distance in the relationship, one pair offered "probably things would get better if we just spent more time together. I'm not sure we need the group." Couples or individuals may *deny personal responsibility* for their recurring conflict: "I know we're trying to save for a house, but I just happen to have a number of expensive hobbies that are also a priority for me, and you need to understand that."

The Workshop

We now know the content of our evaluation. We need to grasp each couple's fight, to assess the partners' psychiatric acuity, their motivation for treatment, and their general maturity and capacity to hold a realistic perspective on themselves and on their partner. In what format should we gather this information? Budman and Gurman (1988, Chap. 10) point out that the best indicator of group behavior is group behavior. We agree. The cotherapists evaluate two prospective couples at a time in a "minigroup," 1-hour workshop. The workshop is so similar to the actual couples group that people who can work effectively in the former will be able to navigate the latter as well.

First we ask couples their reasons for seeking treatment. What is the fight? As each pair describes its recurring conflict, we react supportively and attempt to draw parallels between the two situations, "both women feel their husbands need to control." As the interview continues, we take the opportunity to evaluate the exclusionary criteria for emotional and behavioral disturbance and to assess motivation.

Of equal importance, we can observe four clients in interaction. Some prospective group members are tongue-tied, others bombastically monopolize the small group or vociferously blame the spouse. We gently call attention to this behavior and wait to see if the patient can shift toward a more constructive direction.

At the close of the 1-hour meeting, much has been accomplished. A pair of couples gets to know each other surprisingly well. The therapists have gathered a great deal of diagnostic and background information and have assessed, first hand, how each of the four clients behaves in a small group. We point out that the actual group will be very similar to the pregroup and ask if the clients have questions or reservations. We respond to these in straightforward fashion, "No, the group will not include structured exercises." "Yes, we have led previous couples groups." If we intend to screen out a couple, we don't do so publicly but call the pair the next day.

Since the couples group is brief, any pair that drops out midway can cause a major disruption in cohesion (Budman & Gurman, 1988, Chap. 10). The pregroup does not completely prevent later dropouts, but it does significantly decrease them. Patients now grasp the experience to which they are committing, and perhaps as many as 25% decide not to go forward, some at the therapists' urging. Better to have patients leave now than when the group has actually begun. During the 10 years we have used the pregroup workshop, the short-term couples groups, once underway, have suffered less than a 10% dropout rate. Other short-term group therapists report that the pregroup workshop has similar utility (Budman & Gurman, 1988, p. 255). The pregroup workshop is therefore the analog of trial therapy in the Gustafson (1984), Malan (1979), and Malan and Osimo (1992) methods of short-term individual treatment. If a couple cannot manage the workshop comfortably, it makes little sense to offer the pair the couples group.

A cautionary admonition to therapists: Do not be too nice. The success of your group depends absolutely on wise selection at pregroup. If the couple feels to you as if the partners are too mistrustful, too furious, or too infantile, they probably are. Including problematic people in the group does them and the other members no favor. Trust your gut reaction in this regard.

In real life who is likely to be excluded from the group? We are unlikely to accept couples that cannot commit to the schedule for practical or psychological reasons, couples in which one member is so acutely upset he or she would preoccupy the group, couples in which one or both members take only minimal responsibility for the problem or do not believe there is a problem, and couples in which one member has only recently ceased substance abuse. If we cannot accept a couple, we refer the pair back to the original therapist or arrange to treat the couple ourselves individually.

Group Size and Composition: Homogeneity

Four couples represent the most workable size for the group. Three may not provide enough stimulation or variety of viewpoint, and in the case of an absence, the group shrinks too small. Five couples crowd the "air time," and inevitably, one seems to get excluded from the interaction. The Cochés (1990) suggest a similar group size for the same reasons.

Because the group runs only 15 sessions, homogeneity in membership assumes particular importance (Hoyt, 1993). The Cochés (1990, p. 8) also warn against including a "solo outsider" (p. 8) in the group, but can an "outsider" be included, and along what dimensions? Perhaps surprisingly, race and ethnicity do not define an "outsider." Solo black or mixed-race couples working with three white couples usually function productively in the groups. Class appears to be a more significant homogeneity factor than race. Large differences in social class and education among members do retard group cohesiveness. A blue-collar couple can feel quite lost in a group with three professional pairs. Likewise, the therapist should avoid including only one couple with, or only one without, children. Finally, the gap between the oldest and youngest members shouldn't exceed about 15 years. Failure to observe these guidelines can easily lead to difficulties in mutual identification within the group

Because dropouts are so destructive to group cohesion, we ask that the couples all contract for the 15 sessions. If they remain leery, we require a hard-and-fast agreement to a trial of three sessions before leaving. In fact, no couple, to our memory, has departed after the third meeting. At evaluation, we ask if there are practical impediments to the couple's attendance such as regular business trips or evening classes. If it seems that one or both partners may miss more than one session per month, they shouldn't join.

Our last guideline concerns extragroup socialization. We expect couples to speak outside the group with one or more of the other couples. Therefore, we do not forbid such activity; indeed this interaction probably increases cohesion. We do ask couples to discuss extragroup contact in the sessions and never to mention the details of the group to outsiders.

BUILDING THE ALLIANCE

In group therapy, cohesion is the analogue of therapeutic alliance for individual therapy (Budman & Gurman, 1988). Below, I discuss the sequence of group sessions and show how the therapists work very hard to foster group cohesion, particularly in the early meetings. If cohesion is established, then the group will predictably traverse the required stages of group development. If cohesion isn't achieved, then the group will stall, and the curative processes will have no chance to flower. The usual reasons for aborted cohesion are that one or more couples drop out or cannot attend regularly because of unanticipated work or community commitments. If, unfortunately, a somewhat paranoid, extremely depressed, angrily defensive, or controlling and intrusive person has been included, this too can undermine cohesion.

STAGES OF GROUP PROCESS AND CORRESPONDING THERAPIST ACTIVITY

The Cochés (1990) describe the five stages of their 1-year group (p. 73): (1) joining, (2) beginning work phase, (3) group crisis/dissatisfaction, (4) intense work, and (5) termination. MacKenzie (1990) and Budman and Gurman (1988) note similar phases for short-term group work generically. Our short-term couples group passes through stages nearly identical to the Cochés' 1-year group, though in telescoped fashion. We observe (1) pregroup workshop (already discussed but too important a phase to omit), (2) getting acquainted, (3) early engagement, (4) reassessment, (5) passionate engagement, (6) termination, and (7) follow-up/outcome. Not only patients, but therapists as well alter their behavior as the group moves from stage to stage.

Getting Acquainted (Sessions 1–2)

The couples introduce themselves and begin to describe their fight. They usually spontaneously supply important biographical information concerning their personal histories, such as failures of prior marriages, and relate family-of-origin details, including parental divorce, illness, or addiction in parents or siblings. Occasionally, they reveal personal histories of sexual abuse or trauma. These getting-acquainted sessions understandably begin tentatively. The members of the group know only their own spouse and one other couple from the pregroup workshop. Common sense dictates moving slowly.

During this opening phase the leaders contribute actively and grasp every chance to accent commonality between or among couples or individuals. Group cohesion is what we seek, and we need to work for it. "So, John, both you and Cathy have alcoholic fathers." "Ted, 5 minutes ago, Paul said he also was the youngest brother with many older sisters." The leaders assume an active, group inclusive stance. They encourage silent members to talk and reinforce couples who appropriately share the details of their troubled feelings and marital conflicts. In other words, the therapists attempt to prepare the group atmosphere to support the increasing intimacy session by session. The leaders are also modeling constructive group behavior: high participation, reaching out to others, expression of feelings. As MacKenzie (1990) and Yalom (1990) note, at the start of a group, the therapists need to capitalize on the early stage curative group factors: hope, acceptance, self-revelation, and universality (MacKenzie, 1990, pp. 126–128) in order to build cohesion.

Early Engagement (Sessions 3–7)

Now more comfortable with each other, the members begin to describe their recurrent fight in richer detail and with deeper affect (Step 1 in the phases of treatment). The couples still engage with limited commitment in this process, because most remain in the mutually blaming phase, an initial stage of marital conflict, but one that can last for decades.

Session 5

RICHARD (49-year-old carpenter): You say I don't communicate feelings with you, but every time I do try to talk to you about something serious, you say you're too upset from work, and you leave the room. I chase you around the house.

KAY (45-year-old nurse): You're so vague that I don't know when you're saying something important, and besides you always choose the most impossible times.

The leaders attempt to enlist the other couples as psychotherapeutic detectives in helping this couple to step back from their conflict and investigate the affects underlying each role and the possible family origins of the problematic behavior (Step 2). Richard must have good reasons from his own family history to pursue Kay so ambiguously. What of his identification with his father? In what way is he conflicted over his anger? Kay apparently literally runs from direct communication and involvement. What family experiences may be responsible for her ambivalence over dependence? What can Richard do to reassure her so that tentative communication could start? The other group members may have faced similar issues in their own relationships and here begin to demonstrate their remarkable capacity to help one another by asking incisive questions and offering useful suggestions. The leaders may give homework assignments (Gurman, 1992). "Go out to dinner alone once a week, if even for just a pizza." Some couples give homework to themselves by experimenting with behavior change outside the group and reporting on the results the following session.

PETER (40-year-old business executive): We were lying in bed. I was too tired to talk, but this time I didn't just go to sleep. I knew you wanted to talk so I just listened, and it seemed to help.

JANE (39-year-old teacher): Yeah, it did. I could tell you were there. I didn't feel so lonely.

By the end of the early engagement phase, Session 7 or 8, nearly all the couples have acquired a crucial insight. They now grasp that their fighting makes psychological if not practical sense; it isn't random in pattern, and it fulfills important emotional needs for both. They begin to be convinced that the seeds of the fight were sown a long time ago in their original families and that neither of them bears all the blame (Step 3). Usually the couples haven't managed effective changes yet, but the decision to frame the fight in psychological versus blaming terms offers the conceptual context within which change can be constructed in the second half of the group.

The first half of the group therefore concentrates on Steps 1, 2, and 3 of the therapy template: describing the fight, introducing the triangle of focus, and describing the interlocking defensive solution that underlies the fight. Obviously these concepts aren't introduced in a heavy-handed way but arise naturally out of the group interaction. The therapists need to guide the discussion back to these issues when it begins to wander.

Group cohesion now usually becomes palpable.

Session 7

MARIA (42-year-old artist): It was hard missing the group.

DAVE (40-year-old teacher): I saw that we fought in a different way. There seemed to be less bitterness to our fighting.

PAULA (34-year-old secretary): I'm glad that Dave and Maria are back. We feel like a whole group again.

DAVE: I care about how the others do here. I want to see all of us make some changes.

Reassessment (Session 8)

The Cochés (1990), Budman and Gurman (1988), and MacKenzie (1990) all describe a clear phase of group crisis, marked by disillusionment with the leaders and conflict between the members, after which group cohesion usually deepens. Curiously we find little evidence of dramatic "crisis" midway through our groups. Possibly because the affective bonds are within the couples and not with the leaders, our patients, at midgroup, rarely express bitter dissatisfaction with the therapists or with the other group members outside their own dyad.

There is a definite pause and reevaluation in Session 8, however. The couples are aware of the time. When we announce, "This is Session 8. By the end of tonight, the group will be more than half over," a worried silence descends. Members often stare ahead blankly or voice despondence that meaningful change can happen in the few remaining sessions of this very short group. Sometimes at our urging, sometimes before we have a chance to urge, the couples struggle to assess where they have come in the group and what work they have left to do. Are they cooperating better? Do they argue as heatedly? Has the sexual relationship improved? Is their particular fight any closer to resolution? The building intensity of the group levels off for this, and perhaps part of the next session, as the members pull back and reflect. Here the therapists need to be quietly, realistically optimistic in their comments. They need to acknowledge and encourage the stocktaking and the worry that change will never happen but to actively redirect this fear back to the goal of understanding the couples' recurrent conflicts, crystallized so completely in the fight. Yes, problems still remain but so do 7 sessions to work on these problems.

Passionate Engagement (Sessions 9–14)

Perhaps the confrontation with the clock increases motivation. Perhaps the patients now unconsciously grasp that the leaders cannot deliver all the necessary curative wisdom. Perhaps it simply requires 8 sessions for any group to achieve working cohesion. I can't say. Whatever the causes, after the lull of Session 8, Sessions 9 to 14 usually ignite with intense therapeutic power. Attendance becomes nearly 100%. The couples grapple, at far greater depth, with their own marital issues and those of the other members (Step 4). Tears, rage, recollections of physical and sexual abuse, and terror of abandonment regularly make their appearance.

Now is the time for affective breakthrough (Step 5). The group experience takes on the quality of revelation. In his or her state of psychological openness, each member of the couple may suddenly perceive as a gestalt the multileveled, multimeaning conflict that leads to the fight. Individual, interpersonal, family-of-origin, and group process issues, however entwined, momentarily come into crystal clear focus for the members and the leaders (Steps 4 and 5).

The couple's relationship to their fight usually starts to shift at this point. The partners begin to accept realistic, limited, personal responsibility for their role in the conflict. They also undertake productive, independent steps toward change (Step 7). For example, couples may report calling "time outs" in attempting to interrupt and work at the process of their fight rather than to win it.

The group feels different for the therapists as well. Earlier, the leaders sensed the necessity to pull (or pummel) patients toward a reflective, constructive stance, but now in "passionate engagement," the patients assume more initiative and draw on the therapists as consultants. When they do intervene, the leaders can do so with great force since the group atmosphere can now support a strong interpretation. In general, the therapists feel excited and involved with little effort; the 90 minutes fly by. Both MacKenzie (1990) and the Cochés (1990) have explored this dramatic second-half shift in group atmosphere and its curative significance for the members.

During "passionate engagement," not all of the couples achieve this heightened state of sensibility and maintain it for each of the final sessions. Couples absent for one, and particularly for two, of these crucial meetings appear to have missed the train and to stand bewildered at the station watching the group roll down the tracks without them. Bad luck? These couples usually were the least involved all along and unconsciously may have arranged their absence at key meetings.

The second half of the group thus roughly represents Steps 4, 5, and 6 in the couples group template outlined earlier. The passionate insights occur because anxiety is mitigated and defenses lifted. Once this step is in place, the possibility to develop "tools" (Step 7) for dealing with the fight becomes a practical reality. Couples then naturally move in the direction of exploring techniques to interrupt and work at their fight. Because the members have achieved a state of openness, they can now listen to each other and to the therapists more genuinely. For example, the therapist can offer, "If you're mad at her, so you're mad, so say it right now" and actually expect an affective response from the husband or wife.

Termination (Session 15)

The intensity of passionate engagement doesn't continue unabated into the closing moments. Beginning in the second half of Session 14 and continuing to the end of the group, the participants usually decrease their activity and withdraw slightly. They "debrief" themselves from the experience by recalling what they've learned and step back from one another preparing for separation. At this time, the therapists emphasize the "tools" the couples have learned and encourage them to refer directly to these when they find themselves slipping into the fight in the future as they inevitably will, reinforcing Step 7.

Follow-Up (Session 16)

As the group closes, the members often clamor for either an extension of weekly meetings or a future reunion. Partly in response to these requests, we've experimented with scheduling a follow-up session 3 to 6 months after Session 15. This additional meeting allows us to gauge the sustained effectiveness of the group and to reevaluate each couple's need for further treatment.

Although we lack formal outcome data for the group, in these follow-up sessions, we observe that often one or two couples out of the four has retreated toward its status at initial interview. We usually suggest further treatment for one or both members of these couples. The therapy could be couple or individual work as appropriate. Two or three of the couples seem to have internalized a psychological understanding of their fight and to be continuing to use the methods developed in the group to unravel the conflict-laden issues before they reach incendiary levels. Despite the improvements, members of these pairs may wish or need some additional therapy, which we arrange.

Clients themselves often arrange their own follow-up by continuing to meet after termination as a leaderless group. These sessions usually occur monthly at group members' homes over dinner and may continue for a year or longer. If we reencounter a couple in further treatment, the members usually communicate very few details of these follow-up meetings, although they often attend religiously and seem to find them valuable. Cohesion evidently doesn't end with Session 15, nor does the group collapse without the therapists. Since we are never present, we can't report on the group process or on any further benefits from these meetings.

CORE TECHNICAL MANEUVERS

The crucial skills for therapists in short-term couples group therapy somewhat deceptively number only three. The first, a general skill, is high therapist activity. The group moves very fast, and eight people can talk a great deal. Do not be afraid to interrupt and push assertively for more affect. "Your wife, Susan, just reached over and touched your hand. How do you feel about that?" The second skill has been mentioned and illustrated above: building alliance and cohesion in the group and, most particularly, choosing the right group members.

The third set of core maneuvers has to do with skillfully plying the triangles of focus and conflict. The therapists need to know what they're looking for, and they need to know when forcefully to articulate the focus and when to leave the patient alone.

Session 3

The Triangle of Focus: The Fight → Family of Origin → Character Trait

BEATRICE (40-year-old, teacher, adult child of an alcoholic): When we get ready to leave the house, I'm always rushing around to clean up, and he says, "I'm ready. Let's go." *No matter how many times I'm hurt about this pattern, you don't seem to care. I'm just furious.* [the fight]

KEN (45-year-old sound technician): Well, there's two sides of it. *You're never ready.* [the fight]

THERAPIST 1: Does this remind you of anyone in your family who is kind of daffy, always complaining? [family-of-origin inquiry]

KEN: No one like that. My mother always persevered and got it done. She was a hypochondriac, though. [family of origin]

THERAPIST 1: Oh?

KEN: She always had some physical problem.

THERAPIST 1: Oh, always complaining about something?

KEN: My wife's always complaining; similar pattern, I guess.

THERAPIST 2: What does it feel like when your mother is like that?

KEN: Annoying; you don't listen.

THERAPIST 1: You can kind of make a pattern of that. Problems come by from whatever source. You kind of turn away. Can't stop the music, whatever you do. Does that happen in other parts of your life as well? [character clarification, questioning about relationships with other past and current persons]

When the work with the triangle of focus and the triangle of conflict has productively taken hold, then the patients can begin the task of excavating themselves from their triangles and begin to fashion their own concrete techniques to dismantle their conflict.

Session 15

The Triangle of Conflict: Defense → Anxiety → Hidden Feeling

WILLIAM (40-year-old consultant): Tools we learned. Tools we're beginning to use. [Step 7—new solution] I have occasional slippage, but now I recognize the problem I have. Why it annoys Barbara. What surprises me is that I'm focusing on how my father communicates with my mother. [insight into foreclosed solution in family of origin] What strikes me is that it's the exact problem that I have in communicating with Barbara. It does help to see the connection and to understand where I developed the habit. [Step 2—cognitive and affective breakthrough in triangle of focus; the fight → character feature → family of origin]

THERAPIST 1: How does he communicate with your mother?

WILLIAM: When he disagrees, he doesn't admit a legitimacy to her points. He tries to win the argument by being louder, attempts to assert total authority. He ends discussion. "Let's forget it," is a phrase he uses. [foreclosed solution in family of origin] Mother usually just gives in. [William has been waiting in vain for Barbara to give in.] Understanding where habit develops is helpful. [Step 5—insight softens triangle of conflict]

   Earlier I would deny [defense against recognizing condescension] I was using a superior tone of voice to Barbara. [Step 5—insight softens triangle of conflict, anxiety over control tolerated, defense relaxed] Now when she points it out, I usually acknowledge it. [hidden feeling = wish to communicate honestly and cooperate; anxiety reduced, hidden feeling expressed] I think about it [cognition] and acknowledge [affect] what I do, which I really didn't do before. [argumentative defense relaxed, genuine communication takes place]

   I used to anticipate remarks Barbara would say in the past, led me to disregard her point. [Barbara probably played into the dismissal by offering predictable rejoinders; projective identification is afoot = old solution] Catch myself right there. [projective identification broken] *I change my response.* [Step 7—behavioral tools used to anticipate and avoid fight] Not "Will *you* please call Doctor _____ about the baby's cough?"

BARBARA (37-year-old social worker): When he acted that way, *it made me feel I'm not doing my job as a mother.* [Step 1—the fight] Now he'll say "That's not what I meant. Could you do this tomorrow because I can't." We're at this place, not at the place where we started the group. [Step 7—new, nondefensive solution]

The heart of the couples group can be found in these dialogues. Therapists and patients must focus on and work with the intense affect found first in the triangle of focus and then in the triangle of conflict. Experience has taught me that this therapeutic action is both necessary and sufficient for each couple to gain substantially from the group.

CONCLUSION

In summary, the couples group attempts to teach the participants to dare a crucial shift in their interaction, to stop fighting the fight and to begin working at processing it. Wile (1981) illustrates this point superbly in his version of "nontraditional" couple therapy. He encourages the partners to view the fight as a comment on their relationship. Both feel trapped, deprived, and powerless in their interaction and need to begin to experience the fight as a healthy attempt to draw attention to this fact and to alter it (see Chapter 9). For example, William and Barbara above feel frustrated and isolated in their control struggle. Both want to become closer and more cooperative. The fight expresses and comments on this need. Exploring all their feelings about the fight and its historical antecedents with the group and with themselves helps William and Barbara to see it as a struggle toward the positive goal of mutuality and not as an antagonistic melee.

The short-term couples group is certainly efficient. The 17 group sessions (including evaluation and follow-up meetings) fit within many managed care mental health benefits. More than one patient is treated at once, and the group may carry preventative significance for any children in the home.

Is it effective, though? To answer this, we must ask, effective in comparison to which realistic alternatives? We can establish the effectiveness of short-term groups in general (Budman et al., 1994), but we are still in the midst of gathering hard outcome data on short-term couples groups specifically. The subjective benefits seem remarkably high. As group after group staggers from the office following Session 15, the cotherapists usually stare at each other and mumble something akin to, "How did these eight people become so honest about so much hurt and longing, and how did they ever change so much in so short a time?" This therapist has had few professional experiences so moving and so clearly productive.

REFERENCES

Budman, S. H., & Gurman, A. S. (1988). *Theory and practice of brief therapy.* New York: Guilford Press.

Budman, S. H., Simeone, P. G., Reilly, R., & Demby, A. (1994). Progress in short-term and time limited group psychotherapy: Evidence and implications. In A. Fuhriman & G. M. Burlingame (Eds.), *Handbook of group psychotherapy: An empirical and clinical synthesis.* New York: Wiley.

Coché, J., & Coché, E. (1990). *Couple group psychotherapy.* New York: Brunner/Mazel.

Donovan, J. M. (1987). Brief dynamic psychotherapy: Toward a more comprehensive model. *Psychiatry, 50,* 167–183.

Donovan, J. M., Steinberg, S. M., & Sabin, J. E. (1991). A successful fellowship program in an HMO setting. *Hospital and Community Psychiatry, 42,* 952–953.

Donovan, J. M., Steinberg, S. M., & Sabin, J. E. (1994). Managed mental health care: An academic seminar. *Psychotherapy, 31,* 201–206.

Gurman, A. S. (1992). Integrative marital therapy: A time-sensitive model for working with couples. In S. H. Budman, M. F. Hoyt, & S. Friedman (Eds.), *The first session in brief therapy.* New York: Guilford Press.

Gustafson, J. P. (1984). An integration of brief dynamic psychotherapy. *American Journal of Psychiatry, 141,* 935–944.

Hoyt, M. F. (1993). Group psychotherapy in an HMO. *HMO Practice, 7,* 127–132.

MacKenzie, K. R. (1990). *Introduction to time limited group psychotherapy.* Washington, DC: American Psychiatric Press.

Malan, D. H. (1979). *Individual psychotherapy and the science of psychodynamics.* London: Butterworths.

Malan, D. H., & Osimo, F. (1992). *Psychodynamics, training and outcome in brief psychotherapy.* Oxford: Butterworth-Heinemann.

McCullough, L. (1993). An anxiety reduction modification of short-term dynamic psychotherapy: A "theoretical melting pot" of treatment techniques. In G. Stricker & J. R. Gold (Eds.), *Comprehensive handbook of psychotherapy integration.* New York: Plenum Press.

McCullough, L. (1994). The next step in short-term dynamic psychotherapy: A clarification of objectives and techniques in an anxiety regulating model. *Psychotherapy, 31,* 642–654.

Rutan, J. S., & Smith, J. W. (1985). Building therapeutic relationships with couples. *Psychotherapy, 22,* 194–200.

Weiss, J. (1993). *How psychotherapy works: Process and technique.* New York: Guilford Press.

Wile, D. B. (1981). *Couples therapy: A nontraditional approach.* New York: Wiley.

Yalom, I. D. (1990). *The theory and practice of group psychotherapy* (4th ed.). New York: Basic Books.

4

–◄○►–

A CONTROL MASTERY APPROACH TO SHORT-TERM COUPLE THERAPY

RICHARD VOGEL

In the course of both courtship and marriage, certain behaviors emerge between men and women that alienate one member of a couple from the other. Provocative interactions, such as the overt expression of hostility directed toward an innocent spouse, overbearing criticality, and rejection of affection, are all common sources of conflict among couples who might otherwise yearn for intimacy. Confusion typically reigns in such mutually unfulfilling destructive interactions. Often, the partners comprising these couples are at a loss to account for the underlying motives that give rise to such behavior, which has the effect of alienating one spouse from the other, and which reduces the desire for intimacy to a grumbling, accusatory tirade.

CONTROL MASTERY THEORY: CONCEPTUAL AND TECHNICAL APPROACH

Control Mastery, a psychological model developed by Joseph Weiss, provides an effective vantage point from which to understand such dysfunctional and potentially devastating interactions. Control Mastery theory holds that the motive underlying the experience of self-imposed suffering, which typically occurs when one member of a couple alienates the other through the enactment of maladaptive behavior, has as its basis an acting out of a pathogenic belief. Pathogenic beliefs are acquired by inference and from actual day-to-day, childhood experience, or from traumatic events.

Weiss, Sampson, and the Mount Zion Psychotherapy Research Group (1986) suggest that a child may develop a pathogenic belief when he or she

> first attempts to gratify a certain important impulse or to reach a certain important goal and then discovers that by such attempts he threatens his all-important ties to his parents. The child then develops a pathogenic belief that causally connects his attempts to gratify the impulse or to reach the goal with the threat to the parental ties. As a consequence of the pathogenic belief, the child represses the impulse or the goal in order to retain the parental ties. He fears that if he does not repress these motivations, he will act upon them and so endanger himself. (p. 71)

While pathogenic beliefs may stem from various dynamics, this chapter focuses on those acquired in relation to possessive or suffering parents and/or siblings—beliefs associated with separation guilt or survivor guilt. For an adult, these beliefs and the guilt associated with them dictate that enjoying one's life, work, and spouse is a form of neglect of the suffering, possessive parent or the disadvantaged sibling. It then becomes necessary to dismantle, spoil, and undo any circumstances that bode well for the individual—as in the case of a person whose potential for happiness is undermined by his awareness of his or her parents' unhappy marriage. In this instance, such an awareness, and the guilt associated with it, mitigate against this individual allowing him- or herself a better marital experience than his or her parents had. This person is predisposed to sabotage any attributes—such as warmth, empathy, or affection—that might contribute to marital fulfillment. In effect, for such a person (i.e., one who has grown up in a household where parents or siblings manifested profound suffering and/or excessive neediness), a taboo exists that prevents one from enjoying his or her experiences while significant others are suffering. The repeated manifestation of self-destructive behavior that serves to alienate individuals from their partners is the mechanism by which they remain loyal to the belief that they have no right to happiness while others are in need.

The Control Mastery approach is especially well-suited to a short-term therapy format. It assumes that each of the partners and the couple as a unit enter treatment with an unconscious plan for disconfirming various pathogenic beliefs emanating from childhood that prevent them from achieving happiness in their relationship (Zeitlin, 1991).

Couples may hold various pathogenic beliefs in common. For example, they may erroneously believe that, because they argue frequently, they are unsuited to each another. One partner may harbor a pathogenic belief, stemming from having experienced neglect in his family, that he is not entitled to affection in his marriage. Another partner may harbor the belief that because her parents were unhappy in their marriage, she has no right to happiness in hers.

Couples in treatment attempt to disconfirm such beliefs in accordance with an unconscious plan: (1) by testing the beliefs in relation to their therapist; and (2) by using the therapist's interpretations to become cognizant of these beliefs and to realize that they are false and maladaptive.

"Separation" and "survivor" guilt have been identified by Weiss et al. in *The Psychoanalytic Process* (1996) as the culprits that engender maladaptive pathogenic beliefs destructive to harmonious relations in marriage. While marital discord is caused by beliefs other than those associated with separation or survivor guilt (i.e., beliefs based on shame, rejection, childhood physical or sexual abuse, etc.), this chapter focuses on difficulties that arise from pathogenic beliefs based on these two forms of guilt.

SEPARATION GUILT

According to Weiss (1986), separation guilt

> is rooted in the belief . . . , which the child infers from his experiences, that if he becomes more independent of the parent he will hurt the parent. As regards the part played by real experiences in the acquisition of separation guilt, a child whose mother appears to be deeply upset by his attempts to become more independent of her is, all else being equal, more likely to develop separation guilt than a child whose mother is unhurt by his attempts to become more independent of her, or is proud of his capacity to be independent. (p. 50)

Children who learn that they are *not* responsible for their parents' happiness are free to pursue and enjoy their own aspirations and are better able to tolerate and embrace success than are those who are tormented by the belief and associated guilt that to do so would harm their parents. As adults, such individuals feel free to prioritize their own needs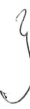

and aspirations, tolerate success, and embrace and reciprocate kindness from their spouses. They are not inclined to undo intimacy, as are adults who have grown up in an atmosphere where they were made to feel responsible for their parents' well-being and guilty for craving their own happiness. In this connection, Firestone (1990) remarks:

> Parents who respect the individuality of their children refrain from treating them as possessions or property. They do not attempt to live their lives through their children or feed off their achievements. When adults try to live vicariously through their offspring, the children grow up with tendencies to withhold their good qualities and special capabilities in a manner that seriously limits them in their adult lives. (p. 178)

Parents who foster separation guilt directly or indirectly indicate to their children that to the extent that they have a life of their own, the parents feel excluded and hurt. In this scenario, the children are coerced into believing that their parents' happiness is contingent upon the children remaining in physical proximity to, and in accord with, whatever it is that the parents identify as satisfying their desires, rather than the children's authentic needs.

According to Weiss et al. (1986), "A child whose mother tells him he must sacrifice for her (even though he consciously repudiates this idea) may come to believe unconsciously that he should sacrifice for her. Moreover, he may behave in accordance with this belief" (p. 51). In marriage, such sacrifice might include rejecting loving entreaties from one's spouse, or inadvertently, and for no apparent reason, provoking her resentment. Such behavior, to the extent that it undermines intimacy, serves the function of maintaining allegiance and psychic proximity to the needy and discontented parent.

The potential for pleasure with one's mate intensifies the separation guilt toward the parent from whom the individual feels he or she is becoming independent, which in turn sabotages the goodwill and intimacy in the romantic relationship. This is achieved by the individual—say, a husband—behaving in ways (e.g., withdrawing, criticizing, or overcontrolling) that have the effect of angering his wife, who previously was demonstrably affectionate. Her anger in turn produces an inclement atmosphere in the home, which is experienced by the husband as punishment for his perceived disloyalty to and abandonment of his needy and discontented parent. This punishment, however, serves to assuage his guilt.

The following vignette illustrates how the presence of separation guilt in one of the partners can have a detrimental effect on a marriage.

On their honeymoon, a married couple, Ted and Rachel, received a frantic call from Rachel's mother, who claimed to be experiencing an attack of vertigo. Rachel knew, however, that this was just another one of her mother's ploys to control her. This had been a pattern ever since Rachel's childhood, when her mother would become depressed whenever Rachel expressed any form of individuality. Each day of the honeymoon, and much to her husband's annoyance, Rachel, though desirous of distancing herself from her mother, was motivated by guilt to call her. To atone for the guilt induced by her mother's insinuation that Rachel was neglecting her, Rachel deprived herself of her husband's affection and goodwill. Rachel's guilt for daring to enjoy her life with her husband while her mother manifested such intense, though contrived, suffering, required her to subvert her good intentions toward him. This included rejecting his sexual overtures on the evening of the phone call.

Firestone (1990) alludes to the phenomenon of separation guilt to explain the behavior of women like Rachel, who sexually reject their husbands:

Each step in a woman's development toward sexual maturity is filled with conflict. She is torn between expressing her love and sexual desire in relation to a man, which separates her from her mother, and holding back these responses, which affirms the maternal connection. Furthermore, as she matures, the daughter may actually fear retaliation from the mother for seeking adult sexual fulfillment. (p. 145)

In couple therapy, I asked Rachel how she felt about her mother's interference at a time when Rachel should have been accorded the opportunity to celebrate her marriage.

Rachel replied that for as long as she remembered, her mother had behaved selfishly toward her, placing her voracious need for attention above her daughter's right to a life independent of such manipulation. Rachel recalled depriving herself of friends, hobbies and a close relationship with her father in response to her mother's incessant plea for her daughter's undivided attention. She described her mother as a needy, unhappy woman who, rather than create a life for herself, was living vicariously through her daughter.

An example that Rachel gave of her mother's intrusiveness that was especially humiliating was her habit of giving Rachel frequent enemas until she was ten, under the pretext that these prevented illness.

Rachel's husband reported numerous instances when his mother-in-law attempted to subvert their marriage. He believed that

Rachel's mother would be happy with him out of the picture. Rachel understood that by succumbing to her mother's selfish and unreasonable demands, she would be placing her marriage in jeopardy.

On one occasion, Rachel posed an unconscious test for her therapist. The purpose of this test was to disconfirm her pathogenic belief, acquired in relation to her mother, that her autonomous strivings were injurious to others.

Rachel's test took the form of her announcing her intention to enter a weeklong couples retreat with another therapist as an adjunct to her couple therapy. Unlike her mother, who denied and denigrated Rachel's attempts at individuating, I encouraged Rachel to proceed with her plan, agreeing that it would be useful to her marriage.

In a subsequent session, Rachel vividly recalled a childhood experience of being kept out of a ballet class by her mother, who chided Rachel for being "too chubby" to succeed in such an endeavor. Rachel felt relieved that I, unlike her mother, responded to her attempts at individuation nonpunitively and with encouragement. Rachel's husband added that by supporting Rachel's independent strivings, I had provided him with role modeling that he intended to replicate on those occasions when he, like Rachel's mother, tended to be controlling of his wife.

Rachel's awareness of the dynamics underlying her relationship with her mother, combined with my (her therapist's) passing of her test, provided Rachel with the motivation to challenge and overcome her belief that her autonomous strivings were harmful to others. This enabled her to affiliate more comfortably with her husband and resist the temptation to experience intimacy in their relationship as disloyalty to her mother.

Rheingold (1964) counsels women in Rachel's situation as follows: "A woman may bring any number of assets to marriage—compassion, wisdom, intelligence, skills, an imaginative spirit, delight-giving femininity, good humor, friendliness, pride in a job well done—but if she does not bring emancipation from her mother, the assets may wither or may be overbalanced by the liability of the fear of being a woman" (p. 451).

In *The Good Marriage*, Wallerstein and Blakeslee (1995) caution that for a marriage to flourish, partners are required to separate psychologically from their families' "emotional ties":

> Psychological separation means gradually detaching from your family's emotional ties. . . . You must shift your primary love and loyalty to the marital partner. . . . (p. 53)

Separation is particularly tricky for women because the ties between mother and daughter, made up of strands of compassion, love, and sometimes guilt, are so powerful. . . . Marriage may be particularly hard for the daughter whose mother is lonely and unhappy or is caring for an ill sibling or spouse. (p. 55)

SURVIVOR GUILT

Niederland (1981) describes a persevering guilt complex that affected survivors of the Holocaust. The survivors' symptoms included depression, anhedonia, psychosomatic conditions, and anxiety. Niederland viewed these symptoms as identifications with family members who had not survived. Underlying them, he believed, was a pervasive and intense sense of guilt, which he referred to as survivor guilt. According to Modell (1971), survivor guilt stems from a biologically based concern for and sensitivity to the pain of significant others, making it difficult to be happy if others are not.

In view of Weiss et al. (1986), survivor guilt "is based on a belief . . . that by acquiring more of the good things of life than parents or siblings [had], he has betrayed them. The person believes that his acquisitions have been obtained at the expense of his parents or siblings" (p. 52).

Survivor guilt might arise when individuals attempt to excel in areas where their parents and/or siblings were deficient, as in the case of a young man whose business acumen posed the likelihood of his becoming materially more successful than his father. The experience of outdoing one's parents or siblings in areas where they experienced minimal success intensifies the guilt, resulting in self-destructive behaviors that serve to undermine success. Zeitlin (1991) comments: "An individual burdened by survivor guilt may appease his conscience by 'leveling' himself with the family by self-sabotage, renunciation, making himself miserable in the face of good fortune, or making himself envious of those who actually have less than he does" (p. 206).

In a similar vein, Firestone (1987) comments: "Guilt in relation to other people who are self-denying takes the joy out of achievement. . . . Most people unconsciously deprive themselves of much of what they value in life because they fear going beyond a significant person in their background" (p. 229).

Engel and Ferguson (1990) state that the crime of *outdoing*

stems from two irrational, unconscious beliefs. The first is that by having the good things in life (happiness, success, love, and affection), you are using them up, not leaving any for your less fortunate parents or siblings. The second is that by achieving your occupational and personal goals, you are showing up those family members who were unable to achieve their own. (p. 42)

For example, a man who has the unconscious belief that enjoying his mate would be outdoing his parents, whom he experienced as having had an unhappy marriage, will be predisposed to undermine his marriage in order to assuage his guilt for doing better than his parents. To accomplish this end, he might, for instance, precipitate an argument with his wife over some inane issue. It is extremely difficult for such an individual to allow himself to be close to his wife, even though he has an authentic desire for such intimacy. Until his unconscious belief of having no right to a better marriage than his parents' can be made conscious and subsequently overcome, this man will feel compelled to placate his suffering parents by depriving himself of pleasure in areas of his life where they failed.

In the novel *The Prince of Tides* (Conroy, 1991), the hero's moodiness and rejection of his wife's affection are manifestations of survivor guilt associated with his brother's violent death and his sister's confinement in a mental hospital. In response to her husband's despondency and self-deprecation, Tom's wife, Sally, implores him to give up his sorrowful ways and be more demonstratively affectionate. She remarks: "You've been so self-pitying, so analytical, and so bitter since what happened to Luke. You've got to forget what happened and go on from here, from this moment. Your life isn't over, Tom. . . . Why do you want to throw even the good things away?" (p. 26).

Tom's hopelessness is evident in his response, "Because they aren't so good to me anymore, because I don't believe in my life anymore" (p. 27). This is the voice of survivor guilt speaking, which echoes Tom's refusal to accept his wife's invitation to a happier life. He simply cannot allow himself pleasure in the wake of his siblings' tragic lives.

Concerning the detrimental effects of survivor guilt, Firestone (1988) comments: "The person who is alive to his experience may unconsciously hold back his enthusiasm, sensing that his vitality might threaten a person who is more self-denying . . . We have observed that people are very susceptible to negative social pressure from unhappy or self-sacrificing family members" (p. 266).

The following vignette illustrates how the presence of survivor guilt in one of the partners can have a destructive effect on a marriage:

Janet and Lew entered couple therapy feuding about Janet's perception of her husband's treatment of their newborn girl. On one occasion, upset by the child's continuous crying, Lew cursed out loud and, in Janet's perception, held the infant too tightly while changing her diapers. Janet accused Lew of being insensitive, implying that his outburst and manner of handling their child bordered on being abusive. During our first couple session, Janet intimated that she was considering divorce. Lew acknowledged that his behavior was out of line, apologized, and promised never to do it again.

Janet disregarded her husband's apology and continued to berate him throughout the days that followed. In the interest of defusing their feud, their therapist interpreted Janet's reaction as exemplary of her maternal instinct to protect their infant. Lew responded positively to this interpretation. He viewed Janet as a compassionate, caring woman—character traits that were influential in his decision to marry her. At the same time, he remarked how difficult it was for him to be repeatedly accused of abusing their child, and that no matter what he did to rectify his error, Janet's rancor did not diminish.

Lew contended that this one occasion on which he appeared to be losing control was an anomaly. He prided himself on being impeccably attuned to his child's needs. Acknowledging Lew's overall sensitivity to their child, Janet surmised that perhaps there might be other factors contributing to her exaggerated response.

Janet's sister, who could not have children, had been visiting at the time this episode took place. Janet felt guilty for being able to conceive a child while her sister could not. Her sister's complaint that Janet had "all the luck" made it even more difficult for Janet to talk about the pleasure she received from her infant. Janet was aware of subduing her feelings and expressions of enthusiasm in relation to her child while in her sister's presence. She remained unaware, however, of the insidious effect on her marriage that her sister's forlorn attitude was creating. Juxtaposed with her good fortune, her sister's unhappiness became the seed of an inner discontent that eventually manifested as an overreaction to her husband's relatively benign and remediable error.

The presence of unconscious guilt for surpassing loved ones or attaining in life what these loved ones were unable to achieve often manifests as self-sabotaging behavior by the more fortunate individual. Janet's bickering with her husband was meant to convey to her infertile sister that although she appeared to be happier and the recipient of more good fortune, this was not really the case, as was evidenced by her marital conflict.

Zeitlin (1991) comments on the role of survivor guilt in promoting marital discord:

> Survivor guilt is a ubiquitous force in modern life; almost all of us have experienced it to some degree. Yet in therapy it can be very elusive. Patients suffering severely are often totally unaware; it is simply the atmosphere they breathe. It is a "great imposter," and many couple conflicts, apparently due to other issues, are actually fueled by survivor guilt. Initially patients may be able to see only the footprints and cannot give more than intellectual credence to the concept. Some patients resent this interpretation at first, feeling disqualified and robbed of the certainty of their conscious feelings. Actually experiencing the guilt as the underlying pathogenic beliefs are explicated is both relieving and painful. (p. 226)

Janet's recognition of her guilt, attained in therapy, enabled her to communicate her feelings in a more even-tempered manner. She now viewed her husband as an ally in protecting their child's well-being. Rather than divorcing him, she was determined to react more reasonably to disagreements that inevitably arise in the course of child-rearing.

UNCONSCIOUS TESTING OF THE THERAPIST

Control Mastery theory pays particular attention to ways in which patients test their therapists. This phenomenon has been alluded to by clinicians from other theoretical perspectives. For example, Angyal (1965) states:

> The patient may, with increasing boldness, test the therapist's sincerity—his attention, memory, sensitivity, his respect for the patient's autonomy, his tolerance of criticism and of other forms of attack . . ., his firmness in not yielding to excessive demands, and his readiness to take a stand when this is necessary to prevent extremes of destructive or self-destructive behavior. . . . In putting the therapist to a severe test, the patient yields to the same compulsions that complicate his relations with people in general. . . . Most important is that the experience with the therapist should turn out differently from the past fiascoes. . . . If the therapist passes all the tests . . . the patient's trust grows. (p. 308)

According to Weiss et al. (1986), unconscious testing of the therapist is a means by which patients attempt to solve their problems. By provoking the therapist and monitoring his or her response, the patient is able to determine whether certain of his or her unconscious beliefs are really true. Both "transference" and "passive-into-active" testing occur throughout the course of treatment. Engel and Ferguson (1990) describe the "transference test" as one in which "the client invites or provokes the therapist to treat him in the same negative way that he was treated by his parents. If the parent was critical, the client invites the therapist to be critical. If the parent was controlling, the client invites the therapist to be controlling. . . . To pass these tests, the therapist must refuse these invitations" (p. 202).

What the patient unconsciously desires, in Engel and Ferguson's (1990) view, "is for the therapist to demonstrate that he will not criticize her, or control her—even if given the opportunity," thus allowing her to "overcome her unconscious beliefs that she deserves these inequities" (p. 203).

In a "passive-into-active" test, Engel and Ferguson (1990) note,

> the client mimics his parents' behavior and treats the therapist in the same way he was treated as a child. He *actively* inflicts on the therapist . . . the same abusive behavior that he *passively* endured as a child. If a parent was critical of the client, the client will be critical of the therapist. . . . If a parent was depressed, hopeless, and inconsolable, the client will copy this behavior. . . . In posing a passive-into-active test, the client is attempting to answer the question, If I treat my therapist the same way my parent treated me, will she [the therapist] assume something is wrong with *her,* as I assumed that something was wrong with *me*? To pass a passive-into-active test, the therapist must be able to endure the traumatic treatment that the client is dishing out, without being traumatized by it. . . .
>
> If the client is critical, the therapist must avoid being defensive or overly apologetic. . . . If the client acts in a guilt-inducing way, the therapist must avoid feeling unduly responsible. . . . Once a therapist passes a passive-into-active test, the client is able to use her as a kind of role model—a role model who does not experience irrational self-blame. (p. 205)

Spouses often pose passive-into-active tests to each other. This occurred for Franz Kafka, the famous novelist, with his fiancée, Felice Bauer. Kafka grew up with a meddlesome and possessive mother, who worried endlessly about his eating and sleeping habits, his work, and his courtship behavior. For example, writing to Felice without informing her son, she revealed her apprehension that he was not taking proper care of himself:

> I have known for many years that he spends his leisure hours writing. . . . But he sleeps and eats so little that he's undermining his

health. . . . I am afraid that he may not listen to reason until, God forbid, it is too late. I would therefore very much like to ask you if you could somehow draw his attention to this fact. . . . On the other hand, he must not suspect that I have written to you. (Heller & Born, 1973, p. 46)

As a child and adult, Kafka passively endured his mother's possessiveness and was traumatized by it. He reenacted his mother's possessiveness by enacting a passive-into-active test in his relationship with his fiancée. The following letter is a poignant example of his infliction upon Felice of the introjected version of his mother as he confesses his jealousy of Felice's relationships with anyone other than himself:

Your second letter today made me jealous. . . . Yes, jealous. All letters in which as many people are mentioned as, for example, in today's letter, make me helplessly jealous. . . . I want to start a fight with them all. . . . To drive them away from you. . . . To read only letters that are concerned solely with you, your family, and the two little ones, and of course, of course, me! (Heller & Born, 1973, p. 120)

Kafka's fiancée eventually left the relationship rather than endure Kafka's acting out his mother's possessiveness in the passive-into-active testing behavior. Unfortunately, this is an all too common occurrence for spouses who unconsciously reenact controlling behavior of their parents by turning passive into active and becoming possessive themselves.

PATIENT SELECTION

I readily accept into short-term therapy most couples who appear to want to improve their relationship. I exclude individuals who abuse alcohol or drugs and refuse to stop. I accept individuals who are willing to confront their substance abuse and who, in the course of treatment, commit to abstinence. I integrate their attempts at sobriety into the couple work, and I praise and acknowledge their efforts to give up their destructive habits. I encourage submissive spouses who have tolerated their partners' addiction to voice their concerns.

In some instances, in conjunction with the couple therapy, one or both partners may be referred for individual therapy. Self-absorbed husbands who are receptive to learning more about how they resist, neglect, or verbally abuse their partners often benefit from the perspective that individual therapy offers about the origins and consequences of such behavior. Submissive women who inhibit their expression of discontent, yet harbor resentment toward their spouses, often benefit from their individual therapist's encouragement to assert their concerns. The input that partners receive from their individual therapist often lends greater depth to the couple work, particularly if the couple therapist compares notes with the individual therapist.

FINDING THE FOCUS

To establish the focus in the context of a Control Mastery perspective, the therapist attends to what the couple makes explicit about what will help both members mediate their immediate conflict(s). Also, the therapist needs to be aware of the unconscious plan of each of the partners, their goals and their obstacles to attaining them, their individual pathogenic beliefs, and the beliefs they hold in common that are preventing them from achieving a more harmonious relationship.

With regard to inferring patients' goals, Rappoport (1996) states:

> Goals, and the priority in which they are pursued, are always the patient's to determine. The therapist's task is to infer the patient's goals, since the patient usually cannot convey them directly. However, people do everything they can to give the therapist this information by describing their current life situation, by giving history, and implicitly by the nature of the relationship they establish with the therapist. All of this is orchestrated, largely unconsciously, by the patient for the purpose of furthering their [sic] therapy. (p. 5)

In the case that follows, the husband, Ray, felt omnipotently responsible for his unhappy parents, suffered from separation/survivor guilt toward them, and therefore tended to sabotage his marriage. He gambled compulsively and provoked his wife, Sharon, by repeatedly leering at and commenting on other women's attractiveness while disparaging hers.

Sharon, as a result of her childhood experience with a disabled brother, whose needs took priority over hers, had a pattern of sacrificing her own desires and therefore believed that she was unentitled to better treatment from her husband. In order to help the couple overcome these beliefs within a brief-therapy format, the therapist would have to offer interpretations about the origins of the beliefs, and also pass the patients' transference and passive-into-active tests. This could be achieved with Ray by encouraging him to refrain from gambling, thus passing his transference "safety" test. This would have to be done without succumbing to Ray's tendency to worry, particularly in response to his parents' despair, thus passing his passive-into-active test. With

Sharon, the therapist would have to encourage her to expect better treatment from Ray, thereby disconfirming her belief in her own unentitlement.

The therapist's formulation of the couple's unconscious plan and of their individual and commonly held pathogenic beliefs, though tentative in the initial phase of therapy, provides a good guide to technique for the duration of the therapy.

I formulate the joint unconscious plans of couples and the separate unconscious plans of each partner by listening closely to what they make explicit and keep implicit. I look for subtle inconsistencies and nuances in their descriptions of their relationship that contradict their pessimistic, all-or-nothing perceptions of each other. I am particularly alert to beliefs emanating from their childhood experiences with unhappy parents or siblings that predispose each or both of the partners to experience separation or survivor guilt of sufficient intensity to incline them to sabotage their current union.

For example, if a woman describes her mate as angry and controlling, and he reluctantly confirms this, I look for indications in his behavior that he has a capacity for empathy and tolerance. These indications can be found both in the sessions and in the pair's descriptions of their relationship at home. Their stated desire to repair their relationship, along with remnants of affection that still surface, as well as subtle intimations by the wife of her husband's transient kindness, lead me to infer that their goal is to enlist my support in finding contradictions to the stigmatization of the husband as incapable of tenderness.

The wife, who grew up with a suffering, neglected mother who constantly berated the father, would be inclined, in deference to her survivor guilt and her fear of outdoing her mother, to selectively retrieve information that confirmed a similar view of her own husband. Her tendency would be to obscure and diminish her husband's attempts to be more responsive to her needs so that she could remain loyal to a version of her husband that agrees with her mother's description of her father as neglectful. The wife's therapeutic goal would be to enlist my optimistic support, as opposed to her mother's pessimism in relation to her father and men in general, to help her identify and embrace behaviors of her husband that counter her belief in his malevolence.

In such cases, I am especially attentive to instances when the wife has effectively intervened to modify her husband's provocative behavior. Often, I will ask the wife what it is like to be more effective with her husband than her mother was with her father, and if she can tolerate feeling so effective, considering her mother's failure to achieve similar results with her father. In doing so, I am in accord with the wife's unconscious plan to disconfirm her all-or-nothing view of her husband, which accords with her mother's critique of the father, thus lending a note of optimism and hope for the future of the relationship.

BUILDING THE THERAPEUTIC ALLIANCE

Couples typically enter therapy with what narrative therapists describe as "problem-saturated descriptions" of their relationship (White & Epston, 1990). They overly identify and affiliate with what's wrong and are oblivious to what's right—for example, strengths that coexist with the flaws in the relationship. The couple may be encumbered by the maladaptive and fallacious belief that simply because there is conflict in their relationship, it is doomed to fail. Conflicts between partners are bound to occur, for no two people are alike. Differences of opinion and temperament often foster disagreement. Such differences do not imply incompatibility any more than similarity of viewpoint guarantees compatibility.

The belief that conflict implies incompatibility must be aggressively challenged by their therapist to provide the couple with motivation to overcome its grim implications. To achieve this end, a therapist must empower the members of the couple early in treatment with a sense of hopefulness by responding to the more positive conflict-free zones that exist in their relationship. The therapist needs to acknowledge and point out the couple's creative efforts to resolve its conflicts, which are indicative of the partner's goodwill toward each another. This response will enable the individuals within the couple to supplant their pessimism with a more optimistic outlook. This will have the added effect of strengthening the therapeutic alliance. Zeitlin (1991) remarks "It is important for the therapist to have an optimistic attitude, but not aspire to omnipotence. Couples often present as demoralized and depleted. The therapist needs to provide energy and encouragement to work and explore" (p. 223).

In order to strengthen the therapeutic alliance regarding the couple's erroneous belief that conflict implies incompatibility, the therapist can inform the couple of research that challenges this premise. For example, Gottman (1994) comments in *Why Marriages Succeed or Fail*: "Much more important than having compatible views is *how* couples work out their differences. In fact, occasional discontent, especially during a marriage's early years, seems to be good for the union in the long run" (p. 28). Couples are typically relieved to discover that their conflicts are not unique and do not necessarily portend the demise of their relationship. In this regard, Schnarch (1991) comments:

It is paradoxical that what many couples take as an indication of a bad relationship is actually the potential hallmark of a good one. If the couple can weather the storm, it paves the way for profound and relatively stable levels of intimacy not possible until projective identifications are withdrawn from the partner and "owned" as a part of oneself.

Living through the head-butting, the threats and ultimatums, the yelling and crying, partners develop *begrudging* respect for each other. (p. 177)

By providing "pro-plan" interpretations—that is, interpretations that are responsive to the couple's conscious and/or unconscious aim to overcome their destructive patterns—the therapist can help the pair to disconfirm their pathogenic beliefs, thus enhancing the therapeutic alliance.

Couples are instinctively repelled by and disengage from therapists who consistently demonstrate insensitivity in the form of anti-plan interpretations that confirm rather than challenge their pathogenic beliefs. This occurred in a previous couple therapy for the wife in the following example. The wife, Sharon, who, as mentioned earlier, had a disabled brother, was made to feel guilty for wanting attention from her parents as a child. Their response was to accuse her of being "selfish" for placing her needs above her brother's. Her unconscious plan in couple therapy was to disconfirm her belief that she was unworthy of better treatment from her husband. Her previous couple therapist advised her to expect less from her husband in the hope that she would receive more from him. Experiencing her therapist's admonition as similar to that of her parents (i.e., that her needs were unimportant and she should settle for "less"), she abruptly left therapy. My response, in contrast to that of her previous therapist, was to encourage her to expect *more* from her husband—the effect of which was to disconfirm her belief that she was unentitled to better treatment.

The Management of Anger

The expression of hostility and the attribution of malevolent intent toward one's partner exacerbates conflict and endangers the relationship. There is a difference between the clear assertion of one's position without rancor and the ranting and raving that typically occurs in the transactions between hostile partners. Cognitive therapist Aaron Beck (1988) comments:

Although expressing anger has become something of a shibboleth in marriage, I have found that it usually seems to do more harm than good. The accumulated hurts from being scolded, vilified, and cursed lead the victim to see the attacking spouse not only as an adversary, but also as an enemy. . . . The compelling fact is that there are more efficient ways for partners to settle disputes than by screaming at each other. . . . People can practice simply stating their wishes in a straightforward way, and use finesse and explanations rather than attacks. . . . It is possible to use self-assertion without depending on anger to fuel their assertiveness. (p. 184)

In a similar vein, Dreikurs (1974) stated that "constructive changes do not require hostility. On the contrary, hostile actions generally disturb more than they improve, because they result in more friction and disagreement" (p. 104). There is a lot to be said for demonstrating restraint—that is, knowing when not to respond to inflammatory remarks directed against oneself by one's partner in the heat of an argument. While one cannot necessarily control or convince an ill-tempered mate of the error of his or her ways, by demonstrating self-restraint devoid of retaliation, one can prevent a further escalation of the argument. This is not always easy to do, however, especially when one's instinctive reaction is to steadfastly adhere to and defend one's position regardless of facts to the contrary. Partners who chronically respond to each other from this defended position are habituating a pattern of relating that, if kept up indefinitely, could lead to the ultimate dissolution of the relationship.

Some couples view the catharsis of anger as an end in itself. These individuals may be reenacting scenarios from their childhood that demonstrate their allegiance to hostile parents. Or the individuals may be taking license with behaviors learned in therapy formats (e.g., encounter groups) that postulate the acting out of aggression as cathartic and curative. In Control Mastery terms, couples who reenact such aggressive scenarios in therapy are posing "protection tests" to their therapist in the hope that he or she will actively intervene to contain and moderate their unabashed expressions of hostility. Zeitlin (1991) emphasizes that "there are times when it is important to intervene strongly and oppose or defuse a particular line of discussion, most frequently when retraumatization appears imminent" (p. 225). Therapists who intervene in this way promote an atmosphere of safety that is conducive to strengthening the therapeutic alliance. Therapists who sit back placidly while partners attack each other fail this crucial test. In many instances, the patients then leave the therapy.

Gottman (1997) advises therapists to intervene in couple's arguments *indirectly* by teaching the individuals techniques (such as breathing) that will self-soothe and modulate their anger. He advises against intervening *directly,* since he views such behavior as "state dependent":

> That is, unless we permit a couple to become as emotional in our ther-
> apeutic office as they do at home, when they leave the office they may
> not have access to the important learning we have offered. . . . Part of
> the philosophical assumptions of this therapy is that the therapist
> should give the couple a "tool" to work with and change their marital
> interaction patterns when the couple is emotional. This is in contrast
> to calming the couple down, then providing the insight and the new
> tool, and then asking them to continue their interaction. Even if this
> procedure goes perfectly, they probably will have less access to the
> tool when they become emotional again. (pp. 76–77)

My experience with *volatile couples* contradicts Gottman's premise
about the therapist's intervention. I often hear from such patients how
my admonition to demonstrate restraint has preempted escalation of
their conflicts at home. It appears that they have learned from their therapist how to substitute rationality for raw aggression. This is in contrast
to what they learned as children from their angry parents.

On the other hand, *conflict-avoidant couples,* many of whom grew
up with conflict-avoidant parents, are typically encumbered by the belief
that it is dangerous to express hostility in any form. From a Control
Mastery perspective, a pro-plan intervention by such a couple's therapist
would be to allow for the couple's expression of anger during the sessions. For such individuals (and here I agree with Gottman), it would be
contraindicated to intervene in a manner that would suppress hostile
emotions. Permitting hostility to emerge in such couples' therapy
disconfirms their belief that their expression of anger presages the
demise of their relationship. Gottman's (1994) research demonstrates,
however, that regardless of a couple's fighting style, it is imperative that
the therapist intervene aggressively to inform the couple of the potentially devastating effects to their relationship of hostile exchanges rife
with contempt, criticism, defensiveness, and stonewalling.

The Use of Interpretations

I have found that the majority of my patients are receptive to interpretations that explain in separation- and survivor-guilt terminology behavior
that is disruptive to their relationship. This is so for two reasons.

First, receptivity is enhanced when the interpreting therapist simultaneously passes transference and passive-into-active tests posed by the
patients. Individuals tend to feel more confident with clinicians who
demonstrate sensitivity to their needs in the form of pro-plan interventions, and are less inclined to resist or to discount their interpretations.
Therapists who respond credibly to their patients' testing and whose

behavior is congruent with the messages implicit in their interpretations are more likely to exert a positive influence than are therapists whose behavior is inconsistent with the intent of their interpretations. For example, a therapist who encourages a husband to be less critical of his spouse, yet who responds defensively to his patient's critique of him, fails a crucial passive-into-active test. In this instance, no matter how accurate his interpretation is—for example, that the patient's criticality derives from his identification with his own critical father—the therapist's explanation will fall on deaf ears, as he is according his patient the same criticality that his interpretation is intended to modify.

Second, a patient is typically inclined to accept interpretations that imply altruistic intent toward his or her unhappy parents or siblings to account for behavior that is undermining the current relationship. In this regard, it is crucial to convey to both members of a couple that while separation- and survivor-guilt provide an explanation for such disruptive behavior, this explanation should not be construed as a justification to continue it.

Lack of receptivity to separation- and survivor-guilt interpretations typically occurs for the minority of patients whose cultural background or extended-family ties preclude cogent discussions of family-of-origin issues during the early phase of treatment—particularly, interpretations that imply faulty parenting. By not insisting on his or her interpretation, no matter how accurate, the therapist gives the patients the freedom not to comply with the prescriptions of an authority figure, as they had to do with their parents. In this way, the therapist passes a transference test that enables the patients to maintain their autonomy, the result of which may be to incline them to be more receptive to family-of-origin interpretations later on in the therapy. In this regard, Balint (1969) writes: "Though the patient is in need of an environment, of a world of objects, such objects—foremost among them the analyst—must not be felt as in any way demanding, interfering, intruding, as this would reinforce the old oppressive inequality between subject and object" (p. 180).

In certain instances, I use anecdotes (Erickson, 1982) to illustrate the ubiquitous effects of separation- and survivor-guilt, employing material about one couple to enlighten another whose conflicts are similar. On the value of using anecdotes in therapy, Zeig (1980) comments: "Anecdotes are nonthreatening; . . . anecdotes are engaging; . . . anecdotes foster independence: the individual needs to make sense out of the message and then come to a self-initiated conclusion or a self-initiated action; . . . anecdotes can be used to bypass natural resistance to change; . . . and anecdotes tag the memory—they make the presented idea more memorable" (pp. 33–34).

An anecdote that I often use when I work with a couple in which one of the partners harbors intense jealousy toward the other goes as follows. A 30-year-old bachelor who has a possessive mother visits his parents for a week. One evening, when he returns from a date, his mother throws a temper tantrum, accusing him of being out too late. Five years later, the man, now married, turns passive-into-active by throwing a similar temper tantrum with his wife when she returns from an evening out with friends. At this point in the story, I ask the couple what they think will happen if the husband keeps this behavior up indefinitely. I enthusiastically concur with their insight that the wife will most likely leave. I then ask who the first person will be that this man will call after the breakup to bemoan his fate. Once again, I emphatically concur with the couple's insight that it will be his mother. This anecdote conveys to the couple in a benign but poignant way how this man's unconscious separation guilt concerning his mother prompted him to undermine his marriage. Partners readily identify with the protagonist in the story and creatively utilize the information imbedded in it by vowing to refrain from reenacting such behavior with each other.

GAMBLING WITH A MARRIAGE

Sharon and Ray requested therapy after reading a newspaper article that I had written entitled "The Grass Is *Not* Always Greener," in which I had alluded to a common concern of women whose husbands are experiencing difficulty committing to the relationship. Such men are captivated by the notion that there is or must be something—or *someone*—more enticing just around the corner. At least, that is how they rationalize their ambivalent involvements with their spouses. From reading my article, Sharon felt that I knew something about this problem, which had plagued her marriage from the onset.

Sharon was an attractive 30-year-old, college-educated woman with two children, ages 2 and 4, from a previous marriage. Ray was a 32-year-old man with a Master's degree in business, who had originally majored in music. He had one child from a previous marriage.

Sharon was troubled by many of Ray's behaviors. She described him as a compulsive gambler who continued to lose large sums of money by betting on sports events. She herself was a recovered alcoholic, who combined information from her AA program with insights from her personal therapy with another therapist to attempt to exert a positive influence on her husband. She feared that if she took too strident or punitive a stand by putting their marriage on the line, Ray would refuse to even consider the ramifications of his gambling.

I asked Sharon how she responded to her husband when he gambled. "I try to ignore it," she said, "hoping it will go away." Ray interrupted, "It never does. I'm unable to stop gambling. I've lost hundreds of thousands of dollars in the last 10 years. I quit for short periods of time, only to begin again."

I asked Ray how he felt about the way his wife responded to his addiction. He said that her even-tempered approach was the right one, because he viewed himself as resistant to either/or positions. "I typically rebel," he said, "when people tell me what to do, even when it's in my best interest. When my first wife threatened that she would leave me if I didn't give up gambling, I gambled more than ever."

One side effect of Ray's gambling was his tendency to withdraw from Sharon, particularly after losing money. During such extended periods of self-imposed isolation, he became extremely critical of Sharon's behavior and rejected her affection, acting as if he were being held captive in a relationship that, when he was in a better frame of mind, he claimed to enjoy. Sharon was particularly offended when Ray leered at other women and then provoked her by saying how attractive he found them. Nevertheless, Ray never actually had an affair with anyone.

I asked Sharon how she felt about Ray's faultfinding and how she coped with his ambivalence. She described herself as being of two minds. "At times," she said, "I confront his mean-spiritedness and total disregard of my feelings. At other times, I overlook his behavior, hoping that it will eventually go away." Then, turning to Ray, she said, "You know, I'm tired of having to walk on eggshells with you. What makes you think you can go on disregarding my feelings forever?"

I felt that this direct confrontation with Ray was partly Sharon's attempt to convey to *me* the intensity of her despair.

"See?" he said with a smile, looking at me. "She *can* assert herself sometimes."

I asked him if he saw any advantage to this, since he had said earlier that he liked her to be nonaggressive.

"I'm not so sure," he said, "that by making it easy on me to continue my behavior, she's helping either one of us."

Sharon responded brusquely, "Yes, but when I stand up to you, you withdraw and become hostile."

To this, Ray became mute. Clearly, Sharon was damned if she did and damned if she didn't. While Ray usually bristled at Sharon's attempts to put limits on his acting-out, I surmised from his body language and his words that he secretly would welcome a less tolerant approach, both from her and from me. Frequently, when Sharon was describing her permissiveness with Ray, he would look at me as if to say, "See what I get away with?" On one occasion, he actually used these exact words. This was Ray's way of *coaching* me to develop a pro-plan interpretation of this dynamic that would encourage Sharon to take a more self-assertive posture in response to his gambling, which placed them both at risk. Rappoport (1996) says of such coaching: "Patients . . . coach the therapist to convey the attitudes and display the abilities which will help them to progress. Patients work collaboratively with the therapist at the deepest level, despite appearances which may be to the contrary" (p. 2).

I inferred from Ray's coaching, in this and other contexts, that his *unconscious plan* was to utilize his couple therapy to develop an incentive to refrain from his self-destructive behavior and to salvage his marriage. My hypothesis was confirmed during the next session, in which Ray provided information about his family that helped to explain the etiology of his gambling addiction and his ambivalent relationship with his wife.

During that next session, I inquired about each partner's family of origin. Ray stated that his father, a Holocaust survivor, was away on business throughout most of Ray's childhood. His mother, left to care for Ray and his sister, was often anxious. At times, for no apparent reason, she would lash out at her son. Ray expressed sadness and regret that he had spent so little time with his father during his childhood. Whenever he alluded to his father's unavailability and aloofness, he became teary-eyed, giving the impression of a forlorn and suffering man who still craved the affection denied him in his youth. Ray believed that many of his fears and insecurities as an adult were remnants of his having been deprived of an intimate relationship with his father.

In college, Ray majored in music, wanting to become a composer. His parents chided their son for his "eccentric" interest, preferring that he take up a career in business, so that he could "make some money." When I asked if Ray continued to be involved in his music, Sharon responded by praising his great musical talent. I asked Ray how he felt about his wife's support of his talent. My intervention was aimed at identifying pockets of goodwill between him and his wife to counter their "problem-saturated description" of their relationship. Ray replied in a somewhat halfhearted and self-abnegating manner that while he appreciated Sharon's acknowledgment of his talent, he did not consider himself "much of a musician." Rather, it was his father, who had recently taken up painting, who was "the real talent in the family."

Sharon challenged Ray's self-denigrating comments by informing me that it was typical of her husband to defer to his father, even when doing so was unjustified. Then to Ray she said, "You always compare yourself unfavorably with your father. You're too quick to put him on a pedestal. He's not a god, you know. Anyway, you've got more integrity than he has, and you're a much better father to your kids than he was to you."

"I feel like a cheap imitation of my father," Ray said. "He's achieved success, while I've thrown away my money by gambling. I'll never be able to compete with him or attain what he has."

Sharon once again interrupted her husband's self-denigrating comments, reminding him that while his father had achieved material success, he was lacking in moral fiber, as was evidenced by the ongoing extramarital affair he had been involved in for many years.

Ray peered down at the floor, receded back into his chair, and with a teary look, revealed the facts surrounding his father's affair and inability to sustain an intimate relationship with his mother. Ray then said that the onset of his gambling addiction occurred some 10 years earlier, after his father burdened him with the existence of the extramarital affair.

"My father told me," he said, "that my mother was unresponsive to him sexually, but that he was a very sexual person and needed an outlet. He told me that he had met a woman who was emotionally responsive, and they were having an affair. He swore me to secrecy. I don't know if it's still going on, but I worry that it is. At family get-togethers, everyone acts as if we're just one big happy family. But I know different. I notice my father flirting with women all the time. He charms them, gives the impression of being shy. They just love it."

I said to Ray, "I wonder what it's been like for you to be aware of your father's affair and to have to keep it a secret."

Ray was near tears. "It's been terrible," he said. "Keeping the secret makes it difficult for me to face my mother. And not knowing if it's ended makes it even worse."

Clearly, Ray's heartfelt description of his father's behavior, combined with his obvious need to idealize his parent, were determining factors in both the etiology of his gambling addiction and his incapacity to commit unambivalently to his own marriage. In Control Mastery terms, Ray's clandestine gambling represented an identification with and a reenactment of the circumstances surrounding his father's affair.

In this regard, it is not uncommon for male pathological gamblers to refer facetiously to their preoccupation with gambling as "the other woman in my life" (McGurrin, 1992). Ray's inability to achieve happiness with his wife, who was openly affectionate and desirous of a mutually fulfilling marriage, emanated from his pathogenic belief that to do so would be disloyal to his parents' dismal relationship. By making himself more available for an intimate relationship with his wife, he would be outdoing and showing up his father—who, rather than work on *his* marriage, chose to act out in an affair. At the same time, Ray was worried about his mother, who was either oblivious to or in denial about her husband's infidelity. Ray's mother was a personification of the archetypically wounded parent who enlisted her son as her confidant to compensate for her husband's neglect. In short, Ray was encumbered by survivor guilt toward his father and by both separation guilt and survivor guilt toward his mother.

I asked Ray if he had confronted his father with his feelings. He replied that he had not, fearing that if he did so, his father would become angry and reject him. He added that he didn't want to expose his father to ridicule, which was typical of Ray's inclination to protect his father from the consequences of his actions.

Instead of rejecting parental attitudes and behaviors detrimental to their happiness, individuals like Ray often adopt and reenact those very same attributes. By maintaining their allegiance to their parents' shortcomings, they are unconsciously protecting and providing redemption for their parents' flawed personalities. Fishel (1991) elaborates on this phenomenon in *Family Mirrors*: "From childhood forward we will make a huge effort to prove our parents right, even if it means making ourselves wrong. . . . We may maintain our childhood loyalty to our parents by continuing the . . . abuse, ensuring that we will not outdo our parents as parents" (p. 84).

It was obvious from Ray's dejected countenance that he continued to bear the brunt of his parents' unfair recruitment of him as a repository for their unresolved feelings associated with their marital discord. Sharon intervened, noting that Ray's parents had an accommodated marriage. Both of them had told Ray that they slept in separate bedrooms, rarely spent time together, and were openly hostile to each other in private, though they put on a facade of conviviality in public. Sharon added that it had been harmful to Ray for his father to confess the affair to him. She described numerous instances when Ray's gambling (and his withdrawal from her) intensified when he returned from being with his father.

As had been typical in previous sessions, Ray once again attempted to protect and restore his father's honor, suggesting that his mother's anxiety and short-temperedness justified his father's looking elsewhere for sexual gratification. This was one of many instances when Ray's rationalization and defense of his father's acting-out radically contrasted with his own torment over having to bear the burden and negative consequences of his father's behavior.

At this juncture, I suggested to Ray that he appeared encumbered by the consequences of his father's affair and the reality of his parents' dismal relationship. I emphasized that his mother's unhappiness, and her attempt to use Ray to compensate for her husband's neglect, intensified Ray's guilt on those occasions when he and his wife were enjoying each another. At such times, Ray's gambling and his denigration of his wife caused Sharon to distance herself from him. Ray experienced his wife's response as punishment for the potential of their relationship being more successful than the one between his parents.

According to Weiss et al. (1986), individuals who, like Ray, are susceptible to survivor guilt inflict punishment on themselves to atone for their attainment of a more prosperous existence than their despondent parent had: "He may, by identifying with the parent toward whom he feels guilty, acquire certain of the parent's most self-destructive behaviors or traits . . . , for example, ruin his marriage by raging at his wife as his father ruined his marriage by such raging" (p. 51). I suggested to Ray that it was neither in his nor his wife's interest to hold himself responsible for his parents' dilemma or accountable for the repair of their marriage. Ray appeared relieved by this.

In a personal communication, Dr. Joseph Weiss compared Ray's experience of his parents' marriage to being on a sinking ship that he felt it was his responsibility to keep afloat. The impossibility of doing so contributed to his feeling of hopelessness and his grim belief that his problems were insoluble. Both in therapy and in his marriage, Ray worked to change his belief that he was responsible for his parents by testing it through turning *passive into active*. He did this by making *me* responsible for his happiness. During periods of intense despondency, he attempted to persuade me that the couple therapy was getting nowhere, that his gambling was as pervasive as ever, and that his situation was hopeless. I passed these tests by demonstrating my concern for his dilemma but without accepting the responsibility that he was imparting to me. In doing so, I was able to provide Ray with a role model of someone who did not feel omnipotent, as he was inclined to feel in relation to his need to solve his parents' problems.

My response was instructive to Sharon, toward whom Ray posed similar passive-into-active tests by reenacting some of his father's maladaptive behaviors—for example, aloofness, criticality, and flirtatiousness. I understood that her unconscious plan was to stand up to and set limits on her husband's unreasonable behavior. To achieve that goal, she would, like me, have to remain unencumbered by her husband's despondency and manipulative attempts to make her feel guilty (as her parents had done earlier) for entitling herself to a better life.

According to Weiss et al. (1986):

When a test is passed, the patient may become unconsciously less anxious and more relaxed than he had been. He may, moreover, while relaxed, become more insightful. He may, for example, bring forth a previously repressed memory. . . . He may, in addition, keep the memory in consciousness without coming into conflict with it and use the insight he gained from it to attain a better understanding of his problems. (p. 106)

In a similar vein, Zeitlin (1991) comments:

When a test is passed, the patient takes a step toward disconfirming the pathogenic belief. He typically becomes less anxious, bolder in exploring the material of the session, and more relaxed and positive. He may also bring the pathogenic belief closer to consciousness, begin to overcome certain inhibitions or symptoms, or lift repressions formerly maintained in obedience to the belief. (p. 207)

In a subsequent session, in response to my passing his test, Ray recalled formerly repressed material—a dream that he had had some 10 years earlier, after his father had told him about the affair. In the dream, Ray provided his parents with an aphrodisiac elixir, indicating his omnipotent belief that it was his responsibility to sexualize his parents' relationship.

At home, Ray and Sharon, somewhat less adversarial now as a result of the progress made in therapy, began to disconfirm their pathogenic belief that they were incapable of meaningful communication. They discussed how Ray's father had used his Holocaust experience to brainwash his son into believing that achievements devoid of suffering are worthless. Ray's unconscious compliance with the content of his father's message took the form of his feeling undeserving of his accomplishments, particularly when these came easily and involved any kind of pleasure.

The torment over his gambling addiction was another way that Ray colluded with his father's grim admonition. Ray's inability to enjoy his marriage, especially with a woman who was so ready to be affectionate with him, exemplified his survivor guilt.

It is typical of couples like Ray and Sharon, mired in their difficulties, to harbor a mutually held pathogenic belief that their conflicts are insoluble and a sign of their incompatibility. As has been noted above, the therapist needs to challenge such beliefs in order to instill a more hopeful and optimistic outlook. To accomplish this, I concurred with the couple's insights regarding Ray's self-destructive behavior in relation to his father's Holocaust indoctrination. My intervention was intended to convey to them they were obviously in possession of skills and attributes conducive to a harmonious relationship.

My response was informed by the optimism of clinicians who view conflict as an inevitable occurrence in the lives of couples in the process of transforming their relationship to a higher level. As Erich Fromm (1956) stated:

> Just as it is customary for people to believe that pain and sadness should be avoided under all circumstances, they believe that love means the absence of any conflict. . . . Real conflicts between two people, those which do not serve to cover up or to project, but which are experienced on the deep level of inner reality to which they belong, are not destructive. They lead to clarification, they produce a catharsis from which both persons emerge with more knowledge and more strength. (p. 93)

In Control Mastery terms, I passed a crucial *transference test* by acknowledging Ray and Sharon's collaborative efforts, which implied a capacity to utilize their conflicts as a vehicle for their mutual growth.

During this phase of the therapy, I was interested in learning more about Sharon's upbringing in order to understand her reticence to hold her husband more accountable for his behavior. Sharon described having grown up with a disabled brother whose needs took priority over hers. The parents were inclined to minimize Sharon's needs while indulging her brother's, to compensate for his disability. "Even when I excelled," Sharon said, "I got no response. When I confronted my parents about their neglect, they accused me of being *'selfish.'* "

I asked Sharon if she saw any relationship between the way she responded to her parents' treatment of her and the way she responds now to Ray's treatment of her.

She eagerly replied, "My parents led me to believe that I shouldn't expect much from them and that I wasn't entitled to more attention than my brother got. I suppose I'm doing the same thing with Ray— deferring my needs to his, feeling undeserving of being treated any better. God, how I hate my parents for instilling that attitude in me!"

Then, looking puzzled, she asked me, "So *now* what do I do?"

Turning to Ray, I asked how he would answer Sharon.

Rising to the occasion as he had done in previous sessions, and instead of defending himself, Ray said, "Maybe you shouldn't be so tolerant of my crap—my taking cheap shots at you."

Sharon sighed. "But as I've complained in here so often," she said, "when I defend myself, you punish me—either by withdrawing or getting angry."

"It sounds to me," I said, "that Ray wants you to be more self-protective. He seems to be receptive now to facing up to the role that he plays in provoking your unhappiness. He needs you to set limits on what you'll accept from him and what you won't."

I further suggested to Sharon that from what we knew about the abusive way that Ray's father treated his mother, Sharon should not accept similar behavior from Ray.

Before I could finish my sentence, Sharon said excitedly, "Oh, so when I indulge Ray, I'm behaving just like his wimpy mother. God, I never thought of that. The two of us are reenacting his parents' relationship. Ray identifies with his father's acting-out, and I assume the role of victim, like his mother."

Ray concurred with Sharon's remarks, reflecting that he typically felt more responsive to his wife when her behavior contrasted with his mother's victimization.

By setting limits upon her husband's acting-out, Sharon would, in effect, be challenging her survivor guilt, acquired in childhood, that she was undeserving of attention and fair treatment from significant others. At the same time, she would inadvertently be passing Ray's passive-into-active test—namely, his reenactment with her of maladaptive behavior acquired in relation to his parents, injurious both to his self-esteem and the well-being of their marriage. By asserting herself, and thus passing her husband's test, Sharon would be providing Ray with a role model (as I had done previously in response to his testing) of someone who did not feel guilty for prioritizing her authentic needs for fair treatment. This might enable Ray to do the same in relation to being burdened by his father's extramarital affair and disconfirm his belief of being responsible for his parents' happiness.

Sharon began the next session in tears, describing an episode at a movie theater when Ray once again ogled other women and verbally denigrated Sharon's attributes in relation to theirs. "It was too much for you, wasn't it, Ray?" she said. "The fact that we had been getting along better after the last session. I felt closer to you than I have in months. Our sex was great the evening after our session. Guess you couldn't take the closeness—you really blew it with your stupid comments. God, I'm fed up!"

Firestone (1988) noted, after observing couples over an extended period of time:

> Many men and women reported a deterioration in their personal relationships following periods of unusual intimacy and tenderness. These events precipitated a flow of negative thoughts, some self-critical and others critical of their partner. Both parties tended to hold back, on an unconscious level, shared pleasurable activities, sexual responses, or special traits and behaviors that had been admired by the other. . . . It

was generally observed that critical, "picky" thoughts and misperceptions of one's mate were activated following a time when the partners had been especially close, both sexually and emotionally. (p. 43)

It would not be helpful for a therapist to inform a couple that their problem is simply one of sustaining intimacy. Nevertheless, that is precisely what many couples therapists convey to their patients—especially those patients who are in the midst of a downward spiral because one of the partners has done something provocative to sabotage the other's goodwill. In response to such a generic interpretation, couples feel inadequate, and the provocative partner learns nothing about what factors contributed to his withholding affection from his spouse. There is more to be gained from helping partners to identify the circumstances that rekindle their guilt—for example, outdoing significant others who have been denied similar pleasurable experience.

Intending to help Ray and Sharon identify factors that had precipitated Ray's undoing of their loving feelings, I asked Sharon how she had responded to Ray's flirtatious behavior. She replied that in this instance, unlike in the past, she had confronted him, attributing this assertive response to the encouragement I had given her to prioritize her needs rather than submit to her husband's provocative behavior. "I told him in no uncertain terms," she said, "that if he continued, I'd go home alone—he'd have to take the bus. That it was his wandering eye or me. He couldn't have both."

I asked Sharon what accounted for her newfound ability to stand up for herself. She said: "In the past, I would have avoided confronting Ray, afraid that he'd become angry and leave. This time, I felt different. I knew I deserved better." In Schnarch's (1997) terms, Sharon's new assertiveness is an example of "self-validated intimacy," which

> relies on a person's maintaining his or her own sense of identity and self-worth when disclosing, with no expectation of acceptance or reciprocity from the partner. One's capacity for self-validated intimacy is directly related to one's level of differentiation; that is, one's ability to maintain a clear sense of oneself when loved ones are pressuring for conforming and sameness. Self-validated intimacy is the tangible product of one's "relationship with oneself." (pp. 106–107)

Impressed with Sharon's self-assuredness, I seized the opportunity to ascribe a positive connotation to her behavior. I asked Ray what it was like to be with someone who had sufficient self-esteem to prioritize her needs in response to his acting-out—unlike his mother, who suffered the inequities of his father in silence.

Once again, Ray rose to the occasion by acknowledging the power in his wife's response. "Yeah, she really meant business," he said. "She wouldn't let me get away with it. You know, it's probably good when she does that. I feel relieved when she sets limits. When I'm left to my own devices, I end up hurting both of us."

In an attempt to consolidate material from previous sessions having to do with Sharon's survivor guilt, I asked Ray if he understood, considering his wife's childhood, why it was so important for her to expect more from him. Acknowledging the detrimental effect on Sharon of the survivor guilt she harbored in relation to her brother, Ray said to Sharon: "Whenever we visit your brother, I notice how his needs come first and how dismissive your parents are of you. Now that I'm more aware of this, I'm inclined to give you what you deserve. I really hate it when your parents treat you that way." Ray's insightful, compassionate response to his wife's dilemma demonstrates how patients can creatively integrate separation- and survivor-guilt interpretations that enable them to empathize and collaborate with each other to meet their personal and relationship goals.

I asked Ray if he understood why, with his leering, he had been predisposed to undo the closeness that had developed between the two of them after our last session.

Sharon chimed in, "It's his Mama again! She called and told Ray how unhappy she was with his father, who continues to pay more attention to his business and hobbies."

"And other women," Ray added.

"She was lamenting how lonely she is," Sharon continued. "She wanted to have lunch with Ray to 'get a little pleasure out of life' with the time she has left."

Instead of responding defensively to his wife's tirade, Ray confirmed her hunch about the role that his mother's phone call had played in the resurrection of his self-destructive behavior. "I felt lousy after the call," he said. "I took it out on Sharon, I guess for the reasons we've talked about here—that I had no right to be happy while my mother's so unhappy."

Firestone (1988) refers to the deleterious effect of guilt activated in proximity to or induced by one's less fortunate and/or envious family members: "Many patients . . . regress when they have contact with original family members, particularly if members of their family either actually manipulate them to activate their guilt feelings or indirectly foster guilt in the patient because of the negative quality of the family members' lives" (p. 229).

It was blatantly apparent to Ray, Sharon, and me that by acting out, Ray had incurred his wife's wrath as punishment for not being able to rescue his mother or repair his parents' marriage. I reminded Ray that it was neither in his nor his wife's interest for him to feel so omnipotently responsible for his parents' happiness—that he had not caused their problems, nor could he magically salvage their marriage by undermining his own.

I emphasized that it was Ray's choice to continue his provocative actions, but that, given Sharon's newly acquired self-confidence, Ray's behavior might presage the eventual dissolution of the marriage. "Is that what you want?" I asked.

"No, not really," he replied. "I love Sharon. I even respect her more these days. I can't say I always like it when she confronts me, but I understand how much courage it takes for her to stand up to me. I'm not the easiest guy to live with."

I asked Sharon how she felt about what Ray just said.

"It's good to hear him acknowledge that I can have a good effect on him," she said.

I told her how impressed I was with her ability to demand better treatment from Ray—especially since, in her childhood, she had been made to feel that she always had to "settle for less." My aim was to model for Ray respectful behavior toward his wife to counter his unconscious belief in her inadequacy—an irrational belief that did not conform to the reality of Sharon's persona. Nevertheless, if Ray maintained this belief, it would provide him with a rationale to abandon a relationship that in fact had the potential to enormously stimulate his emotional development. In that case, he might never disengage from the shadow of his parents' miserable marriage.

In the following session, Ray revealed that he had decided to stop gambling. His belief was that doing so would make it more likely that he would be "more alive and responsive to Sharon" and less critical. Ray was apparently relieved by my support of Sharon's feelings during the previous session and by her bold initiative to curtail his various forms of acting-out, which were motivated by his survivor guilt in relation to his parents.

While Ray would have liked to have had an effect on his father's behavior similar to what occurred for him in response to Sharon's confrontation, his repeated attempts to censure his father's acting-out were to no avail. His worry about his parents' marital dilemma led to his feeling omnipotently responsible for them. His belief that they were unable to alter their dysfunctional lifestyle led to his feeling hopeless, convinced that he could never attain happiness. Ray inferred from my encouraging his wife to assert her legitimate concerns that I believed him capable of better treatment of her.

Sharon passed Ray's passive-into-active test by setting well-defined limits to his provocative behavior. Setting limits on others was something he had difficulty doing, especially in response to people who took advantage of him (e.g., his father, his ex-wife, bookies, etc.). The combination of his wife's and my responses provided Ray with healthy role-modeling and the motivation to be more protective of himself and his marriage.

As has been mentioned previously, when a test that is posed to one's therapist or spouse is passed, the patient or marital partner posing the test becomes less anxious and more assertive in his or her attempts to master difficulties. This occurred for Ray in his decision to quit gambling.

To increase the likelihood that he would overcome his gambling addiction, and in response to both his wife's and my encouragement, Ray joined Gamblers Anonymous. To provide momentum for the gains that were occurring during this phase of therapy, Ray decided to stop making himself available to his father's complaints about his marital discontent and his denigration of Ray's mother.

"Every time I listen to him complaining," Ray said, "I take it out on Sharon, as we've discussed here so often. It's a pattern that's got to stop."

I acknowledged to Ray that it made sense for him to set limits with his father, as the latter had been presumptuous in burdening his son with the never-ending details of his marital dissatisfaction. I reminded him how, in a previous session, he had used the word *restless* in relation to Sharon, following a meeting with his father, who had once again burdened Ray with how "restless he was feeling" in his marriage. Prior to his meeting with his father, Ray and Sharon had been getting along well, and he had spoken of her in glowing terms.

Acknowledging that he had picked up the theme of restlessness from his father, Ray recognized the negative implication to himself and his marriage of his compliance with his father's dysfunctionality. He was no longer willing to assume the role of the identified patient in his family. His gambling addiction provided his parents with something to talk about, whereas at other times they hardly spoke to each other. With regard to being identified as the patient or "sick one" in a family, Firestone (1990) comments:

> Generally, psychologists agree that many dysfunctional families are "held together" through the process of designating one family member, usually a child, as the "sick one," the "bad one" ("scapegoating"), or the "mentally ill one." By focusing negative attention on a particular child, the family is able to maintain a semblance of stability and continue to function as a cohesive unit. On another level, the

"sick" child is aware that he serves this function and that, by remaining ill, he is, in effect, saving his family from dissolution. (p. 47)

To muster the strength, without feeling guilty, to set limits on his father's usage of him as a receptacle for his dissatisfaction, Ray posed a passive-into-active test to his therapist. He and Sharon had missed a previous session without giving notice. Ray objected to my charging him for the session, accusing me of being unfair, unconcerned for his well-being, and interested only in receiving the fee. His accusations were meant to make me feel guilty, though, unconsciously, he hoped I would remain undaunted by his recriminations. He needed me to role-model behavior—namely, self-assuredness, devoid of guilt—which he could then reenact with his father. By remaining firm without feeling guilty in my decision to hold Ray to our initial agreement regarding missed sessions, and thus passing his test, I provided him with a template that he could incorporate in his subsequent confrontation with his father. A few days later, Ray informed his father that while he would continue to relate to him, he could not condone his father's affair, nor should his father expect him to continue to listen to his marital discontent or his demeaning of Ray's mother.

In the remaining four sessions of couple therapy (I saw them a total of 20 times over 8 months), I continued to encourage Sharon to stand up to Ray. She was especially successful at this in response to Ray's ex-wife, Joan, who was dismissive to Sharon when making arrangements for Ray's 4-year-old boy to visit him. A relationship triangle (Guerin, Fogarty, Fay, & Kautto, 1996) existed among Ray, Sharon, and Joan that was exerting a detrimental effect on the marriage. Triangles of this sort are often fueled by survivor guilt. Such triangles need to be acknowledged by the couple and their therapist and countered by them with strategies designed to ameliorate their insidious effects.

Ray experienced intense survivor guilt over Joan, who continuously lamented her unhappiness with her current boyfriend and her experience of being burdened in her role as a single parent. She insinuated to Ray, despite facts to the contrary, that he did not do enough for her or his son. As Joan observed Ray's resolve to quit gambling becoming stronger, and as she saw him becoming happier in his marriage, her interference grew in intensity. This took the form of enlisting Ray's assistance at all hours of the day or night, regardless of his responsibility to his wife and stepchildren. Joan's insistence that Ray be available to her beyond the scope of their divorce agreement and in spite of his dedication to his child's well-being was extremely destructive to Ray's relationship with Sharon, who experienced herself as an outsider to these events. The problems in the marriage were exacerbated by Joan's exclusion of

Sharon in the plans for Ray's child. Instead of including Sharon in scheduling school activities and visitations, Joan would communicate unilaterally with Ray, who was indulgent of this, even though he understood that Sharon felt hurt. Ray's passivity was predicated on remnants of guilt from his divorce, for which he felt inordinately responsible, and on the survivor guilt he experienced in response to Joan's constant complaints. Ray's tolerance of Joan's insatiable demands and his inability to stand up to her were facilitated by Sharon's initial reluctance to confront Ray about establishing more appropriate boundaries with Joan, a residual of Sharon's survivor guilt in relation to her disabled brother.

During our discussion of these dynamics, I conveyed to the couple the ubiquitous presence of such triangulation in the lives of blended families and the need to address these issues if the relationship were to flourish. In this regard, Guerin et al. (1996) comment: "Remarried parents need to have realistic expectations of each other as stepparents. Therapists must make the ghosts of ex-spouses explicit and get the family to deal openly with them. This demands an acceptance of the fact that the bond between former spouses is never broken when the marriage has produced offspring, but lives on for generations to come" (p. 220). A similar idea is expressed by Kirschner and Kirschner (1986): "An important priority in the treatment of stepfamilies is to create clear psychological boundaries around the marriage. Primary loyalties need to be cultivated in the direction of the current spouse and away from the former spouse. The practitioner guides the couple toward a strong and united relationship" (p. 220).

In order to strengthen the marital dyad, I encouraged Sharon to voice her objections to being excluded from the decision-making process regarding Ray's child. I suggested to Ray that Sharon's concern was intended to protect him from Joan's unfounded criticisms and to promote the well-being of the marriage. Although Ray initially defended Joan, he subsequently rose to the occasion by agreeing to set more appropriate boundaries in response to Joan's intrusiveness. He accomplished this by informing Joan that from now on he and Sharon would make decisions together about his child's visits, rather than making these decisions unilaterally with Joan. In their general demeanor, and by demonstrating affection for each other in Joan's presence, Ray and Sharon conveyed to Joan that she could no longer exert a divisive effect on their relationship.

Both Ray and Sharon had been involved in prior couple therapy formats, which included behavioral interventions as well as prescriptions in the form of homework assignments designed to stop Ray's gambling and engage the couple in more intimate dialogue. Ray and Sharon were unsuccessful in these endeavors and failed to establish a therapeutic alliance because, in their words, they had "no inkling" of what was fueling their self-destructive behavior.

One aspect of my interventions that led to a successful outcome with the couple consistent with Control Mastery theory was my encouraging them to view their parents' inconsiderate treatment of them realistically, without minimizing the ramifications of that treatment. Well-meaning therapists who regard family-of-origin dynamics as irrelevant and who encourage premature forgiveness by patients of the inequities meted out by their parents run the risk of invalidating the patients' accurate perceptions of their real experiences, thus repeating a scenario that occurred frequently for them during their childhood. Ultimately, this impairs the therapeutic alliance and exacerbates the couple's conflicts. Such individuals are entitled to and benefit from role-modeling by their therapist that in no uncertain terms validates the role of their real experience in relation to parents and siblings who fostered their separation- and survivor-guilt. In this regard, I am in agreement with Firestone (1990), who asserts that to reinforce an idealized image of a patient's parents while denying his or her real experience is counterproductive:

> Some clinicians consider it questionable to disrupt a *false* positive idealized view of parents. . . . These psychotherapists directly and indirectly support idealization, to the detriment of their patients over the long term.
>
> This is not our position. The anxiety, anger, and guilt aroused after exposing the truth about parents is an essential part of therapy. We feel that these reactions must be worked through in successful therapy. In general, we are opposed to the reinforcement of any process of self-deception. Defenses and illusions distort life experiences and cause many unnecessary problems and pain in relationships. (pp. 133–134)

Harold Sampson (1992) makes essentially the same point:

> If we interpret as resistance patients' criticisms of their parents, we may interfere with their reality testing, that is, with their right, and hence their capacity, to see their parents through their own eyes rather than as they believe their parents (and parental surrogates such as the analyst) would prefer to be seen. . . .
>
> Patients who criticize us or their parents in exaggerated and implausible ways may be unconsciously testing us. They may be inviting us to show them the untenability of their criticisms or to tell them that they are "overreacting." They have probably heard that they are overreacting before ever meeting *us*. It means to them that they are being petty or oversensitive to react so strongly and that they have lit-

tle, if any, genuine grievance. The patient often already believes *that* (unconsciously). Therefore, it is better to resist the patient's invitation and, in doing so, to resist interfering with the patient's attempts not to have to comply with parental blaming, put-downs, rejections, and abuse. If we fail this test, we may make it harder for the patient to become aware of, and to take responsibility for, his own *real* feelings and wishes. (pp. 525–526)

TERMINATION AND FOLLOW-UP

In the final session, the couple reported an overall improvement in their relationship, more enjoyment of their shared experiences, and an enhancement of their sexuality. Ray continued to abstain from gambling, receiving warm support and encouragement from Sharon.

During termination, I informed the couple that I would be available to them at any time if the need arose. Earlier in treatment, I had told Ray that once his gambling stopped, it would be worthwhile to enter a men's group. I added that I thought this would be a good idea so that he could develop relationships with men other than the bookies and ne'er-do-wells he had been associating with in relation to his gambling. My hope was that Ray's pathogenic belief in his own unworthiness, combined with the shame he harbored about his father's affair, would be challenged and disconfirmed in the safe confines of a men's group.

Ray did in fact join a men's group led by another therapist. Initially, feeling that he didn't belong, Ray was critical of his peers, another manifestation of his allegiance to his family of origin. He experienced the support he received from his peers as encouraging his separation from his parents—something he both desired and feared.

A turning point occurred on the day that Ray brought one of his music tapes to the group, for which he received much praise and acknowledgment. Ray's realization that his initial criticism of the group members only served to maintain his loyalty to and protection of his parents enabled him to challenge and transcend this self-imposed limitation. Now, as one of the other members of the group put it who was in recovery for alcohol addiction, Ray could affiliate with "higher companions" rather than continue his dysfunctional association with the "lower companions" who encouraged his self-destructive behaviors. In response to Ray's portrayal of Sharon, the group as a whole consistently reminded him of the strengths of their relationship, and passed his "protection test" by cautioning him not to impetuously "throw away a good thing."

In a follow-up couple session a year after terminating couple therapy, Ray reported in Sharon's presence that he was maintaining his abstinence from his gambling addiction, was comfortable in his men's group, and was enjoying his marriage. He understood that it would be unrealistic and contraindicated for him to intrude himself in his parents' marital strife. Sharon reported that she and Ray were talking about having a child—something she had desired from the beginning of their relationship but had concluded would be virtually impossible until their relationship changed for the better. That change had now occurred.

The case study referred to above illustrates the importance of attending to family-of-origin dynamics in the treatment of couples who are experiencing marital difficulties. Control Mastery theory provides an optimal vantage point from which to understand the origins of such conflict, as well as a format and vocabulary that allow for a myriad of effective therapeutic interventions to resolve and ameliorate such difficulties. The therapeutic milieu fostered by this approach pays particular attention to each partner's and the couple's proclivity to test their therapist by repeating traumatic patterns from their past. They do this in the unconscious hope that the therapist will respond with more integrity than those who originally enslaved them to self-defeating beliefs and agendas. The significance and meaning of such repetitions are perhaps most meaningfully expressed by Fishel (1991):

> We repeat in an unconscious effort at mastery and control. We repeat the painful episodes of our childhoods in the hope of making sense of them now. We are in a sense doing research into our own pasts. With our repetitions we are asking questions that may remain cruelly unheard for another generation. But our questioning may also lead us to new and healing answers and interventions from a sensitive partner or therapist—or even from a courageous child whose response shows us a new direction. . . . We also repeat to make the passive active, to *do* instead of *be done to*. We repeat in order not to feel out of control. This time we hope we'll magically create the happy ending we so yearned for as a child. (p. 85)

REFERENCES

Angyal, A. (1965). *Neurosis and treatment: A holistic theory.* New York: Wiley.
Balint, M. (1969). *The basic fault: Therapeutic aspects of regression.* Evanston, IL: Northwestern University Press.
Beck, A. T. (1988). *Love is never enough.* New York: HarperCollins.
Conroy, P. (1991). *The prince of tides.* New York: Bantam.
Dreikurs, R. (1974). *The challenge of marriage.* New York: Hawthorn/Dutton.
Engel, L., & Ferguson, T. (1990). *Imaginary crimes.* Boston: Houghton Mifflin.

Erickson, M. H. (1982). *My voice will go with you: The teaching tales of Milton H. Erickson, M.D.* New York: Norton.

Firestone, R. W. (1987). *The fantasy bond.* New York: Human Sciences Press.

Firestone, R. W. (1988). *Voice therapy.* New York: Human Sciences Press.

Firestone, R. W. (1990). *Compassionate child-rearing.* New York: Plenum Press.

Fishel, E. (1991). *Family mirrors.* Boston: Houghton Mifflin.

Fromm, E. (1956). *The art of loving.* New York: Harper & Row.

Gottman, J. M. (1994). *Why marriages succeed or fail.* New York: Simon & Schuster.

Gottman, J. M. (1997). *A scientifically-based marital therapy: A workshop for clinicians.* Seattle: Seattle Marital and Family Institute.

Guerin, P. J., Fogarty, T. F., Fay, L. F., & Kautto, J. G. (1996). *Working with relationship triangles: The one-two-three of psychotherapy.* New York: Guilford Press.

Heller, E., & Born, J. (1973). *Franz Kafka: Letters to Felice.* New York: Schocken Books.

Kirschner, D. A., & Kirschner, S. (1986). *Comprehensive family therapy: An integration of systemic and psychodynamic treatment models.* New York: Brunner/Mazel.

McGurrin, M. C. (1992). *Pathological gambling: Conceptual, diagnostic, and treatment issues.* Sarasota, FL: Professional Resource Press.

Modell, A. (1971). The origin of certain forms of pre-Oedipal guilt and the implications for a psychoanalytic theory of affects. *International Journal of Psycho-Analysis, 52,* 337–346.

Niederland, W. (1981). The survivor syndrome: Further observations and dimensions. *Journal of the American Psychoanalytic Association, 29,* 413–423.

Rapport, A. (1996). The structure of psychotherapy: Control mastery therapy's diagnostic plan formulation. *Psychotherapy, 34,* 1–10.

Rheingold, J. C. (1964). *The fear of being a woman: A theory of maternal destructiveness.* New York: Grune & Stratton.

Sampson, H. (1992). The role of "real" experience in psychopathology and treatment. *Psychoanalytic Dialogues, 2*(4), 509–528.

Schnarch, D. M. (1991). *Constructing the sexual crucible: An integration of sexual and marital therapy.* New York: Norton.

Schnarch, D. M. (1997). *The passionate marriage: Love, sex, and intimacy in emotionally committed relationships.* New York: Norton.

Wallerstein, J., & Blakeslee, S. (1995). *The good marriage.* Boston: Houghton Mifflin.

Weiss, J., Sampson, H., & the Mount Zion Psychotherapy Group. (1986). *The psychoanalytic process.* New York: Guilford Press.

White, M., & Epston, D. (1990). *Narrative means to therapeutic ends.* New York: Norton.

Zeig, J. (1980). *A teaching seminar with Milton H. Erickson, M.D.* New York: Brunner/Mazel.

Zeitlin, D. J. (1991). Control–mastery theory in couples therapy. *Family Therapy, 18*(3), 201–230.

PART II

◄○►

THE SYSTEMIC
APPROACH

In the opening chapter, I observe that couple therapy has an uncertain paternity but is often thought the child or stepchild of family therapy. Given this parentage, I find it fascinating that only four approaches here are frankly systemic—focusing on the network of the couple or family rather than on the individuals. Even so both Cohen's and Budman's models represent a hybrid melding of psychodynamic and systemic approaches.

Guerin and his group, true systemic therapists from the Bowenian school, offer us a crucial insight. Whenever we cannot understand an interaction between two people, search for a *third* person who may be playing a key unacknowledged role. Unstable dyads make themselves into triangles, and only by including all three points of the triangle in the treatment can we hope for resolution. For instance, a young man becomes engaged but then develops debilitating anxiety attacks. The relationship with this fiancée seems solid. How to make sense of the sudden panics? Perhaps a look to the young man's relationship with his mother. Is he afraid of deserting her or that she'll be angry about his choosing another woman? Guerin and co-workers show us step by step how to identify the crucial triangles and how to reverse the flow of energy within them to free the participants toward a more satisfying adjustment.

If the system is the focus, then the work will concern the boundaries around the system and between the individuals in that system. Nichols and Minuchin teach us, as few could, how to seek boundaries enmeshed as the nexus of the couple's conflict. In the case they present,

101

the 13-year-old son is overinvolved with his mother, who in turn is underinvolved with her husband. This enmeshment leads to chronic arguments between husband and wife.

The partners in Cohen's older couple also illustrate enmeshed boundaries, this time with each other. Each partner feels compelled to manipulate the other to take responsibility for the relationship. Angry conflict erupts seemingly hourly. Cohen demonstrates sound strategies to forestall this vicious cycle drawing upon interventions both at the systemic and the individual, psychodynamic level. "Integration" has become the watch word in nearly every sector of contemporary psychotherapy. Cohen illustrates just how complex, difficult, and powerful real conceptual and technical integration can be in everyday practice.

Budman wants most of all to interrupt his couple's protracted argument, so that they can move on to their own productive dialogue. What Budman knows is that couples do not change in one fell swoop but according to a sequential model of change and that different couples enter treatment at different points in that sequence. He shows us how to gauge the intervention to the couples present stage of motivation. Once he has braked the fight, he will address how each partner feels afraid and deprived, which ignites the snapping between them. Budman intervenes at the systems level first and concentrates later on the pressing individual issues. If the couple is stuck in the pattern of simply trading accusations, that stand-off must be addressed before affective uncovering can begin.

JAMES M. DONOVAN

5

<o>

BRIEF MARITAL THERAPY

The Story of the Triangles

PHILIP J. GUERIN, JR.
LEO F. FAY
THOMAS F. FOGARTY
JUDITH G. KAUTTO

BRIEF THERAPY AND TRIANGLES

Brief therapy is defined in different ways by different groups of clinicians. As best we can tell, every group's definition is based on that group's theoretical perspective and clinical methodology. The Guerin group's tradition is to base all psychotherapy, whatever its duration, on a systemic theoretical base with an integrated clinical methodology. Thus, our main text on marital therapy (Guerin, Fay, Burden, & Kautto, 1987) is divided into two distinct parts, one devoted to an explication of our theory and the other to an elaboration of its corresponding clinical method. It's clear from that book that, in dealing with intense marital conflict of longer than 6 months' duration, we prefer to allow 18 months to accomplish symptom relief as well as rehabilitation of the damaged relationship bond.

However, the reality of the present clinical marketplace often makes our preferences irrelevant. To remain viable today, it is important for therapists to have a less intensive clinical approach, which requires a minimum of contact hours. In shaping our model of brief marital therapy, we borrow a format used by Bowen as early as the mid-1970s. Bowen would see individuals and couples in distress infrequently, but over longer periods of time. For example, he might see them once a month for 2 to 3 years. In our model, we begin with a session once every 7 to 12 days for the first 2 months and then meet monthly over the next 12 to 18 months. The entire treatment usually lasts less than 20 sessions.

For clinicians to use this brief model (or its lengthier cousin), a working knowledge of triangles is essential to success. Therefore, this chapter focuses on interventions based on triangles. These are meant to be combined with interventions on a dyadic and individual level. For further understanding of the integration of these three levels, we refer the reader to *Working with Relationship Triangles: The One-Two-Three of Psychotherapy* (Guerin, Fogarty, Fay, & Kautto, 1996).

At the very beginning of your life, as soon as your conception became known, either your father, your mother, or both may have experienced you as an intruder. The fact of your existence may have overjoyed your father and presented a threat to your mother's career, making your father too eager for your arrival and your mother too anxious. Even before your conception, not-so-subtle pressure from your maternal grandmother may have led the campaign for your existence. At your birth, the genetic map on your face was probably the stimulus for all kinds of loyalty-driven distinctions by well-meaning relatives. "He looks just like George's mother," says George's mother's sister.

From this perspective, we can see life not so much as a series of paths to be chosen but as a maze of triangular shoals and reefs to be navigated around. As if this weren't difficult enough, you decided to become a psychotherapist—a professional sailing instructor. In every clinical presentation, every patient faces a mass of these triangular crosscurrents, and you're volunteering to help. Most systems psychotherapists have a mental file of their own experience of wrestling with relationship triangles. Whether you use a short-term solution-focused approach or a long-term growth model, the triangles are there, affecting your outcome.

MARITAL TRIANGLES

Guerin, Fay, Burden, and Kautto reported on their clinical experience with marital conflict in 1987 (Guerin et al., 1987). *The Evaluation and Treatment of Marital Conflict* is about the theory and treatment of marital dysfunction and was the result of many years of wrestling with the difficult work of sitting with bitter couples and trying to help them. They found that, in marriages with a modest degree of conflict of short duration and relatively low intensity, work on the dyad itself was usually sufficient to produce good results. However, in cases of severe marital conflict, with long duration and high intensity, the therapist almost always must locate, define, and resolve the triangles surrounding the marital relationship. Otherwise, in the highest percentage of cases, treatment either fails or produces only short-term improvement with rapid recycling and, perhaps ultimately, disintegration. In fact, it was this discovery about triangles in treating severely disrupted couples that motivated us to look at triangles across the whole spectrum of clinical practice (Guerin et al., 1996).

Work on triangles in marital therapy makes sense to many clinicians, especially in cases where extramarital affairs or interfering in-laws are the presenting problem. Often, however, marital triangles aren't as easy to see or to work with in treatment as are those mentioned above. Therapists find themselves bogged down in the morass of dyadic wars. They are unable to grasp or alter the triangles that are reinforcing the wars and making a negotiated settlement difficult. People do displace unresolved conflict. Husbands and wives can (and do) displace unresolved conflicts from their own families into the marriage. (Take the example of the wife who is convinced, with compelling evidence, that her parents and siblings don't love her and never have. She gives up on them and then fights the battle of "You don't really care about me" with her husband.) Similarly, a spouse can displace anger, resentment, and bitterness toward the other spouse onto a child, making that child the issue between them. ("She should just be stricter with our son instead of excusing everything he does," for example. Or, "He should be more understanding of our daughter.") The marital treatment is going to fail unless those unresolved issues are dealt with *in the relationships where they belong.*

THE CLINICAL CENTRALITY OF TRIANGLES

Lasting success in therapy usually depends on some resolution of the central triangles surrounding the presenting marital problem. The relevance of relationship triangles to brief marital therapy is based on six factors. Picture the following case. Mary and John D developed creeping distance in their relationship over time, partly from his silence and her need to express everything. Mary drew closer to their children, and John ended up in the outsider position in that triangle. The outsider position produced feelings of loss and loneliness in him that led to difficulty in concentrating, loss of energy, oversleeping, and overeating. His down mood became a mild clinical depression (*factor 1:* Triangles promote the development of symptoms in the individual). John wasn't in enough difficulty to motivate anyone in the family to seek therapy. He gradually started to alternate between sulking in his withdrawal and depression and moving toward Mary in angry conflict over the triangular issue of how to raise the children. All this confrontational behavior escalated when he really wanted more love and attention from her and equal primacy with the children (*factor 2:* Triangles support the chronicity of symptoms in an individual and of conflict in a relationship).

Much of the trouble in John and Mary's marriage began when they were first married. Mary had great difficulty separating from her father and making her attachment to John the primary one in her life. Mary's underlying problem of attachment to her father placed him on a pedestal and allowed no room in her heart for her husband. Once they had children, she got overly attached to them, too, leaving John in the outside position in both triangles. John, on the other hand, had never dealt with his mother's emotional intensity, and so he had cut off from her and had clung to Mary as his emotional lifeline. John's failure to develop a mature relationship with his mother was a serious difficulty. If the family doesn't recognize these complexities, the issue may get defined as Mary being too lenient with the children and John being too strict. Then they don't identify or address the underlying emotional entanglements (*factor 3:* Triangles work against the resolution of toxic or conflictual issues in an individual or a relationship).

John isolated himself from his children, Mary took refuge in her closeness with them, and the parent–child relations became stuck in distance and overcloseness. The marital relationship was fixed in conflict (*factor 4:* Triangles block the functional evolution of a relationship over time). The therapist found Mary's sympathetic situation more understandable than John's strict one but didn't want to side with one or the other. If the therapist has no knowledge of triangles, she or he may try to get the parents to agree on a mutual approach to the children. This will result in an endless series of compacts between the parents to handle one situation after another by agreement. The number of situations will be interminable and the agreements poorly operated and forgotten. Therapy will continue until all members are exhausted or run out of money (*factor 5:* Triangles can create or support the therapeutic impasse).

Both John and Mary were caught in primary parental triangles in their families of origin and never got free enough from them to form their own relationship. Thus the relationship difficulties in their families of origin got displaced downward onto the marriage, and John and Mary were caught in in-law triangles. Once the couple had children, the conflict in the marriage got displaced downward again, onto the children, the spouses became caught in triangles with their children, and the way they were caught in these triangles drove their behavior. John and Mary didn't have any autonomy or control over that behavior, and the triangles set the behavior in concrete (*factor 6:* Triangles get people "caught," depriving them of options). Let's look at these six factors in more detail.

The Mechanism of Symptom Activation

Triangles promote the development of symptoms in the individual. Being caught in a triangle is stressful and kindles feelings of helplessness and hopelessness. For example, Billy, a child drawn into a triangle because of his sensitivity to emotional upset in his mother internalizes her emotional arousal and begins to underachieve in school and isolate from his friends. Ben, an adolescent in developmental turmoil, threatens the already shaky truce in his parents' dysfunctional relationship. Triangles refortify the fragile bond by joining Ben's parents in concern for and criticism of him. His response is to feel angry and justified in stealing the family car. Harriet, a 52-year-old woman dealing with decades of pressure and criticism from her husband and mother, has the noose of the triangle tightened when her 75-year-old mother comes to live with them. Her frustration and hopelessness over the situation trigger an episode of clinical depression. (However, being caught in a triangle doesn't *always* feel stressful. The wife who feels exhilarated about her new affair, and the adult child who feels special when his mother complains to him about his father are examples. Eventually, though, the negative consequences of this willing complicity in being caught in a triangle will show up, feel stressful, and activate one or more symptoms.)

A person emotionally trapped in a triangle is likely, just by virtue of being trapped, to suffer some loss of function. Being caught in a triangle arouses emotional reactivity to the point where the reactivity constrains behavior, and the person can't imagine any options. Consider, for example, a little girl whose mother develops an anxious attachment to her in response to her husband's distance. As a result the father then becomes very critical of the girl. In response to her position in the triangle, the child may refuse to go to school, or her asthma may get much worse. The intervention here would be to get the father to decrease his level of criticism and move toward his daughter to spend relationship time with her (*not* time for shaping her up). Simultaneously, the mother can be encouraged to focus less on her daughter and more on other, neglected areas of her own life. Perhaps she needs to narrow the distance between herself and her own mother. As the triangle shifts, the marital issues may emerge and treatment can then be directed at them. Anyway, working on the triangle at least frees the child and provides relief from her symptom.

The Chronicity of Symptoms

Triangles support the chronicity of symptoms in an individual and of conflict in a relationship. A 48-year-old executive named Bob M was passed over for a promotion at work, and he became irritable at home, more demanding of sexual attention from Terry, his wife, and much more easily wounded. The loss had activated a mild depression. Terry, anxious about their financial well-being, began to avoid sex, especially in the face of Bob's irritability and babyish behavior. She withdrew from him and looked for a job to provide security in case he were to lose his position. Then Bob felt justified in starting an affair with his divorced neighbor who drove to work with him every day. As long as the milk and honey of the extramarital affair were flowing, Bob wouldn't face his performance at work, his depression over the lost promotion, or the conflict and sexual problems in his marriage that preceded the affair. Four years later, the problems were chronic and remained camouflaged.

Once symptoms have appeared, or conflict has begun, being caught in a triangle heightens stress. Stress is a pivotal factor in the persistence of symptoms and conflict. Symptoms in an individual or relationship, which might otherwise be amenable to management or even change, sometimes become entrenched and resistant to direct intervention. Often when this happens it is because the therapy left unaddressed a relationship triangle. For example, a middle-aged woman had a depression that did not respond to trials of several medications. It stayed intractable as long as both her husband and her mother were allied in defining her as sick and trying to get her to "pull herself up by her bootstraps." In working with this couple, the therapist made the alliance between husband and mother-in-law explicit. This put the wife's reaction to it on the table, and the therapist coached the husband how to take a different position in the triangle. Shifting the structure and changing the process in the triangle addressed the underlying cause of the woman's depression. If medication is prescribed now to help alleviate the symptoms of depression, the problem is less likely to recur than if medication had been employed without addressing the relationship imbalances that led to the depression (or exacerbated it once it was in place).

The Resolution of Toxic or Conflictual Issues

A triangle can, and very often does, allow the relationship system to continue without change and without resolving issues that need to be resolved. For example, an extramarital affair makes it "unnecessary" to address the sexual immaturity of a couple in which one spouse is sexually demanding and the other sexually constricted. The lover is meeting the demands of the spouse having the affair, and that takes the pressure off the constricted spouse, who therefore feels less pressured. If the therapist persuades the spouse having the affair to end it, the sexual issues within the marriage are likely to become explicit and can be dealt with in treatment. If the unfaithful spouse stops the affair, that person will experience three reactions: feelings of loss of the relationship and the emotional and sexual perks that went along with it; anger directed at the spouse for having to suffer this loss when the spouse's behavior was the justification for the affair in the first place; and discouragement about the sexual incompatibility that may be driving the distancing and the acting out. A therapist without a knowledge of triangles will get caught by these reactions into being judgmental about the affair or justifying it based on the betrayed partner's behavior. In either case, the therapist is caught, a new triangle is formed with the therapist, and the process gets displaced into the therapy triangle rather than provoking an examination of the marital problems that led to the affair.

The Functional Evolution of a Relationship

Triangles block the functional evolution of a relationship over time. They keep relationships frozen in the same old quarrels and issues and don't allow relationships to grow and change as circumstances change and as the life cycle progresses. Bob's extramarital affair had put the marital relationship on hold for four years. Because the affair hadn't stopped, and the married couple hadn't dealt with the underlying problems and their fallout, the evolutionary maturing of their relationship remained arrested. Their marriage began to deteriorate into the chronic distance of an emotional divorce. The next developmental crisis might well cause the final fracture of the marriage.

It is natural and desirable that relationships grow and mature over time. As a son or daughter grows up, for instance, his or her relationship with parents should go from childlike dependence to an adult relationship. Triangles can retard this development, as in a triangle where a mother is overclose with her child and father is in the distant position. The relationship between mother and child won't evolve appropriately as the child grows older, and the child may remain infantilized, even as an adult. This adult may come to therapy because of his or her difficulty in forming romantic attachments. If the therapist thinks that the patient's position in his or her primary parental triangle is at the root of the problem, the therapist would coach the patient to shift the triangle.

The patient does this by finding ways to move toward the father and to behave in a less childlike way with the mother.

Therapeutic Impasse

Triangles can create or support the therapeutic impasse. An unaddressed triangle is a vehicle for voluntary noncompliance with treatment or is a reason for involuntary noncompliance. When a patient suffering from depression fails to respond to the most sophisticated combination of drugs and psychotherapy, look for a background triangle that you can't easily see. The same is true for a marital conflict that defies intervention. First review to see if the therapist is caught in a triangle with the couple. If not, search for a background triangle that is supporting noncompliance with therapy. (The individual therapist of one or both spouses may be one place to look.)

A therapeutic impasse is most often caused by noncompliance, misdiagnosis, or a mismatch between the patient's abilities and the type of therapy being used. Triangles play a role in creating or supporting the impasse. When therapy is stuck, it can often be unstuck if the therapist stops to look for and work on unresolved triangles. These triangles may be embroiling the patient, blocking the therapy, or both.

When mental health professionals trained in a psychodynamic paradigm are faced with a therapeutic impasse, they think about the patient's defenses, resistance, or problems in the transference. After reviewing these factors, they consider possible countertransference problems. For instance, an analyst might be puzzling over why a 50-year-old woman hasn't yet developed a therapeutically useful negative transference in spite of lengthy therapy. The analyst might be speculating that her apparently obsessive curiosity about his marriage represents a resistance to developing the transference. This might be the problem, but in this particular case, the problem is a therapy triangle. The patient's husband is suspicious that the therapist is turning his wife against him and developing an attachment to her, and so he keeps insisting that she find out the therapist's marital status.

A psychiatrist may be treating a patient with a major clinical depression that isn't responding to antidepressants. The first step is to check that the patient is complying with the prescribed program of treatment. If the patient is compliant, the psychiatrist then searches for a different drug to which the patient might have a better response. In addition, the psychiatrist might profitably check on whether a family member with influence over the patient is negative about medication in general or psychotropic medication in particular. Consider, for example, the case of a 27-year-old married woman with early-morning awakening, loss of appetite and libido, difficulty concentrating, and a preoccupation with thoughts of death and dying. The psychiatrist tried several serotonin reuptake inhibitors without much change. When he asked about the woman's compliance, he found that the patient was "forgetting" to take her medication about three times a week. The physician asked to see the woman's husband and learned that the possibility his wife could become addicted to the medication frightened him, and he told his wife so every day. The psychiatrist educated this man about the biochemical aspects of depression and about how antidepressants work, including their nonaddictive nature. He explained that depression was at the root of his wife's recent behavior (including loss of libido), that medication was likely to relieve her depressive symptoms, and that the drug chosen wouldn't complicate her libidinal problems. The husband was relieved by both pieces of information and agreed to encourage his wife to comply with the medical regimen. She did, and her symptoms improved markedly within a month.

Getting Caught

Triangles get people "caught," depriving them of options and insuring that their behavior will continue in the same dysfunctional rut. For example, people can experience therapy triangles as supportive when in fact the only things they are supportive of is the chronicity of the symptoms around which they were formed.

In active triangles, people are never free. Their responses to events are constrained and predictable. They are unable to consider alternatives. Even if they can think of something different to do, they are afraid to risk the consequences. They fear that they or someone else will get hurt or angry with them or leave. Joseph P, a 30-year-old man in marital therapy, was working hard on controlling his tendency to shout at Linda, his wife. His therapist asked him who else he has shouted at like that and whether anyone had shouted at him. These questions made it possible for him to link his anger with the feelings he used to get as an adolescent. His mother would complain to him about her life and, he thought, expect him to make it all better. When he couldn't, his mother would act disappointed in him, and he would feel helpless and inadequate. Then he would become withdrawn and rebellious, and his father would yell at him and call him names. When Linda criticized him or made demands on him, he would feel helpless and inadequate all over again, and get furious with her "for making him feel that way."

Joseph agreed that he had never found a way to deal with his mother's complaints and demands so that he was disconnected from them while staying in touch with her. Every time she complained or demanded, he tried to fix things or reassure her that everything would be all right. Inevitably, he failed. He then got angry with his mother for "making him feel inadequate." In therapy, Joseph couldn't think of any other way to approach these situations (except to avoid his mother). When the therapist suggested various experiments to him, he found himself unable to try them in the field, although they "sounded terrific" to him in the therapy room. One problem Joseph had with these experiments was that he continued to have the uncomfortable feelings he usually got with his mother, even though he expected not to if he tried something different with her. As soon as he started to feel uncomfortable, he assumed that the experiment had failed even before he tried it. He had hoped that having a different plan would prevent those feelings. The reality is that the *feelings* will continue to come for a while. The first step for Joseph in getting "uncaught" is to manage his feelings and not be determined in his *behavior* by them. This will insure that his emotions won't drive him into a set of predictable actions. The next step for Joseph is to monitor what happens inside himself when he refrains from getting angry with his mother. Is there a new feeling, a vacuum, or what? This kind of self-control and raised consciousness is the beginning of change. The next step is to observe what happens to Joseph's mother when he behaves differently. It's predictable that she will escalate her efforts to bring Joseph back into his usual pattern of behavior. If he can get past that, if he can see what is happening and hold his position without showing his resentment, eventually his feelings will change too. At that point he will have become detriangled, and he will have a much better chance of controlling his anger at his wife.

METHODS OF MANAGEMENT OF RELATIONSHIP TRIANGLES: A BRIEF COUPLE CASE

Our approach to the clinical management of triangles is best summarized in the following five steps:

1. Find the triangle.
2. Define the triangle's structure and the flow of movement within it.
3. Reverse the flow of movement in the triangle.
4. Expose the emotional process.
5. Deal with the process and move toward improved functioning.

When Dave O met Ann W one summer on the beach, they were both 23. They were a year out of college, tired of the bar scene and its unending string of beer parties. Each of them had an unspoken longing to meet someone special who might turn out to be the "one." Neither of them believed that the chaotic madness of another summer at the beach would provide the fulfillment of these wishes.

Now, 18 months later, Dave finds himself in a place he never dreamed he'd be: a therapist's office. Dave and his family didn't really believe in psychiatry or "any of that mental health crap," but for the past 3 months Dave had been experiencing anxiety attacks at work, while driving to pick up Ann in the city, and even at a professional football game with some old friends. The anxiety attacks included a pervasive sense of impending doom, with no rational stimulus, profuse sweating, heart palpitations, and nausea. All of this was occurring in spite of his job going well and his relationship with Ann building in a beautiful way. In fact, over the past few months, especially around Christmas time, they had begun to talk about the possibility of becoming engaged on Ann's birthday in April.

Dave, concerned that he might have a cardiac problem, had consulted his family physician. The physician examined him and ran the appropriate battery of tests, including an EKG and stress test, before telling Dave that he was physically fit and suffering from anxiety attacks. He prescribed small doses of alprazolam (Xanax), which gave Dave some relief. However, on a follow-up visit, Dave reported awakening at 3 A.M. each morning, in panic over the dream he was having that his mother was in a hospital with terminal cancer. In response to this information, the physician had referred Dave for a psychiatric evaluation.

The therapist discontinued the alprazolam and prescribed moderate doses of imipramine (Tofranil) at bedtime. Imipramine is a tricyclic antidepressant with an excellent track record for controlling panic attacks. The therapist assured Dave that his condition would respond to the medication, if Dave complied with the treatment plan. He also asked some questions about Dave's life, looking for sources of developmental and situational anxiety. In addition, he looked for the relationship processes that might be involved in the formation or maintenance of Dave's symptoms.

Finding the Triangle

In Dave's case, the active triangle (Dave, his mother, and Ann) surrounding his anxiety symptoms was easy to see from the content of his dream and the developmental timing of the symptoms (just at the time his relationship with Ann was moving toward engagement). However, this clear presentation isn't the usual case: Finding triangles isn't always so easy. More likely someone like Dave would present his symptoms oblivious to their connections in time and relationship space. From shame, embarrassment, or denial, he would not mention his relationship with Ann or his repetitive dream about his mother, not seeing them as relevant. If the clinician Dave consulted thought about biology alone, the treatment would consist only of prescribing an appropriate medication. Perhaps the first drug would give only limited relief, and the prescriber would try additional medications, all of which would give the same limited relief.

If the clinician believed in the importance of relationship process, his or her evaluation would include a search for developmental or situational issues in Dave's life. A logical focus would have been Dave's work and love life. Probes into either of these areas would have produced glowing reports from Dave. Only if the clinician had added a systems perspective to his knowledge of individuals and dyads, would questions be directed toward potentially active relationship triangles in Dave's life.

For the fullest possible perspective on Dave, and to catch problems that might otherwise remain invisible, the clinician must be able to think about threes. Once the clinician does this it becomes simple, because the same tracks are followed to look for symptomatic triangles in any clinical case as are used to nail down individual and dyadic factors. The major tools in finding the relevant triangles are exploring the patient's genogram, asking questions about the developmental and situational threats or challenges that are going on and about the triangles in the patient's relationship system that would most likely be activated. The genogram very quickly helps the clinician to visualize the developmental and situational landscape in the patient's life and so directs the flow of process questions. If Dave had presented clinically without making the key triangle explicit, these two sets of tools would do the trick.

But so what? The imipramine would manage Dave's symptoms well enough, and the panic attacks would go away. Dave would feel better and be none the worse off for lack of enlightenment about the cause of his anxiety. Clinically, one could defend this position, especially in light of the constraints of time and money and the demands for rapid symptom relief from our present models of care. This position can be criticized, however, as being medically indefensible. In an analogous scenario, if a young patient presented to an internist with hypertension, it would be irresponsible for the internist to prescribe diuretics and other antihypertensive therapy without inquiring about family history, diet, and aerobic fitness.

In Dave's situation, even without the information about his marriage plans and dreams about his mother's death, a cursory look at the genogram would demonstrate the developmental challenges. A few well-placed process questions would uncover the active triangle. Process questions are formed more easily if the clinician already has a picture of possible triangles in his or her head. With respect to Dave, Ann, and his mother, for example, some process questions might be: "How does your Mom like Ann?" "Did your mother have health problems or any separation anxiety when you or your sister left for college?" "How do you think your mother would do if you and Ann got married and your company transferred you to Europe?" "Does Ann admire the closeness you have with your mother?" "Does she worry about the impact that closeness might have on your marriage?"

Now, depending on how open Dave would have been to this type of questioning, his answers still might not yield much more information than the therapist already had. Even as our society reels through this age of disclosure, psychiatry is being pushed by the edicts of managed care. After decades of probing to uncover internal and relationship conflicts, therapy has entered an age of containment. In the midst of this revolution, though, there remains a place for clinical discernment. Sound clinical judgment calls for at least a modest attempt to cut through denial rather than celebrate the superficial accounts of some patients by accepting their limited perspective and allowing it to dictate the course of treatment. It's worth the effort to take time to look for triangles.

Defining the Triangle's Structure and the Flow of Movement within It

If we track the central triangle in David's life (with Ann and his mother) from the time he met Ann through the triangle's activation, we'd assume that the potential for an active triangle existed from the start. As Dave's relationship with Ann developed over time, the direction and intensity of his movement was increasingly toward Ann and away from his mother. It may have been that when Mrs. O met Ann, in spite of feeling positive about her and pleasure in her internal feeling that Ann was "the one" for Dave, she found herself involuntarily asking Dave critical questions about Ann and their relationship. At this point, the triangle was activated. Its structure, and the flow of movement in it, were largely determined by Dave's developmental challenge to separate from his mother and form a new primary relationship. Dave and Ann are now closer in relation to one another, and Dave's mother is on the outside of their twosome.

There are many variations on this theme that could have occurred. Mrs. O and Ann might have taken to each other and spoken so glowingly about each other to Dave that he might have become uncomfortable and started to wonder if he were doing the right thing. Or, their immediate appreciation of each other might have relieved Dave, as he felt Ann taking on the pressure of his relationship with his mother, and vice versa. In that case, he might have come to believe that he could play golf with his buddies without worrying about demands or criticism from either one of them. In fact, what happened was that Mrs. O reacted with coolness toward Ann and was distant and subtly critical (very much like Maureen O'Hara's character as the mother in the movie *Only the Lonely*). Ann responded by insisting that Dave get his mother under control and that he defend her against his mother, or even that he choose between her or his mother.

The point is that, no matter what the variation, the problem Dave presents clinically will not be successfully resolved unless it's seen in triangular, as well as biological, individual, and dyadic terms. The underlying triangular process is the same whatever form the structure and movement take. It has to do with Dave separating from his mother and forming a new primary relationship. All three twosomes are interconnected and have to be dealt with—both separately and in their interconnectedness. Every new relationship in a person's life is affected by existing relationships. If the new relationship is (or should be) a primary one, it sets up the likelihood of conflicts about the primacy of attachment and the hierarchy of influence between the new relationship and the old ones. Just such an underlying triangular process was at work creating conflict for Dave, Ann, and his mother.

Reversing the Flow of Movement

Once the therapist has a clear idea of the structure and the way the movement flows back and forth within the triangle, the first task is to create an experiment that reverses the direction of the relationship movement. Essentially, such experiments attempt to engage one or more members of the system to stop moving in the direction called for by affect and reactivity and to begin moving in a planned, experimental direction that usually is the opposite of what has been going on.

There are several reasons for employing such a strategy. First, the intervention increases self-focus, the ability to work to see the parts of ourselves that contribute significantly to our own pain and our relationship discomfort. Self-focus increases as people become aware of how difficult it is to do an apparently simple experiment in relationship movement. They begin to see themselves as caught and controlled by their emotions. Second, it gives people the sense that they have options in their behavior. There *are* ways of doing things differently from what they've been doing, which hasn't been working. Third, people's reactions to doing (or even thinking of doing) something different brings the underlying emotional process into the open.

In Dave's case, the medication relieved his panic attacks and took the edge off his inner turmoil. The therapist offered him the option of accepting this as the result of treatment or of moving on to deal with the source of the anxiety that was driving his symptoms. Dave decided on the latter. Rather than deliver a lesson on triangles this early in therapy, which often creates confusion and misuse of the concept, the therapist suggested a relationship experiment. He pointed out to Dave that this was just that—an experiment, not necessarily a solution. While doing it, Dave was to monitor his own internal emotional reactions, as well as the response in the relationship where the experiment was taking place.

He suggested that Dave move toward his mother (the opposite of what he had been doing). He suggested that Dave ask her what she thought about his closeness to Ann and the strong possibility that they might marry. Dave could open up with his mother the feelings he was having about not being so close to her any more and talk to her about how they could stay connected in ways appropriate for a mother and her married son. Dave could also just spend some relationship time with his mother, hanging out with her and talking about old times.

By this time Ann had joined the therapy, and the therapist asked her, too, to perform an experiment. He predicted that she would have an emotional reaction of some kind to Dave's moves toward his mother, and he asked her to monitor it carefully. He suggested she might want to keep a journal of her reactions and bring it into the therapy. Ann did raise objections to Dave's spending more time with his mother, saying that Mrs. O was against her and the marriage. The therapist pointed out that, unless this triangle was resolved in some way, it would remain a permanent threat to their marriage. He said that Dave was doing the experiment for them, and for the long-term health of their relationship, not for his mother.

The goal of Dave's experiment was to face his phobic avoidance of his mother, her understandable anxiety over losing her son, and the effect her anxiety had on him. The therapist offered two choices. One was for Dave to move directly toward his mother and spend some relationship time with her. Eventually he would talk to her about his anxiety, his symptoms, his plans with Ann, even about his and his mother's special relationship, and how they were going to deal with this difficult time in their lives.

A second option was for Dave to move toward his father and to discuss with him how to deal with his relationship problem with his mother. At first glance, this option might appear to the novice triangle doctor as the activation of another triangle. But behavior in an active triangle is driven by emotional reactivity. If Dave is moving toward his father to return the gift of his mother many years later, it's a developmentally appropriate, thoughtful, planned behavior and *isn't* driven by emotional reactivity. (Of course, if Dave's movement were laden with reactive feelings of anger and resentment toward his father, it would in fact represent the reactivation of Dave's primary parental triangle.)

At this point you may be thinking, "Well, if men are from Mars and women are from Venus, the families you see must be from Pluto, if you can get them to do an experiment like moving toward either of their parents." This thinking raises the issue of clinical judgment. Which families and family members are coachable and which will require the direct intervention of getting everyone into the treatment room? In general, coaching as a technique requires highly motivated, high-functioning adults, with significant relationship leverage in their families. It also requires a belief that, through the modulation of anxiety and affect, and by means of relationship experiments, people's behavior in relationships can change. In the absence of some of these characteristics, it can still be useful to attempt coaching a patient through a relationship experiment. If coaching fails, then we can resort to enlarging the membership in the sessions to deal directly with the triangle.

To continue an exploration of the importance of triangle dynamics, let's return to Dave and his dilemma.

Exposing the Emotional Process in the Triangle

Six weeks later, after two more therapy sessions and a cancellation, Dave had yet to move toward his mother. Discussion with Dave uncovered his apprehension and aversion toward making this move. He also revealed that, in talking about this experiment with Ann, she kept saying she didn't "get it." She thought that grown-ups drew boundaries between themselves and their parents. This was the reason she had moved several states away from her own family and kept her visits home to a minimum.

The therapist repeated his earlier point that Dave didn't have to do the experiment. He could just take his medication and forget the project with his mother. However, he also offered Dave a plan to help him make up his mind about how to proceed. He lent him a video copy of *Only the Lonely*, a John Candy film about the struggle of a single, Chicago cop who lived with his mother, to separate from her and marry the woman of his dreams. The therapist suggested that Dave watch the tape with Ann and invite her to the next therapy session.

One of the purposes of a relationship experiment is to bring underlying emotional process to the surface. Just proposing this relationship experiment had revealed the following pieces of process:

1. Dave had an intense relationship with his mother and an inability to open up for discussion between them important issues in his and his mother's life. This lack of openness had forced the anxiety about these issues underground. The anxiety then came out by triggering Dave's biological vulnerability to panic attacks.
2. From his experience over the years, Dave had grave doubts about whether his father could or would be a supportive refuge for his mother as she suffered through the separation from Dave. In addition, his relationship with his father was weak enough that Dave couldn't ask his father to do so.
3. In his apprehension about the experiment, Dave's anxiety had been elevated, with two important side effects. First, there had been a moderate return of his panic symptoms. Second, a therapy triangle had been activated, consisting of Dave, Ann, and Dave's therapist.

It became the therapist's job to establish a plan to neutralize this threefold process.

Neutralizing the Process and "Detriangling"

The therapist had begun Dave's treatment by medically managing his symptoms of anxiety and then moving on to assist him in addressing the symptomatic triangle with Ann and his mother. The relationship experiment, designed with this triangle in mind, did its job by opening up the process described above: Dave's anxious attachment to his mother and his inability to communicate with her about difficult issues; his insufficient attachment to his father; the formation of a therapy triangle around the experiment.

The activation of a therapy triangle almost always calls for dealing with it immediately. Dave's taking *Only the Lonely* home to watch with Ann was the first of a number of steps designed to involve her in the therapy. Perhaps now is a good time to raise a philosophical (and perhaps ethical) question about the methods we're describing. Someone who adheres to a minimalist approach to therapy might argue that all this playing around with Dave's triangles is producing iatrogenic problems, not to mention prolonging the therapy and increasing its cost. Such a critic might add that, if Dave's panic attacks had failed to respond to medication and cognitive techniques, or that, if, after initial relief, he had suffered multiple relapses, the treatment described here could be offered as an adjunct to fortify the primary intervention. However, we believe in a heavy emphasis on patient education and efforts at prevention. Primary care medicine today emphasizes the importance of changes in diet, exercise, and life style in caring for cardiac and cancer-prone patients. In much the same way, we believe that work on relationship triangles is essential to the comprehensive care of anxiety, depression, and relationship conflict. It's important to educate patients about the choices available to them for elective procedures and to allow them to make the choice.

In the case of Dave and Ann, Ann came to the next session and, in a clear and forthright way, stated her thoughts on Dave's situation. She said that they had both enjoyed *Only the Lonely* and, after watching it, had a long discussion about driving to her hometown so that Dave could meet her family. They saw this as a step on the road to getting engaged. At that point the therapist asked Ann about her family and how it differed from Dave's. He also asked her directly if she thought the separation between Dave and his mother might go better by dealing openly with the issues between them rather than leaving them unspoken and having everyone anxious about them. Ann said that she could imagine talking openly about issues but had never seen it work. The therapist asked her to help him by trying to get emotionally neutral about the idea of having a session with Dave and his parents and sitting back and evaluating the results with him. The therapist added that, with Dave's and his parents' permission, he would videotape the sessions with Dave and his parents and allow Ann to study them as a part of her evaluation. If she liked the results, she might even get Dave to take the camcorder along on the trip to her hometown.

Ann expressed the thought that the therapist was even more relentless than her mother, but she agreed to the challenge. Dave agreed to speak with his parents about coming in for a series of three sessions (to be recorded for Ann) to deal with some issues that were important to him.

All these steps were aimed at neutralizing the therapy triangle that the proposed experiment had activated. The therapist depolarized the triangle by decreasing the distance between him and Ann, thereby diminishing the emotional reactivity in the therapy triangle. If the therapist had tried to bring Ann in to lecture her on how she was blocking Dave's therapy, to convert her to the therapist's way of thinking, or to shut her out of the work Dave would do with his parents, the triangle would have gotten further polarized and reactive. Therapy might, in fact, be dead in the water for the foreseeable future.

The therapist hoped that, in addition to neutralizing the therapy triangle, by engaging Ann actively in the process, other good things would happen. If Dave and his parents were successful, enough of a conversion would take place in Ann that she would support the present therapeutic efforts, and the potential for future problems (or at least the fallout from future problems) would be diminished.

With the therapy triangle under control, the work with Dave and his parents could begin. Dave's reluctance when the experiment had been suggested made it clear that coaching him was unlikely to work. Directly involving his parents in therapy seemed the most efficient way to deal with Dave's overly strong attachment to his mother and his weak attachment to his father. The first item on the agenda was making it safe enough for Dave and his mother to talk about the emotional side of their developmental problems. The feelings of loss that go along with children growing up are as predictable as the moon and tides, but they're often handled by angry distance or silent emotional paralysis.

To make the therapy safe, the therapist's questions in the first family session gently and curiously addressed the family's ability to deal with the hard feelings (anger, resentment) versus the tender feelings (loss and longing). Dave and his mother did most of the talking about this in the first session, and they planned to continue doing so outside the therapy. (It might seem that encouraging all this talking and connection between Dave and his mother intensifies and prolongs the separation difficulties. Our experience and our theory predict just the opposite: It's the *failure* to communicate openly and work through these overly close connections that makes separation more of a problem.)

In the second session, the therapist directed the discussion toward the question of whether either side of the family had a tradition of the men being connected to one another in a way that was emotionally supportive. The idea was to plant a seed that might germinate and foster an improvement in the attachment between Dave and his father.

In the third session, the therapist asked Dave's father for his opinion about the first two sessions. Mr. O said he thought they'd been worthwhile; he hoped his son thought so, too. About 15 minutes into this session, Mrs. O somewhat hesitantly said that the first two sessions brought up for her the topic of *her* mother-in-law. She said she hadn't wanted to talk about it then but asked her husband if he would come back to the therapist with her and without Dave to talk about Mr. O's relationship with his mother and the impact that relationship had had on her. Mr. O looked thunderstruck and said that he wasn't sure what his wife was talking about. He agreed reluctantly to a session with her but had great difficulty settling on an appointment time.

Ann came in once more with Dave. She had watched one of the tapes of the sessions with Dave's parents and said that it looked too good to be true but that she'd be willing to keep an open mind. She even kidded the therapist about bringing him along on the trip to her hometown. No further appointments were scheduled, and the therapist told Dave to call if he wanted to do some more work or if his anxiety symptoms returned.

The follow-up of treatment proved satisfactory. With the help of imipramine, Dave hadn't had a recurrence of panic attacks for 6 months. When the therapist saw him at that time, he explained that there were two options—to taper off the medicine or to remain on a maintenance dose for a longer time. Dave asked the therapist to write down the schedule for tapering off and made a follow-up appointment. He canceled that appointment, and the therapist didn't hear from Dave, Ann, or Dave's parents for 4 years. At that time, Dave called for an appointment. Just the day before, on the train going to work, he had had another of those panic attacks. So, he thought he ought to check with his old therapist before the situation got out of hand. Delighted at Dave's intelligent use of therapy, and looking forward to seeing him again and catching up on what had happened, the therapist gave him an appointment. When he came in, Dave reported that he and Ann had been married for 2½ years and were very happy. He also said that things were going well with his mother—she and Ann had been getting along fine, and he had been careful to maintain a relationship with his mother. As the session neared its close, the therapist was feeling puzzled that he could find no trigger for the panic attack Dave reported. On his way out the door, after making an appointment for a few weeks later, Dave smiled and said, "By the way, Doc, we just found out 2 weeks ago that Ann is pregnant."

This was a couple's therapy, but it broadened into a systemic treatment involving four patients. Still the intervention remained brief, with only 12 sessions over a 6-month period.

SUMMARY AND CONCLUSION

This chapter has reviewed the pervasiveness of relationship triangles in people's lives, both personal and professional, and the relevance of these relationship triangles even to brief models of marital therapy. Dave's developmental struggle illustrates the part triangles play in the predictable events of all our lives. All therapists, whatever their theoretical persuasions, have listened to Dave's story and ones like it over and over again in their offices. In their personal lives, therapists have experienced triangles activated by marriage, the birth of a baby, death of a parent, a child leaving home for college.

We suggested six reasons why triangles are important factors in producing and maintaining marital dysfunction, and in making marital therapy more complex. We also presented the five-step method we've developed for managing clinically the triangles that people bring to us and the ones that we create in therapy and in our own lives. Our purpose has been to propose to you, the reader, the usefulness of becoming a "triangle doctor." This chapter, therefore, suggests some of the tools to do that.

It is important to note that, in spite of the potential promise of this model for some couples, in certain clinical situations those couples that present in intense marital conflict often require substantially more contact hours than this model allows, especially in the first 12 to 20 weeks of the treatment. For further consideration of this point, we refer the reader to Guerin et al. (1987).

Finally, we'd like to emphasize a point we made earlier, a point essential to good clinical practice. In order to work skillfully with triangles, a therapist must also be skilled at working with individuals and dyads. This is true because the fabric of any worthwhile and effective psychotherapy is woven out of an integration of individual, dyadic, and triangular factors. You could say that this is the one–two–three of psychotherapy.

ACKNOWLEDGMENT

This chapter is an adaptation of material in Guerin et al. (1996). Copyright 1996 by The Guilford Press. Adapted by permission.

REFERENCES

Guerin, P. J., Jr., Fay, L. F., Burden, S. L., & Kautto, J. G. (1987). *The evaluation and treatment of marital conflict.* New York: Basic Books.

Guerin, P. J., Jr., Fogarty, T. F., Fay, L. F., & Kautto, J. G. (1996). *Working with relationship triangles: The one-two-three of psychotherapy.* New York: Guilford Press.

6

◄O►

SHORT-TERM STRUCTURAL
FAMILY THERAPY
WITH COUPLES

Michael P. Nichols
Salvador Minuchin

What makes couple therapy structural? That it deals, not just with the dynamics of interaction between partners, but also with the boundaries around and between them. *What makes it brief?* An energetic, interventionist approach to helping partners realize that they create, and can change, each other's behavior by their own actions. Both things—the need to understand couples in context and our interventionist style— have generated misunderstandings, which we'd like to address before moving on to more detailed considerations of techniques.

THE NEED FOR A STRUCTURAL
UNDERSTANDING OF COUPLES

Although most family therapists are familiar with the structural model introduced in *Families and Family Therapy* (Minuchin, 1974), many don't see the need to worry about family structure when it comes to working with couples. With only two people in treatment, there may be little indication of the alliances and coalitions that define a couple's context. Besides, most unhappy couples have enough complaints about each other that it doesn't seem necessary to consider who's enmeshed or disengaged with whom. There is some truth to this. But only some.

Problems in couples almost always involve the complicating influence of third parties. Murray Bowen was right.

The first task a couple faces is establishing a boundary to protect them from outside interference. That's why most couples live in their own place and why, even though they spend time with friends and family, they reserve time to be alone, to work out the details of their relationship. But by the time they show up at a therapist's office, the boundary around a couple is likely to have been eroded by competing, or compensating, attachments. Sometimes the boundary around a couple was never very strong in the first place, as was the case with Janet and Keith.

A LITTLE UNFINISHED BUSINESS[1]

It was the third marriage for both of them, and they had the kind of complex arrangement you might expect. Janet's two boys, Bobby (18) and Jeffrey (13), had lived with them for all 3 years they'd been together. Keith's two boys, Chris (21) and David (16), lived with them for the second year of their marriage before moving out, David to live with his mother and Chris to his own apartment. Keith's daughter Andrea (19) had been living with her mother but recently moved in with Janet and Keith. Got it?

After 3 years of adjustments and readjustments, what finally brought the family to therapy was 13-year-old Jeffrey. He'd been "acting out," according to Keith, who tended to talk like that, formal and a little distant. Jeffrey's "acting out" consisted mostly of arguing with his mother and neglecting his chores. (One symptom of enmeshment is coming to therapy with relatively minor complaints about the children.)

"I play the role of the policeman," Keith said, glancing over at Janet. The implication was clear: he did; she didn't.

Janet, a pretty woman who'd put on 50 pounds since marrying Keith, sat next to Jeffrey on the couch. She made the unspoken accusation explicit, describing herself as a poor disciplinarian and admitting that she tended to undermine Keith's attempts to lay down the law. I wondered if this was her own assessment or whether she'd just learned to accept her husband's version of events.

Keith went on. "I'm pretty much at my wits' end. I've done everything I can possibly think of. Those two are so wrapped up together that it almost precludes Janet and I having any kind of relationship. All I hear is *Jeff's doing this, Jeff's doing that.*"

With the kind of reduction that brings clarity at the risk of oversimplification, brief structural therapy can be described as following several distinguishable steps.

1. Consider the Whole Family System in the Evaluation

Although it often makes sense to omit the children when couples seek treatment, imagine how much information and leverage would have been lost if the children hadn't been included in this case. Perhaps a useful rule of thumb is to have a session or two with the entire household somewhere in the first stage of treatment, even if the couple ends up being the primary unit of treatment.

It's possible to meet with one partner first and then to invite the other, but doing so may yield biased or incomplete information, may induct the therapist into a one-sided view of family problems, may create (the reality or illusion of) an unbalanced alliance, and may undermine the missing partner's motivation to participate in treatment. Even if he later shows up, he may begin with the idea that therapy is about helping his partner get more of what she wants from him.

2. Build an Alliance of Understanding with Each Member of the Family

Everyone has a story to tell, and in unhappy families almost everyone feels misunderstood. The first step in breaking the cycle of misunderstanding is for the therapist to offer the empathy family members may not be ready to provide each other. Hearing, understanding, and acknowledging each person's account of the family sorrows provides information and begins the process of releasing partners from the resentment that unheard feelings breeds.

"Joining," as we call this empathic connection, opens the way for the partners to begin listening to each other and establishes a bond with the therapist that enables them to accept the challenges to come.

Joining should not be a strategic pretense, a "technique." A therapist who's just waiting to say, "I understand," doesn't really need to listen. Such formulaic reassurances are the stock and trade of people who master the art of not listening with an air of attention. A genuine effort at understanding is more likely to be expressed in the opposite kind of statement—"I don't understand; tell me more about it."

Having heard from their parents, I turned to the children and asked how the process of reshuffling these two families had been for them.

Two themes emerged, both having to do with diffuse boundaries. When Keith and Janet set up housekeeping, the boys, who'd been used to having their own rooms, had to double up. Chris, Keith's older son, moved in with Jeffrey, Janet's younger son. The other two boys, Janet's Bobby and Keith's David, shared the remaining room. Jeffrey had trouble falling asleep when Chris listened to his radio, and Chris had trouble sleeping with Jeffrey's nightlight on. Bobby and David also got in each other's way. Eventually Keith's two boys moved out. Although the period of adjusting to their suddenly rearranged lives hadn't been more than mildly difficult, things never really got worked out because there was no lock on the exit.

The second story that emerged was Jeffrey's account of his own "acting out."

"My Dad says I'm a master manipulator," he said, trying to suppress a grin. He wore glasses and had on a striped polo shirt. Like his mother, he was considerably overweight. And, like her, he was quick with self-reproach, describing himself as always arguing and trying to get his way.

"What's wrong with that?" I asked.

He looked surprised. Then he went on to explain himself as though from the perspective of a disappointed parent, rather than like any normal, red-blooded 13-year-old who could be expected to try to get his own way.

3. Promote Interaction

Many therapists shy away from enactments because they can be difficult to work with. To initiate a productive enactment, zero in on a specific subject about which both partners have strong feelings. Vague instructions, such as "Why don't you two discuss this," may not overcome the natural reluctance clients have to talk to each other, from whom they don't expect understanding, rather than to the therapist, from whom they do.

The best way to begin an enactment is to ask one partner to respond to something specific the other said, especially a criticism or complaint. For example, "She says you never want to spend time with her, can you respond to that?" It's useful to emphasize the importance of dialogue. "He says you don't care about his feelings; that sounds important. Unless you can convince him that you do care what he's feeling, he's never going to be very eager to talk to you."

In the first session or two when enactments are used to discover what goes wrong when couples try to talk, it's important for the therapist to interfere *as little as possible*. Even if the partners are saying hard things or using ugly language, a conversation is functional as long as the participants are able to keep talking. The important thing to identify is what actually leads to the dialogue breaking down.

In subsequent sessions, when enactments are used more for therapeutic than diagnostic purposes, it may be useful to make suggestions about how the partners might best get through to each other. "He seems reluctant to talk about his feelings. Would you be willing to listen to what he thinks about this?" "As long as she keeps her complaints to herself, she isn't going to feel like getting any closer to you. Can you convince her that you're willing to listen? And can you tell him how you feel about this in such a way that he really hears you?"

Hoping to focus more on their strange blurring of boundaries, I asked Janet and Jeffrey to talk about something they frequently argued about.

Janet looked at Jeffrey, and he looked at her, neither of them sure how to begin. Keith suggested that they talk about Jeff's not doing his chores. I didn't say anything.

Jeffrey's crime was neglecting to fold and put away the laundry after his mother had done the washing. Sometimes he'd just forget; sometimes he'd stuff the clothes into drawers without bothering to fold them.

What bothered Janet more than not getting the job done was Jeffrey's lack of willingness to cooperate. If he were more willing, she'd have less need to assert her authority. She didn't exactly say that, but she did say, "I'm wishy-washy. Keith is more . . . strong, more of a disciplinarian."

I asked her to resume talking to Jeffrey about the chores, and she asked him why he didn't cooperate more, much as one adult might appeal to another. When Jeffrey didn't immediately answer, she asked if he felt put upon, and then she appealed to him to agree that her rules were reasonable.

At this point I interrupted. "Do you always work so hard?"

She gave me a look, like the cat who ate the canary. "You mean controlling?"

"No," I said, and I meant it, "working so hard. Carrying on both sides of the conversation."

Janet was too caught up in the content of her dealings with Jeffrey to notice the process. She wondered what she should say to him. I wondered why she was so preoccupied with him.

"The real problem is that I'm too wishy-washy."

Again Janet described herself as the problem. The drawback of this kind of thinking, from a structural perspective, isn't just self-blame but of an individual isolating herself from her context. It's true that she was indecisive. But she wasn't indecisive all by herself. Like most parents, she was part of a pair.

4. Make a Structural Assessment of How Boundaries and Subsystems Are Organized in a Way That Supports the Presenting Problem

It can be a mistake to assume, just because a couple describes their problems as being between the two of them, that other subsystems aren't relevant. Treating a couple without taking into account the rest of the family is as myopic as treating individuals in isolation. Partners disengaged from each other are almost certain to be enmeshed elsewhere. A therapist who attempts to break through a couple's disengagement without considering competing attachments is working with one hand tied behind his or her back. In other cases, an enmeshed couple's disengagement from family and friends may lead them to put more pressure on their partnership than any one relationship can bear.

Janet went on to say, "I want more peace in the house—I should be a stronger disciplinarian."

"And Keith won't let you?" I asked.

"I think he would like me to be," she insisted.

"I don't know," I said, "I think he needs you to be a buffer for his sternness."

This wasn't an idle comment. Yes, these two parents polarized each other, but they were also a unit, and whatever they were doing seemed to be working. They had managed a very difficult job, the blending of two rather large families, and they had done so with no major casualties.

There was, however, one major unfinished piece of business. Saddled from the start with the burden of raising children and coordinating households, Janet and Keith's couplehood had been submerged in parenting. It was to that unfinished business I now turned.

"Janet, how would you like to change Keith?" I asked.

"Change *Keith*?" This wasn't what she had expected.

Unless you consider them in splendid isolation from their surroundings, couples who come to therapy can be understood as more or less alienated from each other and more or less enmeshed with other interests and attachments, as indicated in Figure 6.1.

Keith and Janet had allowed the demands of parenting to smother their couplehood. Their gradual disengagement sealed off the inevitable

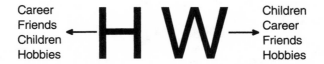

FIGURE 6.1. Emotional distance is supported by outside involvements.

conflicts that go with the formation of any new couple. Rather than address the difference that kept them from being close, Janet found it easier to worry about the children, especially Jeffrey; and Keith found it easier to immerse himself in his law practice and, when he was feeling tense, to go out for a run. Almost invariably, what stands between two people who are disengaged is unaddressed conflict. From a structural perspective, the first two steps in treatment are to draw a boundary around the couple (as indicated in Figure 6.2.) and then push them to address the conflicts, overt and covert, between them (Figure 6.3). We use the term "push" advisedly. Because bluntness has fallen out of favor in family therapy circles, we're going to pause to consider the criticism of a confrontive approach.

THE CASE FOR AN INTERVENTIONIST THERAPY

Somewhere in the mid-1980s a reaction set in against the activist approach to family therapy. Harlene Anderson and the late Harry Goolishian called for a more "collaborative" style (Anderson & Goolishian, 1988) and urged therapists to step down from the stance of expert and

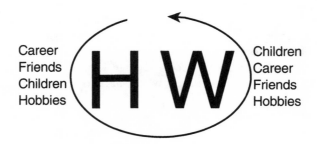

FIGURE 6.2. Reinforcing the boundary around a couple is the first step in closing the distance between them.

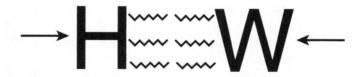

FIGURE 6.3. Breaking through disengagement requires confronting dormant conflicts.

engage in respectful conversation with clients. The narrative approach that emerged in their wake (White & Epston, 1990) emphasizes cognition over action, and, by defining problems as external to families, has gotten away from the notion that family conflicts lie at the root of many difficulties that bring people to therapy. Although it's not always so plainly put, part of what narrative constructionists were reacting against was the aggressiveness of interventionist approaches.

Structural family therapy *is* aggressive. It's hard for unhappy families to face their problems; it's hard for them to face each other. That's why we rely on enactments, to push family members to engage directly with each other, and that's why we challenge people, at times bluntly, to face their role in the problems that plague them. The trick is to challenge families bluntly enough to push them past habit and avoidance but sympathetically enough for them to accept the challenge.

When a therapist says to a husband that he's not doing enough or to a wife that she's pushing her husband away, it may seem combative. But the real enemy is fear—fear of change. For all their uncertainty and vulnerability, some families are rigidly organized and their members afraid to risk change. As helping professionals, we care about people, but as therapists, we aren't content just to "be understanding." With all our hearts, we want to help people break out of their cycles of self-defeating behavior.

What usually goes unnoticed in the debate between restrained and interventionist approaches is another dimension that may be more important: the centrality of the therapist.

One of the things that makes problems between couples seem intransigent, and therapists feel helpless, is the dynamics of polarization (see Lawrence, Eldridge, Christensen, & Jacobson, Chapter 10, this volume). The more she complains, the more he withdraws. The more he withdraws, the more she complains. One unideal strategy for breaking these polarized patterns is for the therapist to dominate the interaction—insisting that partners take turns, getting them to paraphrase what each other says, having extended conversations with each of them, and, in general, controlling the show. (This works fine as long as the couple remains in treatment.)

While it's become popular to see the good therapist as "collaborative," we believe that what distinguishes control from empowerment isn't whether therapists are interventive or laid back, but whether they remain central, controlling the flow of conversation through themselves, or encouraging family members to face each other, face their conflicts, and face their own role in their problems. To be truly transformative, therapists can neither do most of the talking nor ignore the context in which couples are embedded.

"I'M LOOKING FOR A PARTNER, NOT A MASTER–SLAVE RELATIONSHIP"

5. Develop a *Structural* Focus for Brief Therapy

One of the biggest mistakes therapists make is getting caught up in the content of a couple's problems and losing sight of the process and structure that supports such problems. Keith's complaint that Janet wasn't available to him as a partner was embedded in a process in which a husband's control was mirrored by his wife's passivity—*and* a family structure in which a mother's closeness to her son reinforced her distance from her husband.

Janet was taken aback by my strange question—"How would you like to change Keith?" She was used to thinking *she* was the problem: She was "wishy-washy." But I sensed that unrecognized resentment of Keith's imperious manner was keeping her from getting closer to him, and so I pressed. Having drawn a boundary around the couple's relationship, I was going to push them to face each other—and face things they found it easier not to talk about.

"Look at Keith as though you were a sculptor," I said. "He is your clay. How would you like him to be?"

She looked puzzled, indecisive.

"If you don't speak up, he'll tell you how you *should* want to change him."

6. Highlight and Focus on Problematic Interactions

Having Janet and Keith talk to each other about their dissatisfactions brings up the heart of their conflict and puts it between them where it belongs. In addition, because they're talking with each other rather than to the therapist, it's possible to observe what actually happens when they try to get through to each other. Their complementary contributions—Keith's domineering and Janet's subservience—are both obvious and available for intervention. By returning repeatedly to such key dialogues, a therapist can challenge both parties to face their own contributions to unhappy interactions.

Janet turned to face Keith. "I would like you to let your wall down. I feel that there's a wall there. I would like. . ." she started but again got flustered. "I don't know *what* I'd like!" she said, giggling self-consciously.

She turned to me, looking for help. I just waited.

Then came one of those moments that happen once in a while in families, when one person says something and everything shifts.

"I would like you to open up to me more and let me know more of who you are. Share with me. Communicate with me . . . instead of *telling* me all the time—not all the time, but some of the time." All this came out in a rush, but then, as though frightened by what she'd said, Janet laughed nervously. "This is really hard!" She looked at me, ready to throw in the towel, but I continued not to meet her gaze, and she turned back to Keith. "I'd like you to let your guard down. I'd like to get to know you."

She was now at the heart of the matter, speaking with feeling about the gulf that separated these two wounded veterans of divorce. But I wanted to make sure that Keith could hear her and that they could get beyond an expression of feeling to creating real change in their lives.

"Think about specifics," I said. "Think about little things that you would like him to change."

People may live by the stories they tell themselves, but it's the details of their everyday actions that must be changed to create a lasting shift in a relationship.

Janet wasn't sure where to start, and Keith asked for a turn. She said okay.

"It would be important for me," he began, "that you begin to get up earlier in the morning. So that I'm able to share that morning, and we're able to function as if we, the parents, are up when the young people are up." He sounded slightly pompous, but he was sincere.

"We never share the mornings," Janet said.

"I understand that," Keith replied. "One of the reasons is that you aren't up for us to be able to do that."

"Are you talking about my making lunches for the kids or being together as a family?" she wanted to know.

"I want a life-style partner," Keith answered. "I'm looking for a partner, not a master–slave relationship. That means you have to be responsible for yourself." And then he went on at great windy length about what he meant by her being responsible for herself. "I want you to stand up for yourself. I want you to be your own person."

7. Push Interactions Beyond Their Usual Homeostatic Cutoffs

What keeps families from resolving their problems isn't so much not knowing what to do but, rather, not doing it forcefully or consistently enough. Successful change requires pushing past the point where family members are tempted to break off and revert back to the same old same pattern.

If a therapist's goal were merely to help couples express their feelings, getting them to open up would be sufficient. But with Janet and Keith, getting them to go beyond complaining to actually making things change meant pushing them past naming their discontent to insisting that they make clear what things they want to change. (Incidentally, the same tentativeness that keeps family members from following through on good intentions often applies to young therapists. It isn't usually that they don't know what to do but that lack of experience and confidence holds them back from pushing hard enough to make it happen. To be an effective structural family therapist, you must be willing to work with intensity.)[2]

"He is now your teacher," I said to Janet. "Do you like that?"

"No," she said emphatically. "I don't like that!"

"Why don't you change it?" I asked.

"I don't know how," she said, looking pained.

"It's very simple," I replied. "Tell him to stop it."

"Stop it," she said, but then she broke into a nervous laugh.

Again I pushed her. "If you don't like it when he talks to you that way, why don't you change it?"

"I think it has to do with his being so strong; and I'm not."

"No," I said, "that's not true."

He was "strong," she was "weak." He was the "disciplinarian," she was "wishy-washy." These labels handcuffed them. Couple therapy is about unlocking labels and opening up alternatives, more flexible ways of functioning.

"It's not true that you aren't strong," I said. "You have your own kind of strength. And if you don't want him to talk down to you, all you have to say is, 'Keith, how old do you think I am?' But you don't tell him."

"No, I don't," she agreed.

"I can understand that Jeff likes to be close to you. When you feel dissatisfied with Keith's tenderness, Jeff gives you a wonderful opportunity to be tender." I turned to Jeff. "So, you are Mom's teddy bear."

Jeff smiled sheepishly. Then no one said anything, and I could hear the whir of the electric clock on the wall behind my head.

Continuing, I said to Jeff, "I don't know how long you want to be your mom's teddy bear." Still no one said anything. "How old are you, Jeff?"

"Thirteen."

"Well, maybe you will be a 15-year-old teddy bear. Maybe you will be a 20-year-old teddy bear. . . . "

I turned back to Janet. "Maybe you will be a mom playing with a teddy bear—*if* you don't change *him*," I said, looking at Keith.

"I never looked at it like that before," she said softly.

"The truth is, Jeff looks more like a teddy bear than Keith," I said. Janet laughed. "Maybe you can fatten Keith up, and maybe Jeff will lose some weight." I looked at Keith. "Maybe you can soften him up."

They might have been threatened by what I said, but they weren't. Instead they looked at each other tenderly.

8. Promote Empathy to Help Stuck Dyads Get Past Defensive Wrangling

When members of a couple can't get through to each other because their conversation consists of accusations and counterattacks, a therapist can interrupt to block these unproductive discussions by talking to the partners one at a time about what they're really feeling and what they want from each other. By bringing out the hurt and loneliness beneath angry tirades and lending an ear to the unspoken complaints beneath defensive avoidance, a therapist can help partners connect at a more genuine level.

Janet turned back to me. "I find it real threatening when I have to confront him with my feelings on something."

Facing him was hard for her. She was demonstrating that now by continuing to address me. I avoided eye contact and said, "Talk to *him*. Tell him how you want him to change."

"Get down and beg?" she said and laughed. This *was* hard. But nobody else laughed, and she went on: "I find it very, very threatening when I have to tell you how I feel about something that you're doing. I've never been able to tell you when there have been times when you aren't meeting my needs. I've never ever been able to tell you that. I'm afraid you'll totally ignore what I'm feeling—and you'll tell me how I *should* be feeling. Like my feelings aren't valid."

Janet was no longer indecisive, no longer the girlish other half of Keith's stern sensibleness. She was a woman telling the truth about her feelings. To her surprise, Keith didn't seem threatened or get defensive. He listened.

I glanced over at Bobby and Chris and Andrea and then back to Janet. "He treats you like one of the kids," I said. "There are people who like to be treated like that. I don't know, I don't want to ruin your fun."

They all laughed.

"I think when we first got together that *was* what I wanted. I needed a big strong father. But I don't need that anymore." And then Janet spoke directly to Keith. "I don't want that anymore."

Janet made this declaration simply. Her voice had none of that earlier tentativeness, none of that high-pitched girlish quality. Keith listened intently.

At this point my concern was that if he did nothing but listen, Keith's own unvoiced complaints would shut his ears to his wife's statement. And so I said to him, "You said you wanted her to get up in the morning. How will you make that happen?"

"All I can do is request it. She can either do it or not do it. It's her choice."

"That's too soft," I said.

"That's true," he said. "That's all I'm prepared to do. If I want her to stand up and be her own person, all I can do is give her opportunities. If she chooses not to, she chooses not to. If my need is for you to be an independent person, and you choose not to, then you choose not to."

"No," I said. "You can't tell her that. You can tell her what you want from her, but you can't tell her what she should do for herself."

"I'm telling her what I want her to be," he said.

"No," I said, "tell her what you want her to *do*."

Keith's experience was that Janet was unresponsive to his wishes. What he failed to recognize was that the pompous, lecturing way he went about expressing those wishes made her resistant. Most people are resistant to being lectured to.

"You said that you wanted her to get up in the morning so that you could have breakfast together? Why is that so difficult?"

"I don't know," he answered. The implication was clear: it wasn't *his* fault.

"So find out," I suggested. "She's right there."

"Why is it so difficult for you to get up in the morning?" Keith asked.

"I don't know that it's been all that long that I've been sleeping late. My perception is that it's just been a few months."

"My perception is that it's been much longer," Keith said, as though unwilling to cut her any slack.

I broke in. "You want it to happen tomorrow morning?" I asked him.

"Yes."

"So?" I said.

Keith turned to Janet. "Tomorrow morning, will you get up a little earlier?"

"Yes," she said.

"You were right," Keith said to me. "I was lucky."

"No," I said, not willing to let him put all the onus on her. "I think you could have probably changed that weeks ago. People get into ruts, and then you accept to continue like you are."

I went on. "I don't think you will have any problem with Jeffrey moving out of the position of teddy bear . . . if you find a way to change each other, so that *he* becomes more satisfying to you, Janet," I said looking at Keith, "and *she* becomes more satisfying to you," I said to him. "But if you don't do that, Jeff, your destiny is to grow up to be a large teddy bear."

Jeffrey laughed and pushed his glasses up on his nose. He had his mother's ability to laugh at himself.

A SEARCH FOR ALTERNATIVES

In the 1990s we've come to see marriage in more realistic terms. Contemporary couples are learning to give up their fantasies and settle for tolerable instead of terrific. Now that divorce is no longer viewed with such equanimity—especially by couples like Janet and Keith who've lived through its jumble of griefs—partners, especially if they're parents, are surrendering to the real meaning of commitment, as a promise and a pledge. Becoming realistic about the difficulties and responsibilities of marriage and distinguishing it from uncomplicated romantic love are seen as necessary for a union that lasts.

Welcome as this new realism may be, it rests on a partial truth. Lowering unrealistic expectations may be part of what it takes to build a lasting relationship, but you don't build anything with resignation alone. Surrendering to the despair that passes itself off as realism, many disillusioned couples stabilize themselves with fixed and rigid distance. They give up on each other and lead parallel lives.

A more useful attitude than resignation is acceptance. Successful partners learn to accept their differences and realize that while they simply may not be compatible in some ways, they will be in others. So instead of a fixed distance, they choose a selective coming together. Keith may never enjoy going to craft shows with Janet, just as she may never care to go jogging with him. But they probably can find some activities to share happily, perhaps going to movies, or taking walks together, or birdwatching, any of a variety of things that will allow them to enjoy being together.

Relationships succeed when people find a way to live with their differences—and still remain loyal to each other. This doesn't mean some grand and generous capacity for total acceptance. Sometimes it means facing up to the fact that in some areas two people are too different to relate successfully. Rather than battle over these differences, or be untrue to oneself by giving in entirely, wise people avoid certain activities that they don't both enjoy. But instead of drifting apart or insulating themselves emotionally from each other, they find other things they can share. It's a selective union.

If this process of selective coming together sounds simple, consider what most people do. When they discover differences in their partners, they can only imagine two alternatives: One must change the other, or the two must drift apart.

Two other factors complicate the success of a relationship. One is that every relationship needs a boundary around it to ward off undue interference and to keep the couple connected. Couples with too little privacy can't work out the things they must. Couples with too little loyalty, on the other hand, lack the glue to keep them together through the hard times.

Part of what makes for healthy families is learning to accept other family members as they are—not as you want them to be—letting go of trying to change them, and learning instead to live with them. However, in order to accept people and learn to live with them, it's necessary to recognize and accept one's own limits of tolerance. Some things we may not be able to share. The healthy response is not to continue to bang up against these clashing characteristics but to search for alternatives.

"MAYBE HE'S MORE MALLEABLE THAN YOU THINK"

Having seen how Janet and Keith avoided confronting their dissatisfactions by preoccupying themselves elsewhere—Keith, with his work and jogging, and Janet with the children, especially her youngest—I wanted to drive home the point that they could change, but not without help. And this brings us to our ninth suggestion about technique.

9. Challenge Family Members to Accept Responsibility for Their Behavior

We've said it before, yet it bears repeating: Structural family therapy is a therapy of challenge. But challenging people to accept responsibility for their behavior isn't the same thing as telling them what to do. The minute a therapist slides from pointing out what people are doing to pressuring them to change, their attention goes from their own behavior to the therapist's suggestion. When pressured to change, your choices are to comply or resist; and since most of us have had quite enough of people telling us what to do, thank you, the natural tendency is to resist. For this reason, the most effective confrontations point out what people are doing—but stop short of pressuring them to change. Consider the following.

THERAPIST: As long as she continues to feel that you don't care about what's going on in her life, your wife is going to continue to be angry.

HUSBAND: What *should* I do?

THERAPIST: You don't have to do anything. You can continue just as you are.

For a therapist to resist giving an obvious piece of advice ("start listening to your wife") in this way may seem cold. But in fact it's true: the husband *doesn't* have to do anything; he can keep doing what he's always done. (Isn't that what most of us do most of the time?) More important, the therapist's refusal to preach keeps the focus where it will do the most good: on what people are doing that keeps them stuck.

Another way to disarm the natural tendency to resist therapeutic challenge is to discuss other people's reactions rather than continuing to confront the person they're reacting to. Most of us hear better when we aren't busy preparing to defend ourselves.

Having risked the unflattering metaphor of Jeffrey as his mother's teddy bear, I now turned to his older brother. "Bobby, how is it that you managed not to be Mom's teddy bear and Jeff got himself saddled with that role?"

"I don't know," Bobby said. "Maybe he likes being a teddy bear. I don't like—just coming home and getting right in the middle of things with everybody. I like to go out and do my own thing. I'm home as little as possible."

"So, when you're home as little as possible and Dad's home as little as possible, that leaves Mom with Jeff alone?"

"Yeah. They're together a lot."

Should a therapist discuss a couple's emotional distance in front of their children? Wouldn't it be better to reinforce the generational boundary by meeting with the couple alone? Not necessarily.

Although some subjects are private and should be kept that way, it's a mistake to think that boundary making is better achieved by excluding people from the consulting room rather than having them present to explore and challenge cross-generational coalitions.

"Andrea, how long have you been living in this household?"

"About a month."

"And how are things for you?"

"Tolerable. . . . I'm gone early in the morning until the afternoon. I just kind of go through without getting involved."

So. Like Bobby and Keith, Andrea kept her distance. There was a lot of avoidance in this family. Was it a smothering mother Andrea was avoiding?

"Do you have contact with Janet?" I asked.

"Yes." Andrea seemed surprised at the question.

"Is it easy, can you talk with her?"

"Sure. She's easy to talk to."

"What about with your dad?"

"Not the way I want to." Andrea glanced at her father briefly. "I can't talk to him the way I want to."

"Why?" I asked. "What happens?"

"I don't know, I've always had a hard time telling him how I feel." She was leaning over now, worrying a little turquoise ring on her left hand. "I'm always afraid that I'll be talked down to. Somehow I'll be in the wrong, and he'll be in the right."

"Hmm," I said. "You don't have that feeling with Janet?"

"No."

(So much for the "wicked stepmother" theory.)

"That means that whenever you need her, you can talk to her?"

"Yeah."

"So, that's good. Then there will be a time when your father will grow up to be a little bit different . . . or you will grow up a little bit more on his wavelength. But for the moment Janet is available."

So, it seemed that all the children and stepchildren turned to Janet for understanding. Keith was pompous, yes, but rather than deal with him, the children, like Janet, had learned to avoid him. He was an excluded man. His sternness with the children and paternalistic manner with Janet both fueled and were fueled by emotional distance. Which was cause and which was effect? It didn't really matter. The important thing was to break through the distance where it mattered most—at the heart of the family, in the relationship between Keith and Janet.

"YOU JUST TAKE THE RISK AND DO IT?"

Now, nearing the end of my time with this family, I turned back to Janet, who, for some reason, seemed to doubt her power to change things in this family.

"I don't have any doubt that you can change him," I said, glancing at Keith, "if you want to. I don't know if you want to."

"Oh, I do," she said. "I'm just not sure I know how."

"Maybe he's more malleable than you think," I said.

"I really do think I want it to change," Janet said, cautiously substituting the impersonal "it" for the more threatening "him."

"Maybe you will begin to play with Keith instead of Jeff," I said, again emphasizing the triangle that kept this family running in place. "If he's not available, then maybe you will make him more available"—I looked over at Jeffrey—"and she will not need you as much. Do you have many friends?"

"Sure," he said.

"Name three of them," I said.

He did.

"Great! These are people in your class?"

"Several classes," he said.

"And do you visit them?"

"Yes."

It seemed that Jeff was ready and willing to move out more into the world on his own.

Turning back to Janet and Keith, I said, "I don't think Jeff likes to be a teddy bear. I think he wants to be his own man."

At this Jeff sat up a little straighter. But Janet, unsure of herself, wanted more concrete direction. "How do you do it?" she wanted to know.

But of course telling Janet how to demand more of Keith would be one of those paradoxes, like telling someone to be more spontaneous or saying, "You should have more self-confidence!" So I just shrugged.

"You just take the risk and do it?" Janet said.

"Maybe it's not so difficult," I replied.

It was time to stop now, to resist the urge to direct and advise in order to let the fundamental message sink in.

"Keith, do you have any questions?" I asked.

"Do I change—do I attempt to change myself because of something I perceive I should change, or do I wait for a specific request?" he wanted to know.

"I don't think you *can* change yourself," I said. "I don't think that's possible." And then I got up and shook hands with all of them, and we parted.

SUMMARY

Therapy is a place where conversations that should occur at home but don't can take place. Instead of nursing their disappointments in silence, a couple such as Keith and Janet can be encouraged to open up to each other about what's bothering them. But although they might have come in, as many couples do, to work on their marriage, they might not have gotten very far if we'd attempted to address their disengagement without considering their enmeshment elsewhere.

NOTES

1. We selected this case, which was a one-session consultation with Salvador Minuchin, to illustrate how the concepts and methods of the structural model can be applied to the brief treatment of couples.
2. Therapists can add intensity to their work by prolonging enactments beyond the point where family members are tempted to break off and retreat; repeating their messages in a variety of contexts; and emphasizing what's at stake if family members persist in destructive patterns of interaction.

REFERENCES

Anderson, H., & Goolishian, H. (1988). Human systems as linguistic systems: Preliminary and evolving ideas about the implications for clinical theory. *Family Process*, 27, 371–393.

Minuchin, S. (1974). *Families and family therapy.* Cambridge, MA: Harvard University Press.

White, M., & Epston, D. (1990). *Narrative means to therapeutic ends.* New York: Norton.

7

◄◦►

PSYCHOANALYTICALLY INFORMED SHORT-TERM COUPLE THERAPY

PHYLLIS COHEN

Psychoanalysis and family systems are radically different theories of mind and relationship that have traditionally been isolated from one another and often framed in opposition. This chapter argues that a meaningful, clinically effective couple treatment requires a dual approach. Emphasis on interaction alone minimizes the complex contribution of an individual's history and psychodynamics, while exclusive emphasis on individual psychology misses the way in which interpersonal interaction governs a couple's intimate life. The perspective presented here integrates systemic theories and techniques (derived from the theoretical traditions of general systems, cybernetic, and communications theories) with a psychoanalytic focus that incorporates classical psychoanalytic theory and contemporary relational ideas (a perspective that has been called a "two-person psychology").

Many therapies are described as "psychoanalytic couple therapy." Some feature a nondirective psychoanalytic approach that concentrates on the separate psychologies of the individuals, whereas others emphasize a more active and directive involvement by the therapist focusing primarily on the intersubjective field. A psychoanalytically informed couple therapy approach is not just about the joining of individual psychology and couple interpersonal patterns; it also addresses the two-person psychology that emerges when people engage in an intimate relationship.

REVIEW OF RELEVANT LITERATURE

Psychoanalysis

In order to apply an analytic metapsychology to short-term work with couples, we must first agree on a definition of "What is psychoanalytic," an almost impossible task. Not only is there no single theoretical view, there are warring factions among the various contemporary schools and orientations, including drive theorists (Freudians), self-psychologists (Kohutians), interpersonalists (Sullivanians), contemporary relationalists (Mitchell & Greenberg, 1983), object relations theorists (Fairbairn, 1952; Winnicott, 1971, 1975; Scharff & Scharff, 1991), and thinkers in the hermeneutic tradition (Spence, 1982; Gill, 1994; Schafer, 1983, 1992).

In the climate of postmodernism, contemporary psychoanalysis has moved from a one- to a two-person psychology, incorporating the participation of the analyst into the interpersonal field with the analytic dyad as the basic unit of investigation (Aron, 1990; Ghent, 1989; Gil, 1993, 1994; Hoffman, 1983). When a two-person perspective is applied to couples therapy, the focus of the treatment includes how the therapist "creates or co-creates a context with the patient[s]" (Gerson, 1996, p. 67), and how each of the partners co-create the intersubjective field between them.

A psychoanalytically informed couple therapy is based on the fundamental assumptions of psychoanalytic metapsychology including the *topographic* view, that *conscious* and *unconscious* phenomena govern all functioning; the *dynamic* view, that mental phenomena are the result of an interaction of forces in the mind including *instinctual drives, ego* interests, *defenses, conflicts,* and *symptoms*; and the *genetic* view, that incorporates history and seeks to explain why specific solutions have been adopted (Greenson, 1967).

In the psychoanalytically informed method of couple treatment, the therapist applies and teaches relevant psychoanalytic principles to couples thereby helping them understand their own behavior. For example, the therapist teaches that the past is contained in the present and that all thoughts, words and actions are responses to things that came before (*psychic determinism*). In turn, individuals learn that not all behavior can be in their *conscious* control as new meanings and contexts are created. Thus, "family members expand their insight by learning that their psychological lives are larger than their conscious experience, and by coming to understand and accept repressed parts of their personalities" (Nichols & Schwartz, 1995, p. 267).

Other psychoanalytic concepts pertinent to work with couples include: the principle of *overdetermination,* that behavior, thoughts and attitudes have more than one meaning and can be experienced in more than one way; the concept of *defense,* that we do things protectively, though often *unconsciously,* in response to what is felt to be an impending threat; *projective identification,* a defense mechanism whereby a person attributes or projects disowned parts of the self or thoughts or attitudes onto another person, and, in turn, that person is induced into behaving in accord with those projections; the ideas of *primary and secondary gain,* that we may do something for one purpose, while serving another intent; the idea of the *repetition compulsion,* that we may be irrationally compelled to repeat some behavior that is unconsciously connected to childhood experience; the concept of using the *observing ego* to step outside of oneself to look at what is going on; and the concept of *transference/countertransference,* that in reaction to each other, we may unconsciously displace feelings and attitudes that were intended toward someone else. An additional idea with psychoanalytic implications that informs the work is based on the concept of *attribution/perception of causality,* that we respond to others based on "perceived motives and intentions" (Reber, 1985), be they accurate or not.

In working psychoanalytically, the therapist must create an atmosphere of trust to facilitate a willingness on the part of the partners in the couple to expose previously hidden parts of themselves not only to the therapist but also to each other. Nichols (1987) stresses the importance of *empathy* so that a *holding environment* can be created. In addition, *interpretations* are made by the therapist to make *unconscious* and *preconscious* material understandable, and *insights* must be *worked through* until they are transformed into new and more effective ways of behaving and interacting (Greenson, 1967).

The data for the psychodynamic interpretations are often revealed in the couple's "*transference* ridden interpersonal relationships" (Sander, 1997), with each other, with the therapist, and with other family members. These transferences are often unconsciously *enacted* and *reenacted* within the couple's therapy sessions. As each partner *projects* and *projectively identifies,* repetitive dramas are often played out between them.

Over the past two decades, a number of clinicians have combined various psychoanalytic theories with different techniques to work with couples (e.g., Nichols, 1987; Sander, 1979, 1989; Scharff & Scharff, 1991). When an object relations perspective has been added, the interactions of the couple are understood in terms of how the unconscious internal objects of each individual are involved in each partner's perception of and reaction to the other. Internal object relations may reflect dramas rooted in each of their early histories, including the marital relationship of the couple's parents. The goal is to free family members to relate to each other on the basis of current realities rather than on the basis of distortions from the past.

In contrast to an object relations approach, not all psychoanalytic couple therapists believe that the achievement of insight is necessary. From a Kohutian point of view, it may be more important for family members to express their unconscious needs for the other to serve a "selfobject function," than for such self needs to be understood (Kohut, 1984). Livingston states that one of the most important aspects of the self psychological approach to couple therapy is "its stress on the legitimizing of both partner's developmental needs for each other" (1995, p. 431). I believe that, in working with couples, the psychoanalytically informed therapist must do both—foster insight and encourage the communication of conscious and unconsciously derived thoughts and feelings.

Because the psychoanalytic couple therapist is, like any couple therapist, often asked to address immediate life crises (such as divorce, affairs, acting-out children, etc.), there is good reason to be more active and directive. Couples do not usually enter treatment primarily for personal growth as many individual patients do. Many come because their circumstances have become extreme, and some kind of action needs to be taken. Being active and/or directive does not mean that the therapist doesn't allow a psychoanalytic process to unfold; rather, it reflects a task- and problem-focus that is deepened by psychoanalytic insight.

Systems Theory

Systemic theory is based on the premise that the family is a complex whole that is greater than the sum of its individual member parts. It is assumed that since couples and families have superordinate properties above and beyond the psychologies of their members, the family therapist should focus on these metaprocesses—interactions among family members—rather than only on individual dynamics.

Unlike psychoanalysis (where theories are many and complex but techniques are few), in family systems approaches, theories are simple and widely shared, but techniques are quite diverse. Thus, although the field of family therapy is also not a monolithic entity, it is generally more acceptable than in psychoanalysis to use a variety of techniques.

As Braverman, Hoffman, and Szkrumelak (1984) put it, "The sophisticated family therapist needs to be trained in several treatment modes, e.g., structural, intrapsychic, behavioral, and strategic, and be able to choose the most appropriate for the particular case at hand" (p. 30). Even though there are many theoreticians and clinicians who believe that it is a mistake to mix and match theories and techniques because to do so weakens each paradigm, others argue that relational issues are complex and that a combined approach is the most effective. An approach to couple treatment that is psychoanalytically informed draws from both modalities as indicated, and the integration of these approaches is a recent trend in the field of couple therapy (Nichols & Schwartz, 1998).

Many of the concepts from systems, cybernetics, communications, and structural theory are useful in a short-term, psychoanalytically informed couple therapy, such as *homeostasis,* where the relational system, like other nonhuman systems, tends to resist change by recalibrating to maintain itself (Jackson, 1965b); *first-order change,* when the elements of the system shift, but the rules stay the same, and *second-order change,* when the change is a result of a change in the fundamental rules of the system that determine its structure and functioning (Watzlawick, Weakland, & Fisch, 1974); the Bowenian concepts of *differentiation* from family of origin, referring to separation and independence of self from others, and *triangulation,* when the conflict between two people is stabilized by involving a third member (Bowen, 1978); *family life cycle,* refers to the stages of development of family life (Carter & McGoldrick, 1989); *circular causality,* when family interactions are seen as a series of self-reinforcing, repetitive feedback loops that trigger and interact with each other (Bateson, 1972); *subsystems,* when various subgroups in a family join together to perform a function; *boundaries,* the invisible barriers that surround individuals and subsystems and regulate the amount of contact with others; and *symmetry* and *complementarity,* describing the positions partners can take in relation to each other, either equal and parallel in the former, or one-up and one-down in the latter (Jackson, 1965b).

Systemic *techniques* frequently used in this method include: *reframing* or *relabeling* of the problem when the therapist changes its context to make it more amenable to change, and the use of *positive connotations* to address resistance by emphasizing the positive aspects of symptoms and problems (Watzlawick et al., 1974; Selvini Palazzoli, Boscolo, Cecchin, & Prata, 1978; O'Brian & Bruggen, 1985); the use of *enactment,* when the couple is encouraged to demonstrate in the session how they relate on the outside (Minuchin, 1974; Minuchin & Fishman, 1981); *quid pro quo,* the bargaining tactic used by couples and highlighted by Jackson (1965a); and the use of *assignments* and exercises within sessions or at home.

Although most couple therapies deal with here-and-now interactions, psychoanalytically informed therapists also trace family history. Relevant information is either compiled chronologically, as in a time line, or thematically in a *genogram* that organizes the family-of-origin relationships (McGoldrick & Gerson, 1985). In addition, Erikson's concept of *individual life cycles* (1963, 1982) as well as the couple's stage in the *family life cycle* (Carter & McGoldrick, 1989) both need to be considered, since developmental tasks and stressors vary on each level and from stage to stage (Wachtel, 1982).

In a successful marital relationship, the individuals must accomplish the tasks of *differentiating* themselves while separating from their *families of origin* and their current *nuclear families* (Bowen, 1978). At the same time, the couple must avoid cutoffs and connect with their families (Minuchin, 1974). Any change in the system may stimulate a counterforce to maintain *homeostasis,* and such *first-order change* is often temporary or superficial (Watzlawick et al., 1974). Only a true *second-order change* that transforms the system's organization and functioning can be long-lasting.

THE CONCEPTUAL APPROACH: COMBINING PSYCHOANALYSIS AND SYSTEMS THEORY INTO A SHORT-TERM COUPLE THERAPY

The gap between psychoanalytic and systemic theories has been narrowing with the influence of the postmodern constructivist movement. A contemporary psychoanalytic view acknowledges that the analyst–patient dyad consists of two individuals who influence and affect the thoughts, behavior, and development of each other and that the intersubjective field thus created should be the focus of the analytic work (Aron, 1991; Gill, 1993, 1994; Hoffman, 1983). Psychoanalysis is no longer rooted in an empirical, positivist objectivism but, rather, is moving toward a hermeneutic social constructivism. Silverman explains that in the psychoanalytic dyad, "Each participant lends meaning to the other, and our interactions enrich and enhance our mutual understanding" (1994, p. 106). In the field of family therapy these concepts are applied to the couple (Goldenberg & Goldenberg, 1996).

In a psychoanalytically informed approach to couple therapy, the points of convergence between contemporary psychoanalysis and systems theory are emphasized. One point of intersection occurs between Bateson's discussion of repetitive, recursive feedback loops (1972), and Gill's recognition that "the analytic process is a series of episodes of interaction which are highly redundant, that is, recur over and over again" (1992, p. 24).

One way to think about the differing emphases between psychoanalytic and systemic views is that, in general, the couple therapist is trained to deal with the couple's current here-and-now dynamics of interaction with a view toward the future, whereas the psychoanalytic therapist looks to see how unconscious drives, defenses, and derivatives from the past are affecting the current relationship. The genogram, which we traditionally use in family therapy, demonstrates how multigenerational "patterns are stored, transformed and manifested in the present" (Wachtel, 1982, p. 335) to effect a change in the future of the system. Although this distinction may capture one piece of the truth, it is also true that all well-trained couple therapists, whether analytic or systemic, value work in the here-and-now, because this is the domain where insights and interpretations about the couple's enactments and psychic experience have their most powerful emotional impact.

In psychoanalytically informed couple treatment, the focus of the work can shift back and forth over dimensions of time according to the couple's need at any given moment. The therapist and couple may attempt to reconstruct the past, thus giving new meaning to old unresolved conflicts; at other times we may deconstruct the present by asking questions of the data "so that unconscious elaboration can be seen"; or at still other points we may co-construct the future by developing a "joint narrative construction" (Siegert, 1990, p. 168). Furthermore, conflicts can be reconstructed, deconstructed or co-constructed in separate individual sessions and/or in joint sessions with the couple.

Based on the assumption that there is no one way to effect change, Melito attempts to combine psychodynamic and structural therapy. He explains that psychoanalytic insight is achieved on a cognitive and emotional level, which "can result in altered perceptions and attitudes about oneself and others"; yet what is also needed for behavior change is the "translation of new understanding" (1988, p. 37). Thus, change in both attitude and behavior is necessary for any sustained difference, and this can be achieved through the two separate approaches of psychoanalytic and systemic therapy.

In running short-term couples therapy groups, Donovan (1995) explains that insight comes about when the couples understand the psychological and practical sense of their fighting. The partners begin to see that the historical antecedents of their fights started in their families of origin, and Donovan helps them avoid placing blame. Yet this is not enough. Donovan not only uses a psychodynamic approach, but he also utilizes psychoeducational and cognitive-behavioral methods to enable couples to change effectively. Although marital partners are helped when they understand how they consciously and unconsciously attempt to have their emotional needs met within their relationship, they also need to learn and practice new ways of interacting.

In short-term analytically informed work with a couple, there is no time for a transference neurosis to fully develop and be analyzed; instead, the partners are helped to see transference enactments, *in vivo*, in the therapy room and at home. This approach is most effective when both partners are willing to look at their participation in maintaining the symptom. In summary, the therapist uses analytic interpretation to help the partners gain insight into unconscious dynamics, yet the emphasis is on how these conflicts are played out in the system of the present relationship. In addition, the therapist helps the individuals differentiate from each other, while teaching them better ways to communicate their thoughts and needs.

THE METHOD: SELECTION OF PATIENTS, PHASES OF TREATMENT

Short-term psychoanalytically informed couple therapy involves a therapist who works time-intensively with a couple, *both individually* and *conjointly*, to effect a change as quickly as possible. The model has four phases:

Phase 1 is the period of assessment, when the therapist and the couple build an alliance and begin to focus. They also must agree to the terms of working together.

Phase 2 includes setting goals, agreeing on a plan of treatment within the developing therapeutic relationship and clarifying limits of confidentiality.

Phase 3 is the process of working through, when the therapist uses core technical maneuvers to effect change in the system.

Phase 4 is termination, when the therapist and couple review and evaluate the treatment, and they plan a follow-up session.

Selection of Patients

Since this method of treatment requires a focused and intense commitment of effort, time, and money, couples must be highly motivated to make the maximum effort. This usually means that there is a high degree of stress or a crisis that must be addressed. The treatment is most useful to couples who want to stay together. If they have already decided to separate, a conjoint analytic approach might confuse the issue. In such cases, the therapist could be more helpful by serving as a mediator or by referring the partners out for separate individual treatment.

If the partners are already in their own dynamically oriented individual treatment, psychoanalytically informed couple work can enhance the process; however, the use of individual sessions by the couple's therapist could undermine the individual therapy by splitting the transference. In these cases, I might recommend a more problem-focused conjoint approach. On the other hand, Jacobson (1971) has described disastrous results in numerous cases in which only one spouse was being seen in psychoanalytic treatment. Although it is possible that concurrent therapies can increase the therapeutic leverage, involvement with multiple therapists inevitably increases the levels of complexity in an already complex system of treatment (Maltas, 1996).

Ironically, the intensity of the combination of individual and joint sessions in this treatment approach can help enmeshed couples psychically separate and differentiate their individual needs from the couple needs. In contrast, disengaged couples might need more work in separate individual sessions before working together in joint sessions.

Any couple significantly motivated and capable of entering into an insight-oriented therapy could be considered for treatment. Should anything or anyone stand in the path of this work together, the individuals must be willing to clear away these obstacles (such as getting help for a drug problem or agreeing to suspend an affair for at least the time of the treatment). (See section in Phase 2: Building the Alliance and Handling Confidentiality.)

Phases of Treatment

Phase 1: Period of Assessment: Finding the Focus

In the first phase of treatment, the therapist sees the couple with "time intensity" (Budman & Gurman, 1988) in order to identify the problem quickly. At this point a therapist who is trained in more than one modality has critical decisions to make. Will the treatment be individual, for one of the partners, or will the couple be the patient? If the couple is defined as the patient, the therapist attempts to see both members together to determine why are they coming now, what each individual contributes to the problem, and what each must do in order to improve the situation. Wachtel explains, "It is frequently the case with families and couples that getting the individuals to focus on what they would like to change about themselves rather than other family members is a key step in altering rigidified family patterns" (1982, p. 341).

In addition to the importance of forming a therapeutic alliance with each member of the couple, it is imperative that initial work challenge the couple's propensity to blame one another. At this early point the therapist can offer a positive reframe by saying, for example, "With each argument it's as if you're fighting for your life. It's because you care that you get involved in such battles. If you didn't care, you wouldn't get so upset with each other." In addition, when the couple understands that each partner's individual issues are burdening the relationship, both are assured that these will be addressed in the separate individual sessions.

In Phase 1, I assess the current struggles of the partners in their individual and family life cycles in order to determine specific stressors and how the members of the couple are meeting their developmental tasks. For example, if they're contemplating having a baby, are they preparing for this both individually and as a couple? As the dyad shares specific details, I facilitate the construction of a genogram to organize information into a relational framework.

In the early individual sessions I try to determine the nature of each one's commitment to the marriage and whether either has any secrets that might interfere with the goals of treatment (such as an extramarital affair or drug abuse). The individual sessions also enable the therapist to discuss issues that might be explosive in the couple sessions or otherwise might be used as a weapon by one against the other at a later point. Moreover, distortions can be deconstructed in individual sessions, and this can result in a decrease of unconscious enactments with each other, thus facilitating the work in the couple's sessions.

In some cases the psychoanalytically informed therapist works with material in different configurations and from different perspectives. For example, I may work individually to help one partner understand the origins and/or defensive purpose a projective identification may serve. But then with the couple together, I may comment on the dyad's interaction, saying something like, "You don't have to feel worried (angry, upset, etc.). Your partner feels it enough for the two of you."

Case Example. When Sylvia called for an appointment, she sounded desperate. She said she was having serious problems with her husband of 38 years, and she needed "a sounding board." She was taking an antidepressant prescribed by her primary care physician, who had "highly recommended" her to me. I asked Sylvia whether she wanted to come in alone, or with her husband. She said she and her husband needed to come together since they recently had a big blow-up in which he had resorted to physical violence.

I made an appointment for Sylvia and Harry to come in as soon as possible, without speaking to Harry first (perhaps a mistake?). As might have been predicted, the day before the scheduled session, Sylvia called to say that Harry had refused to come. At this juncture, I instructed Sylvia to urge Harry to attend and to tell him that she'd be coming to therapy with or without him, because the situation had become unmanageable.

Sylvia came to the first session by herself. She was impeccably dressed and well-groomed, yet her face looked older than I had expected. She described a history of depression "for all 38 years of my married life." She had participated in individual and couple therapy three times before, and she had twice tried to commit suicide after major fights with her husband. She explained, "I was angry. I was tired of the disrespect. I felt like the maid." She continued, "He says it's all me, that I'm not well. He takes no responsibility for anything, and he's always critical. He manipulates and tries to control me, like I'm a bad child. It gets to the point that I say, 'Why me?' I let it build up until I can't stand it any more."

Together, we constructed a genogram to map the family dynamics. Sylvia explained that she had three adult children, all living on their own; two of them had been married and were now divorced with children of their own, and one was single. She enjoyed seeing her grandchildren, but every visit was filled with fights with Harry over how to handle them.

Sylvia had been a housewife throughout her adult life, and Harry had recently retired from his profession. After Sylvia's father-in-law passed away a few years ago, she took on the task of "looking in" on her elderly mother-in-law.

When left undirected, Sylvia reverted to complaining about Harry. I asked, "Since this has been going on for over 30 years, why seek therapy now (again)?" She answered, "Recently, things really got worse, and I moved out of the bedroom. I'm living downstairs, and Harry is furious. I've also stopped going out with him. I try to ignore him, but he provokes me until I get involved in screaming matches. My marriage has always been a battleground." I asked about Sylvia's role in the fights. She admitted, "I provoke him. I do know how to get his goat, but I didn't expect him to throw me across the room. I hit my shoulder against the wall, and I had a serious bruise. I went to see Dr. S for my shoulder. Then he told me about you. He said you could help us."

Once again I told Sylvia that it was important for Harry to come to the next session, and she said she'd try to get him to come in. I positively reframed her situation in the hope that she could be empowered to bring Harry in: "You've already taken some important steps toward making a change. You've moved out of the bedroom. You've decided not to take any more abuse, and you've come for help."

Within hours following Sylvia's session, Harry called. "I need to see you alone to tell you my side of the story. Sylvia is a liar. You have to give me a chance to defend myself." Having ascertained that Harry had spoken to Sylvia about his calling me, I set up an individual session with the stated plan that the following session would be for the couple together.

When Harry arrived, a totally different picture emerged. He was casually dressed in jeans, and he looked much younger than his 68 years. He began with "the latest incident," which had followed an extended vacation spent with their son and grandchildren, during which time there had been "nonstop fighting." "She reduces me to a lump of clay, and I'm feeling like I'm on the ground, praying that she'll stop. But she's relentless. She constantly interrupts me and criticizes everything I say. She won't stop at anything. She even brings my dead father into it." Harry continued, "My father was a violent person. He used to whip me. I'm not a violent person, but when we fight, I'm afraid I'm going to do something drastic to her or myself."

When asked, "What do you contribute to the situation?" Harry responded, "I know what I should and shouldn't do with her. I don't praise her. This is a way for me to get even with her. She had a privileged life. I grew up in a very poor family after the Depression. We moved around a lot, and I never had much. Sylvia is used to having everything." Harry continued, "I don't know where to turn. We've been to therapists before. It gets a little better, but [then it] only [lasts] for a short time before it goes back to what it was before." He ended the session saying, "I'm getting on in years, and I don't want to be alone for the rest of my life. At least I know her goods and bads."

At the first couple session Sylvia and Harry screamed accusations at each other. At one point Sylvia made provocative snide comments under her breath. This enraged Harry to the point that he jumped out of his seat, pointed his finger inches from Sylvia's face, and screamed, "You're not going to do this to me any more." This didn't stop Sylvia. At another point Sylvia screamed so loudly that she turned red and became physically ill. Watching and listening to this interaction was unnerving. After a short time I tried to defuse the enactment by using humor. I thanked the couple "for showing me how you really interact."

At this early point I needed to decide what type of therapy would best serve this couple's needs and to find a focus for treatment. Neither member of the couple was receptive to the idea of individual therapy, yet each partner desperately needed to be heard. I suggested that we implement a trial period of individual and conjoint sessions. We discussed how we might work together including the number of sessions per week and what ground rules would be established.

The couple needed to acknowledge early in the process that this would be difficult work, especially given the longevity of the problems and the ways in which their interactional style incited each of them to react to the other in a homeostatic circular pattern. I explained that "relationships are created by two people," that "neither one could continue this kind of behavior without the participation of the other," and that "at any point in the loop either one could effect a change."

In working with an explosive situation that can erupt at any moment, the therapist must take control. Thus, I set the following guidelines: First, this would not be a place where they could point fingers and blame each other; they each had to be willing to accept responsibility for their own participation in creating the problems in their relationship. Second, they were not here to rehash 30-plus years of missed opportunities and angers. It would take more than 30 years to do that, and they didn't have that kind of time. Third, when they looked at the other's behavior, they should confine themselves to considering such things as "Why do you think [the other person] did that?" and, "Why does it upset you so much?"

In the confrontational style of Sylvia and Harry, my using gentle persuasion or assuming a reflective psychoanalytic posture was virtually ignored by this couple. I found it necessary to be explicit about the part I would play, including establishing myself as an authority and avoiding being triangled into their destructive patterns of relating. Thus, countertransferentially, I experienced induced feelings of helplessness as well as identification with the aggressor. At times I felt like yelling or giving the couple a stern lecture, yet I knew it was important to convey an empathic position. I explained, "I know how much it hurts. And I know how tempted you are to want to retaliate, to get back at each other when you feel you've been hurt." This kind of *quid pro quo* is very common in symmetrical couples where each partner provokes and defends what he or she experiences as an attack by the other. At this early stage, I made trial interpretations to the couple, such as, "I can see how when she attacks you like that, it brings back the feelings you had as a young child of . . . " and, "I can understand that now as an adult you'd be feeling 'I won't take that anymore.' "

After only two individual and one couple session, I had learned a great deal about Sylvia, Harry, and their relationship. In addition to the long-standing duration of their problems together, there were also the specific stressors caused by their stage of life. As people move up in the developmental hierarchy (Walsh, 1989), roles must be rebalanced, and new adjustments must be made. Following his retirement, Harry was now spending more time at home, while Sylvia was more involved in caring for her elderly mother-in-law. Also, Sylvia and Harry's last child had been recently launched, and finally, grandparenthood had affected their relationship as did the divorces of two of their children.

In the following individual sessions, I learned that Sylvia and Harry had no secrets to divulge (i.e., they weren't involved in any extramarital affairs, weren't abusing drugs, and didn't have any hidden alliances with other family members, etc.). What they did feel was enormous rage toward one another, and both felt a sense of deprivation and disappointment in their lives together. They also both said that their fighting had taken a physical toll on them and that it had to stop, yet neither had any intention of leaving the marriage.

Phase 2: Setting Goals, Planning the Treatment, Building the Alliance, and Handling Confidentiality

In the second phase of treatment, the therapist and couple must agree to the terms of the work and to issues of confidentiality. Together we set specific, and achievable goals, geared to the couple's level of functioning upon entering treatment, such as, "We will work on changing the way you speak to each other," and "You will learn a new way to communicate your individual needs."

The combination of individual and joint sessions typically facilitates the work and enables goals to be reached in as short a time as possible. I plan no a priori number of sessions; instead I assume that the use of a specific focus and the degree of therapeutic intensity will shorten the process. As the treatment progresses, the patients and I determine the total number of sessions on an as-needed basis. The couple also agrees to carry out certain assigned tasks that will facilitate the treatment.

With this method, we can't expect profound penetration of deeply rooted characterological problems, even though each partner will get a chance to relate the present interaction to his or her own family of origin and intrapsychic conflicts. The important element is that, as each one has the opportunity to be heard without being interrupted or criticized, individual issues can recede, thus allowing the dyadic interaction to move to the foreground in the couple sessions. Donovan explains, "If the parallel between past and present can be meaningfully established and if the shards of repressed affects from both time zones can be pulled into consciousness, then each individual will need to project less and comply less with the projections of the partner" (1995, p. 613).

In some cases, it may be desirable to schedule individual sessions consecutively. In the case of Sylvia and Harry, the couple arrived together, and each partner waited while the other had a separate hour. This arrangement implicitly communicated their commitment to each other, their ability to trust the therapist, and their willingness to allow the partner to have needs met without feeling deprived, while knowing that he or she would also have a turn. On the other hand, if trust is undermined and issues of privacy and confidentiality move to the forefront, then this arrangement may not be in the couple's best interest.

Because the individuals are seen separately and together in this model, the therapist must be absolutely clear about "which hat is being worn" and "who is the patient" (Cohen, 1996). Maintaining an equidistant position with the individuals, knowing full well that the patient is the couple, is a juggling act for the therapist. Boundaries must be unambiguous. Each partner must come to trust that I have the interests of both at heart and that I'll respect and uphold confidentiality.

The individual sessions are always couple-oriented, and I examine any emerging theme in the context of its effect on the relationship. Also, any material brought up in either the individual or the couple sessions, and deemed relevant or important to the couple by either partner, can be used in another session. Since I often become the party through which information is passed, before I share anything (either in the joint or individual sessions), the partners must give informed consent. It's usually advantageous for the couple to communicate with each other directly, and I attempt to facilitate this in joint sessions. On the other hand, there may be times when full disclosure may not be beneficial (e.g., in relation to a long-past affair). If either partner has a specific reason for keeping something concealed, I would work on these issues individually.

It is, however, critical that the couple be honest in sharing their present feelings, especially in regard to their intentions in the marriage. In one case, for example, I learned in an early individual session that the husband had secretly been planning to leave his wife after the marriage of their last child. Since their last unmarried child was approaching a marriageable age, it was essential that he share his intention with his spouse. He reluctantly agreed. Although it was painful for the wife to hear this, the couple could now face reality, and in fact, they made a commitment to begin therapy to try to salvage their marriage, while their last child still remained at home.

If at any point in treatment the therapist believes a partner is being duplicitous, couple sessions should be discontinued, or the therapy can be seriously compromised (Gottlieb, 1995). For example, if one partner is secretly using drugs or an extramarital relationship to address needs outside the marriage, unless the individual is willing to commit to ending this behavior, it's dishonest to go through the motions of trying to save the marriage. Taking a position that the affair needs to be ended for the couple work to go forward is not based on a particular moral stance, but rather, it is a technical imperative.

I try to get a commitment of "serious intent" to take a moratorium on infidelity, at least long enough to give therapy a chance. While some therapists won't work with the couple at all, in these cases I take a middle-ground position. In the individual sessions I reintroduce the idea of commitment to the therapeutic process, and I encourage the acting-out partner to work on this in another treatment.

Case Example. After the initial period of assessment, the work with Sylvia and Harry became more focused. The initial goals of treatment with this nonpsychologically minded couple included gaining insight into their enmeshed relationship, diminishing their provocative behavior, and better communication. There had already been several failed attempts to get help, and unless we did something different, the outcome would be no better this time. I stated, "You have some important choices to make. You could continue the way things are, with no assurances that things might not escalate, or you could decide that life is too short to live this way and that you're willing to try once again to make things better." I also gave them time to decide whether they wanted to begin treatment.

Both partners were in great need of being heard and of having the opportunity to understand the multiple meanings of what was happening in their lives. I specified the format of the treatment: time-intensive in the beginning, with weekly couple and individual sessions totaling three sessions per week. We would modify this schedule if there were signs of a positive response to the treatment or if it became apparent that the format was not working. I clarified the rules of confidentiality with the couple, and the couple committed to giving the process a chance, since, as Harry put it, "It's our last hope."

In the third week of treatment, during a joint session, we constructed a timeline of the couple's life together, and we expanded their genograms to reconstruct relationships that had evolved within their extended families. It was particularly important to discuss the families within which each partner had grown up, giving each one a chance to share individual points of view and to confront distortions, projections, and defenses that were burdening the relationship. We also discussed problems in relation to illnesses, children and grandchildren, losses that each had experienced, and issues related to the couple's stage of life, particularly around retirement. For example, Sylvia said, "For over 20 years I took care of a house and children and loaded a dishwasher. Now all of a sudden Harry is home, and he thinks I don't know how to clean dishes."

In the context of the therapeutic holding environment, the couple began to understand the unconscious motivation for their perceptions, reactions, and behavior, and how their destructive interaction was experienced by each one as a narcissistic injury. Up until this point, each member of the couple had often observed, "You're acting just like my/ your father (mother, sister, etc.)." Yet now they began to understand not only that their past relationships were carried into the present, but how and why this occurred. For example, after Harry admitted that he indeed had been "getting back at Sylvia," he showed that he had benefited from a psychoanalytic perspective when he explained that he would have liked to do that with his father. In individual sessions with Harry, he could now see why he was attacking Sylvia, always feeling that he needed to defend himself, as if he were fighting for his life, as he did with his father. On the other hand, as Sylvia acknowledged that she continually found fault with Harry, she realized that she had not adequately mourned her idealized father and that she had been unconsciously resenting Harry. By our working on these issues in the individual and joint sessions, much of the fighting deescalated as the couple began reacting to each other more in the present.

Phase 3: Working Through and Core Technical Maneuvers

Once we clarify the major interactional conflicts (and these may be redefined as the treatment progresses), every incident, every fight, every complaint, and every intervention is related to its effect on the couple. An analogous process occurs in a psychoanalytically informed child therapy. In collateral sessions while parents are encouraged to discuss anything on their minds that they feel is relevant, the therapist continually relates their discussion to the child (Cohen, 1996). For example, if they describe an argument, the child therapist will respond by asking, "How do you think your child is affected by this?" The effectiveness of this position is corroborated in research by Binder, Strupp, and Henry (1995). Their findings suggest that factors most predictive of positive outcome in short-term dynamic therapy include, "precise formulation of a focal problem and consistently addressing clinical material relevant to the problem . . . " (p. 61).

In this third phase of working through, as in other phases, particular attention is paid to the meaning and significance of the couple's interactions, and I continue to teach relevant systemic and psychoanalytic concepts to facilitate the treatment. From a psychoanalytic perspective, the focus is on decoding the multiple meanings of the couple's unconscious behavior including, the defensive purpose and secondary gains of each partner's behavior, the workings of projective identifications, the compulsively driven repetitive processes, and the dynamics of transference enactments with the therapist, the partner or both. I construct tentative interpretations related to the couple's personal and relationship history, such as, "Your tendency to react to . . . in such and such a way . . . seems to be related to. . . . "

Some of my interpretive statements can be summarized in generic terms to convey the essence of a psychoanalytic perspective. They might include:

> "The way you're interacting with each other is influenced by the relationships from your childhood."
> "You're not as yet aware that many of the ways you interact with each other are influenced by your unconscious mind(s)."
> "Much of what you do is self-protective and defensive because you feel so threatened by (and vulnerable with) each other."
> "You're both getting something out of what you are doing together." (in regard to a secondary gain)
> "You somehow manage to get the other person to react in predictable ways." (referring to a projective identification)
> "You know that all of your interactions occur in repetitive feedback loops. You'll keep on responding to each other in the same old way, over and over, until something or someone changes."

Psychoanalytically informed insights are used to enable each partner to try new ways of interacting with the other. To accomplish this, the therapist concentrates on the relational process, not its content. Whether the couple talks about a fight in the car or who cleaned up after Thanksgiving dinner, the issue is *how* they fight or how they talk about their fight, not the subject itself. For example, Harry and Sylvia consistently failed to listen to each other's complete thoughts, probably in ways that they themselves were not heard as children. They often responded to each other nonverbally, by making faces or noises, a clue to the childhood antecedents of the behaviors. This in turn increased the other's anger at being "interrupted," who then screamed louder to get the point across. Thus ensued a recursive loop, "the more . . . , the more . . . . " The result frequently left one partner feeling devalued and worthless, while the other might be feeling enraged and alone.

It is often effective to reframe the context of an interaction so that a new perception of intent is established. Mistaken attributions of intent can result in negative reactions, yet when a situation is reframed, behavior can change accordingly. The same event may elicit different reactions depending on whether it is perceived to be "sick," "crazy," "stubborn," "accidental," or "well intentioned" (Carter, 1984 p. 9). In relation to

Harry and Sylvia, it was helpful to clarify (both individually and jointly), that even though they didn't consciously mean to be hurtful to each other, they did enjoy sadistically getting back at each other in ways they hadn't been allowed while growing up.

I use both individual and couple sessions to work on applying insights gained individually to improve communication patterns and facilitate empathic responses in the dyad. In general, I help each individual think about and bear painful feelings (such as worthlessness and/or alienation), so that each has the opportunity to experience therapeutic empathy and to see it modeled. As a real object in their lives, I provide a new experience for each of them that can increase awareness and understanding of their sad and lonely positions. They can then, in turn, be empathic with their partner.

Deconstructing each one's experience and complaints in the individual sessions prevents many arguments in the couple sessions, while the couple work provides a new opportunity for the dyad to hear each other and behave more supportively. During the phase of working through, the sessions can be spread over longer periods (Budman & Gurman, 1988), and the configuration of the individual and couple sessions can be altered to allow for more focused work with the couple as a unit. In addition, as the treatment proceeds, I redirect the focus in couple sessions, and we begin to work on the development of new skills that can, in turn, create new behaviors.

The therapist specifically works on the following:

1. *Tasks for additional, focused work for between and within the sessions.* In order to maximize the use of time, I actively involve the couple in creating tasks to ensure optimum motivation and follow-through (Budman & Gurman, 1988). For example, in the present case, it was important for each partner to verbalize the destructive impact of not being heard, constantly being interrupted, and not being understood. Following this acknowledgment, it was possible to create an assignment wherein both agreed that they would try at home not to speak until the other said, "I'm finished," or that person asked, "Are you finished?" Initially this mundane suggestion was dismissed as "elementary," but after some practice, it led to a total change in the tone and desperation of the screaming interchanges. Then, once having had the experience of completing a thought while being heard by the other, the partners were able to move to a new level of relating.

2. *Skills to enable the couple to improve communication.* In the case example, as each partner reported a complaint or talked about a fight, I continually reminded him or her to say, "I'm finished," or to ask "Are you done?" Also when they were unable to control their interrupt-

ing, we passed around a tissue box, without which no one, including the therapist, was permitted to speak!

3. *New behaviors, practicing and generalizing.* After the partners mastered allowing each other to finish a complete thought, they were ready to learn specific communication skills, such as "active listening" and "I-messages" (Gordon, 1970). First, each person practiced clarifying what was being said by the other, such as, "What I hear you saying is. . . . Is that right?"; or "You seem to be feeling. . . . " Next they practiced expressing their own feelings and beliefs, such as, "I like [don't like] it when you . . . because it makes me feel. . . . " At that point we created specific exercises for the couple to work on at home, to consolidate the partners' gains and to reinforce their newly acquired communication skills.

In the third phase of therapy, as the couple accomplishes different tasks, I continually highlight the newly acquired strengths of the individuals and the couple (see Friedman & Lipchik, Chapter 13, this volume). The partners can then gain a new appreciation of each other as concerned, mutually suffering individuals who are definitely committed to improving their relationship and who are indeed making progress.

The working-through phase of treatment continues long past the time when the actual therapy sessions take place. As Budman and Gurman explain: "It may be that under some circumstances the therapist may plant the seeds of change, which then lie dormant until developmental or life-change factors 'trigger' the patient [couple] to take some steps toward growth" (1988, p. 300). In summary, during the working-through phase of treatment, the therapist offers the couple the opportunity, both in and out of the sessions, to continue to practice new ways of behaving that may facilitate additional new ways of responding to each other.

Case Example. In the third month of treatment, Sylvia and Harry entered the working-through phase. Although they continued to accuse each other, they did so less frequently and with an awareness that this was destructive to the relationship. They were beginning to internalize the concept that each one had played a role in creating their problems.

During one couple session I constructed a list: "What I Contribute to Making the Relationship What It Is," with a separate column for each of them. This list enabled Sylvia and Harry to take partial ownership and responsibility for their problems. Sylvia listed such things as, "I won't give in," "I interrupt and contradict Harry to get his goat," and "I don't know how to talk to him." Harry offered "I'm always looking to get even, to find fault, to be critical of her," "If Sylvia turned her back, I'd attack," and "I'm too quick to react when I think I've been wronged." I kept the list and later in the treatment referred back to it.

Although each brought his or her own agendas to every session, I continually pointed out that the patterns of these fights were always the same. Neither would let the other finish; each screamed louder and louder; and each appeared to be fighting a far more important battle than the one at hand. Psychoanalytically speaking, they were fighting decades-old unfinished wars with their parents in their present relationship. Harry reacted to Sylvia as if she were his critical, controlling father. As a result, he constantly had to defend himself against her. Similarly, Sylvia repeatedly compared her marriage to an idealized image of her dead father's relationship with her mother. Each time Harry failed to live up to the image, she became disappointed and critical of him. Interpretations like these helped the couple to make sense of their personal struggle. They also provided a focus for the individual sessions in which each one could work through some of his or her personal unresolved past conflicts that had been transferred onto their current relationship.

In an effort to build on the couple's strengths, I asked them to reconstruct the early days of their relationship. Both Sylvia and Harry recalled the very difficult times that each had lived through as the children of immigrant parents. Sylvia said, "I may have chosen him for the wrong reasons, but I loved him, and I still do. He was older, more mature. I didn't want a man who would act like a kid." Harry responded, "You were so young and beautiful. I just wanted to take care of you." I tried to seize every opportunity to help the couple bond and reinforce their positive feelings toward each other. Their reminiscences were reframed into such statements as "How wonderful that you were both able to get what you wanted; you, Harry got yourself a beautiful wife to provide for, and you, Sylvia, a strong man who had his own mind!"

In the individual sessions, each partner had a chance to explore some of the underlying, intrapsychic determinants of his or her own and of the other's behavior while being heard without interruption. These sessions provided the new experience of a nonjudgmental, nonintrusive environment. No matter how much Sylvia and Harry's interactions elicited all kinds of defenses to regulate closeness, they always reacted to each other out of a combination of neediness, rage, fear of abandonment, and the need to control each other.

It was also possible to discuss the prevalent distortions of intent in the individual sessions. For example, in one session Sylvia talked about how they had attended a driving class to lower their car insurance premium. She reported that Harry had said, "Let me fill out the form for you." Sylvia had experienced this as another example of Harry usurping her power and making her feel inadequate. She had never considered the notion that Harry's offer might have been an attempt to actually help her. In an individual session with Harry I asked him why he had offered to fill out her form. He responded, "She had just had a fresh manicure, and I knew she didn't want to smear her nail polish." This was typical of how the couple attributed bad intentions to each other. In the couple's session when we deconstructed the problem, it emerged that each was still afraid of injury by the other. When Harry said, "I never tried to hurt Sylvia!" it was a good opportunity to bring out the list of "What I Contribute to Making the Relationship What It Is" from an earlier session. When I showed Harry his list, he was then able to say, "Oh yes. I forgot. I'm sorry I used to treat you like that. I really didn't mean it."

While the individual sessions were still used to deescalate conflicts by deconstructing distorted attributions, the couple sessions were used to clarify well-meant intentions. In an individual session Harry talked about Sylvia having sent a cleaning person to service his van, "to humiliate me and to relieve her own guilt for not cleaning it out herself." In the couple session, this would have previously triggered a defensive battle; however, when Sylvia was asked about it in an individual session, she said she had felt badly about him driving around in a dirty car and had wanted to give him a nice surprise! The tendency of this couple to misperceive each other's intentions or to attribute a bad intent was profound, and I continually pointed it out.

In the working-through phase of the treatment, the focus was on helping Harry and Sylvia learn and practice a new mode of relating. First, they needed to listen to each other without interrupting. Next, they needed to hear the feelings of the other and to state their own individual needs in a direct way so that their partner could have the opportunity to respond in a more productive manner. As the treatment progressed, each one became more aware of the underlying significance of their interaction.

During the 4th month of treatment, in one couple session, Harry said, "What Sylvia thinks are my needs and what I think my needs are aren't the same. I know that she goes out of her way to please me, but she misses." To this Sylvia responded, "Sometimes I think I have to treat him like a stranger. He takes what I say as a knife that I'm turning inside him." This exchange provided a here-and-now example of their common problems: miscommunication, misattribution, failing to express their own needs, and failing to listen or be responsive to each other.

In order to help Sylvia and Harry become more competent in their basic interpersonal skills, I asked them to talk about what each wanted from the other. Next, I encouraged them to paraphrase what they were hearing, and I helped them work out ways they could fill each other's needs. Finally, I continued to encourage them to practice their new way of communicating.

In another couple session, Sylvia reported that Harry had gotten angry at her for not telling him that she was going to a charity luncheon with her mother and then for going without him. Sylvia said she thought she had announced her plan to attend the event in advance. "If he wanted to attend, he should have told me." She felt she had done her part and that he had "no right" to be angry at her "for nothing." Both felt misunderstood. Harry explained that he would have liked Sylvia to have *wanted* him to accompany her, and she responded, "He never wants to go anywhere with me. I always have to make plans by myself." Tearfully she added, "I'm so lonely and sad all the time." Her tears elicited an empathic response from Harry, who explained, "Yes, it's true that I was never interested in going to these functions in the past, but now I'm not working. I'm home, and I'm lonely too. And I feel that you don't want to be with me" (a "softening"; see Johnson, Chapter 2, this volume).

While working on differentiation, dependency, and defensiveness, the members of this couple were also learning how to communicate their needs in an empathic atmosphere in which both would be appreciated for what they had consciously intended. At the same time, the focus was consistently redirected from blame of the other to self-initiative. For example, Harry began to change from, "If she knows it sets me off, why does she do it?" to "I'm too quick to react when I feel wronged," or "I guess I have to work on changing my behavior, and then maybe she'll change" (a dramatic shift in responsibility and focus).

When Sylvia moved back into the bedroom, the couple resumed having sexual relations and even began to laugh together once in a while. The quality of their lives was changing, and I suggested that they work on enhancing their relationship. The couple felt they could do this by showing more affection, and by making an effort to ask for things that they wanted from each other. As Sylvia and Harry's relationship improved, they were ready to suspend the two weekly individual sessions. Also, we reduced the one couple session per week to every 2 to 3 weeks, to allow the couple time to integrate and practice their new behaviors.

Phase 4: Termination and Follow-Up

The termination phase of therapy often begins when the couple asks the therapist, "How much longer?" or "Do you think we could ever do this on our own?" This phase of treatment requires the collaboration of both partners with the therapist. As a group, we evaluate the therapy to date, including its current status and future focus. Together we review our original goals to determine whether and how they've been met, which ones may still need additional work, and which may require the couple to come back to resume treatment at a future time (Lebow, 1995). The method that began with the members of the couple needing individual sessions in order to be heard and understood is now primarily focused on couple work together. In this ending phase of treatment, the partners have internalized a number of new skills, and both realize they will now have the opportunity to practice and consolidate gains on their own. In the event that the couple treatment has not been successful, other methods of therapy can be recommended.

The method of psychoanalytically informed, short-term couple therapy is based on the primary care model of medicine in which the partners know they may seek additional help at any future time. Budman and Gurman explain that "many patients return for multiple courses of mental health treatment over the span of their lives" (1988, p. 288). During the last session, we make arrangements for a follow-up session. I may also suggest that the couple continue to work on their relationship during the hour that had previously been reserved for the therapy, only now without the presence of a therapist.

There are many differences of opinion as to whether a therapist should continue to preserve his or her position as the couple's therapist after terminating their couple treatment. Some believe that, at termination, boundaries can be crossed and that either partner can be taken on as an individual patient. I disagree. If the therapist is to remain available to the couple for any future work, he or she must remain in a neutral position. In the event that either of the partners should need additional treatment, I believe that the therapist should refer them to separate "individual" therapists.

Case Example. After 6 months of treatment, Sylvia and Harry had shown significant improvement, and we had already phased-out the regularly scheduled individual sessions and increased the time between the couple sessions. They were now showing affection to each other and were beginning to speak about each other in more positive terms. Harry acknowledged, "She's been more thoughtful and holds a grudge less of the time," and Sylvia said, "He's been controlling his anger better, and he doesn't criticize me all the time any more." The couple also reported that things were going better in many other areas. For example, they were communicating better with their children and grandchildren, and they were not embarrassing each other as much while socializing with other couples.

In the termination phase of treatment, we reviewed our previously set goals and acknowledged that we had accomplished a great deal in a relatively short course of therapy. After 38 years of marriage, Sylvia and Harry were beginning a new relationship, and they needed time to practice being with each other in a more supportive way. The tone of their relating had indeed changed.

In the individual sessions, both Harry and Sylvia discussed some of their fears, based not only on their relationship history, but also going back to their families of origin. They both shared how devastated they had felt to have had their intentions misunderstood, so devastated as to have engendered all kinds of defensive behavior.

In the couple sessions we reviewed many of the psychoanalytic insights they had gained. I reiterated some of the basic principles upon which the treatment was based: (1) that both members of the couple had participated in creating their toxic relationship; (2) that both had contributed to a more positive way of relating as they practiced communicating more directly with each other; and (3) that although their behavior patterns had been established many years before, many of their interactions were based on unconscious processes. Through their commitment to each other and to the therapy, they were able to improve the quality of their lives.

When this couple initially came to therapy, their relationship had become so hateful that for many years they hadn't been able to experience any of the joys of being heard, supported, or loved. They had achieved a negative mode of carrying out the tasks of their individual lives as adults, parents, and grandparents, and had long ago given up any hope for achieving intimacy. Perhaps it was a response to the stressors of the retirement stage of life that had brought them to the desperate point at which they were motivated for treatment: Their last child had been launched, Harry had retired and was spending more time at home, and both partners were burdened with the tasks of aging. As the couple's relationship improved and the fighting between them lessened, Sylvia turned more toward Harry, but he, in turn, pulled back and became depressed. At that time, I spoke with Harry about the possibility of his needing a referral for further treatment (either individual psychotherapy or a psychiatric evaluation for medication). He said he'd think about it.

Perhaps if this couple had married in the 1990s, they wouldn't have stayed together for over 30 years. However, they did reach out for help in a desperate state, and although some tough and intense measures were needed to change their deeply entrenched habits, after 7 months of individual and couple sessions, they were ready to practice more positive ways of being with each other, on their own.

We planned a follow-up session for 3 months after the last session, and Harry said he'd consider a psychiatric consultation for himself "if things got worse." When Sylvia and Harry came in for the follow-up, they reported that there were still many problems between them but that things were definitely greatly improved. They were in the midst of planning a child's wedding, and they weren't fighting as much. Harry also said he felt he was "handling" his depression. At that point, I suggested that they might come back to therapy at any time when they would be interested in doing additional work on as yet unresolved problems as well as on enhancing their relationship.

CONCLUSION

In these unstable times, when many people hope for a "quick fix," we often find ourselves in the position of having to treat patients in as short a time as possible, whether for economic reasons or because the lack of quick results would have an immediate negative impact on one or more members of the family or couple. In addition, when people present themselves as failures at one or more attempts to seek help, it behooves us to search for new ways to make a second-order difference as quickly as possible.

Although psychoanalysis and family therapy are based on different assumptions with different ideas about how best to intervene, when the therapist is informed by psychoanalytic and systemic theory, both lenses can be used to view family members as individuals and the couple as a system. In combining approaches and techniques, including using time flexibly, the therapist must "be firmly rooted in a dual theoretical perspective that renders that combination coherent and meaningful" (Melito, 1988, p. 42).

As a couple, Harry and Sylvia were desperate. Their violent and sadistic behavior toward each other had been escalating, and they were possibly facing divorce—for which neither one was emotionally or otherwise ready. Their desire to avoid a final rift as well as their sense of desperation may have contributed to the success of the treatment. The separate individual sessions in addition to conjoint meetings helped to shorten the actual elapsed time of the therapy. This format provided a setting in which the partners could carry out some greatly needed work in as few sessions as possible. By focusing the treatment and by using techniques of psychoanalytic and systemic therapy, the couple benefited significantly within 7 months time.

Gerson (1996) calls for the maintenance of a permeable boundary between psychoanalysis and couple therapy while keeping in mind the need to respect the parameters of both modalities. In this chapter, I frame the treatment as "psychoanalytically informed" rather than "psychoanalytic" because it involves many technical modifications that deviate from a traditional open-ended psychoanalytic position. These shifts toward a more active and directive therapeutic stance are necessary when an approach is short-term and are useful with couples in general, since couples often enter in crisis and are looking for tangible results in specific areas of distress. In a psychoanalytically informed, short-term couple therapy, the individuals in the couple have the opportunity for personal exploration while the dyad can simultaneously revitalize its relationship.

ACKNOWLEDGMENTS

I would like to thank Drs. Mary Joan Gerson, Jonathan Lampert, Susan Shimmerlik, and especially Dr. Virginia Goldner, each of whom read and commented on earlier drafts of this chapter.

REFERENCES

Aron, L. (1990). One person and two person psychologies and the method psychoanalysis. *Psychoanalytic Psychology, 7,* 475–485.

Aron, L. (1991). The patient's experience of the analyst's subjectivity. *Psychoanalytic Dialogues, 1,* 29–51.

Bateson, G. (1972). *Steps to an ecology of mind.* New York: Ballantine Books.

Binder, J., Strupp, H., & Henry, W. (1995). Psychodynamic therapies in practice: Time-limited dynamic psychotherapy. In B. Bonger & L. Beutler (Eds.), *Comprehensive textbook of psychotherapy theory and practice* (pp. 48–63). New York: Oxford University Press.

Bowen, M. (1978). *Family therapy in clinical practice.* New York: Jason Aronson.

Braverman, S., Hoffman, L., & Szkrumelak, N. (1984). Concomitant use of strategic and individual therapy in treating a family. *American Journal of Family Therapy, 12,* 29–38.

Budman, S. H., & Gurman, A. S. (1988). *Theory and practice of brief therapy.* New York: Guilford Press.

Carter, B., & McGoldrick, M. (Eds.). (1989). *The changing family life cycle: A framework for family therapy* (2nd ed.). Boston: Allyn & Bacon.

Carter, E. (1984). *Family therapy: The innocent looking revolution.* Unpublished manuscript from a paper presented at Hunter College, City University of New York, Family Institute of Westchester.

Cohen, P. (1996) *Wearing two hats: On being a psychoanalyst and a family therapist.* Paper presented at the New York University Postdoctoral Program, Project in Psychoanalysis and Family Therapy, New York, NY.

Donovan, J. (1995). Short-term couples group psychotherapy: A tale of four fights. *Psychotherapy, 32,* 608–617.

Erikson, E. (1963). *Childhood and society.* New York: Norton.

Erikson, E. (1982). *The life cycle completed: A review.* New York: Norton.

Fairbairn, W. R. D. (1952). *Psychoanalytic studies of the personality.* London: Routledge & Kegan Paul.

Gerson, M. J. (1996). *The embedded self: A psychoanalytic guide to family therapy.* Hillsdale, NJ: Analytic Press.

Ghent, E. (1989). Credo: The dialectics of one-person and two-person psychologies. *Contemporary Psychoanalysis, 25,* 169–211.

Gill, M. (1992). *Current trends in psychoanalysis.* Heinz Hartmann Award Lecture presented at the New York Psychoanalytic Institute, New York, NY.

Gill, M. (1993). Interaction and interpretation. *Psychoanalytic Dialogues, 3,* 111–122.

Gill, M. (1994). *Psychoanalysis in transition.* Hillsdale, NJ: Analytic Press.

Goldenberg, I., & Goldenberg, H. (1996). *Family therapy: An overview.* Pacific Grove, CA: Brooks/Cole.

Gordon, T. (1970). *P.E.T.: Parent Effectiveness Training.* New York: Wyden Books.

Gottlieb, M. (1995). Ethical dilemmas in change of format and live supervision. In R. Mikesell, D. D. Lusterman, & S. McDaniel (Eds.), *Integrating family therapy: Handbook of family psychology and systems theory* (pp. 561–569). Washington, DC: American Psychological Association.

Greenson, R. R. (1967). *The theory and technique of psychoanalysis.* New York: International Universities Press.

Hoffman, I. (1983). The patient as interpreter of the analyst's experience. *Contemporary Psychoanalysis, 19,* 389–422.

Jackson, D. (1965a). Family rules: Marital quid pro quo. *Archives of General Psychiatry, 12,* 589–594.

Jackson, D. (1965b). The study of the family. *Family Process, 4,* 1–20.

Kohut, H. (1984). *How does analysis cure?* New York: International Universities Press.

Lebow, J. (1995). Open-ended therapy: Termination in marital and family therapy. In R. Mikesell, D. D. Lusterman, & S. McDaniel (Eds.), *Integrating family therapy: Handbook of family psychology and systems theory* (pp. 73–86). Washington, DC: American Psychological Association.

Livingston, M. (1995). A self psychologist in couplesland: Multisubjective approach to transference and countertransference-like phenomena in marital relationships. *Family Process, 34,* 427–439.

Maltas, C. (1996). *Concurrent therapies when therapists don't concur.* Unpublished manuscript, Harvard University Medical School, Cambridge, MA.

McGoldrick, M., & Gerson, R. (1985). *Genograms in family assessment.* New York: Norton.

Melito, R. (1988). Combining individual psychoadynamics with structural family therapy. *Journal of Marital and Family Therapy, 14,* 29–43.

Minuchin, S. (1974). *Families and family therapy.* Cambridge, MA: Harvard University Press.

Minuchin, S., & Fishman, H. C. (1981) *Techniques of family therapy.* Cambridge, MA: Harvard University Press.

Mitchell, S., & Greenberg, J. (1983). *Object relations in psychoanalytic therapy.* Cambridge, MA: Harvard University Press.

Nichols, M. (1987). *The self in the system.* New York: Brunner/Mazel.

Nichols, M., & Schwartz, R. (1995). *Family therapy: Concepts and methods* (3rd ed.). Needham Heights, MA: Allyn & Bacon.

Nichols, M., & Schwartz, R. (1998). *Family therapy: Concepts and methods* (4th ed.). Needham Heights, MA: Allyn & Bacon.

O'Brian, C., & Bruggen, P. (1985). Our personal and professional lives: Learning positive connotation and circular questioning. *Family Process, 24,* 311–322.

Reber, A. (1985). *The Penguin dictionary of psychology.* London: Penguin Books.

Sander, F. (1979). *Individual and family therapy: Toward an integration.* New York: Jason Aronson.

Sander, F. (1989). Marital conflict and psychoanalytic therapy in the middle years. In J. Oldham & R. Liebert (Eds.), *The middle years: New psychoanalytic perspectives* (pp. 160–176). New Haven, CT: Yale University Press.

Sander, F. (1997, September 30). Unpublished response to Dr. Pyles, "Psychoanalysis at the crossroads," New York Psychoanalytic Society, New York, NY.

Schafer, R. (1983). *The analytic attitude.* New York: Basic Books.

Schafer, R. (1992). *Retelling a life.* New York: Basic Books.

Scharff, D., & Scharff, J. (1991). *Object relations couples therapy.* Northvale, NJ: Jason Aronson.

Selvini Palazzoli, M., Boscolo, L., Cecchin, G., & Prata, G. (1978). *Paradox and counter-paradox.* New York: Jason Aronson.

Siegert, M. (1990). Reconstruction, construction, or deconstruction: Perspectives on the limits of psychoanalytic knowledge. *Contemporary Psychoanalysis, 26,* 160–170.

Silverman, D. (1994). From philosophy to poetry: Changes in psychoanalytic discourse. *Psychoanalytic Dialogues, 4*(1), 101–128.

Spence, D. P. (1982). *Narrative truth and historical truth.* New York: Norton.

Wachtel, E. (1982). The family psyche over three generations: The genogram revisited. *Journal of Marital and Family Therapy, 8,* 335–343.

Walsh, F. (1989). The family in later life. In B. Carter & M. McGoldrick (Eds.), *The changing family life cycle: A framework for family therapy* (2nd ed., pp. 312–332). Needham Heights, MA: Allyn & Bacon.

Watzlawick, P., Weakland, J., & Fisch, R. (1974). *Change: Principles of problem formation and problem resolution.* New York: Norton.

Winnicott, D. W. (1971). *Playing and reality.* New York: Tavistock.

Winnicott, D. W. (1975). *Through pediatrics to psychoanalysis.* New York: Basic Books.

8

-◄O►-

TIME-EFFECTIVE
COUPLE THERAPY

SIMON H. BUDMAN

Time-effective couple therapy (TECT) has a seemingly simple goal: to help two people who are behaving in a particular way with one another act differently. The simplicity of this is, of course, illusory. Partners who have maintained a characteristic pattern of relating over years are likely to have fixed and almost immutable interactions. These couples may feel unable to modify their interactions, unwilling to attempt modifications, or unaware of changes that would contribute to improvements in their interactions.

The approach described here comes out of my work over the past 25 years with hundreds of couples and families. My approach is not doctrinaire but, rather, reflects a practical integration of psychoanalytic, behavioral, solution-oriented, and cognitive approaches. In this chapter, I review some of the central aspects of this model and describe ways to evaluate couples for treatment, plan therapy, clarify core problems to be addressed, and discuss the overall stance of the therapist and issues about ending the treatment. Material from a couple whom I call Lisa and Bob will serve to illustrate these concepts.

THE TIME-EFFECTIVE
COUPLE THERAPY MODEL

There are a variety of ways to understand the interaction between partners in a couple relationship. Psychoanalytically oriented couple theorists have assumed that most aspects of couple relationships are based upon transferential issues dating to the early development of the partners. Behaviorists (Jacobson, 1981) view couple issues as related to problems in behavioral reciprocity. Cognitive-behavioral therapists see couples as having cognitive misconstructions about one another (Baucom, Epstein, & Carels, 1992).

TECT draws on a variety of different ideas in the marital treatment area. Since I have always been interested in basing my ideas about therapy on empirical research (Budman & Gurman, 1988) I have tried to draw on the existent data in conceptualizing TECT. Two sets of such interesting and compelling data come from the work of Gottman and his colleagues (Gottman, 1993, 1994; Gottman & Krokoff, 1989) and of Wallerstein (1994, 1996). I lean heavily on their findings in this description of TECT. Both researchers, although working from very different perspectives and with different client populations, offer the therapist valuable concepts in considering how to help couples change.

CENTRAL TASKS OF MARRIAGE

In a series of recent articles, Wallerstein (1994, 1996) focused on the central tasks of marriage. Her data came from longitudinal interviews with 50 urban, middle-class couples who viewed themselves as happily married. Wallerstein described a number of tasks that her study found as centrally relevant in the early years of marriage and then again as the marriage progresses. These tasks include the following:

- Consolidating separation (from family of origin) and establishing a new connection
- Building marital identity: togetherness versus autonomy
- Establishing the sexual life of the couple
- Establishing the marriage as a zone of safety and nurturance
- Expanding the marital relationship to make psychological room for children, while maintaining the intimacy of the marriage
- Building a relationship that is fun and interesting
- The capacity and willingness of each partner to maintain a vision of the other that combines early idealization and present realities

The three most important of these tasks, according to Wallerstein, are maintaining a good sex life, building a safe environment for anger and conflict, and holding a realistic and romantic view of the spouse over the years.

Wallerstein's tasks present a frame of reference for the marital therapist to use when trying to clarify the issues or concerns in a given marriage. I have also found consideration of these tasks helpful when evaluating a new couple. For each of these areas, a few questions can elucidate how the couple is functioning. ("How does each of you relate to your family of origin?" "How do your parents relate to you and your spouse as a couple?" "How is your sexual relationship?" "Do you feel you can talk about the things that you need to in the marriage?") Getting a sense of some or all of these factors is invaluable when considering the treatment plan. The therapist needs to have a clear sense of the specific problem with which the couple is presenting, as well as a broader contextual sense of how this problem or problems fits in with other aspects of their interactions and who they are as individuals, that is, what each brings to the relationship.

One of Wallerstein's most fascinating findings was that many of the partners in happily married couples come from difficult and troubled families. The data did not support the common belief that, in order to establish a solid, stable marriage, one needs to come from a secure and stable family. In Wallerstein's sample, this was true only approximately half the time; many of the people she interviewed came from backgrounds they described as greatly troubled. Some had been severely traumatized as children, coming from families where there was sexual abuse, abandonment, alcoholism, drug use, and severe mental illness. The optimistic message is that when troubled couples arrive for treatment and report horrendous family backgrounds, the therapist need not make the assumption of a poor outcome. It is clear that people from the worst of childhoods can overcome their upbringing and form stable, loving, sustained relationships.

CENTRAL CONCEPTS OF TIME-EFFECTIVE COUPLE THERAPY

The central idea in TECT is that the troubled couple, for whatever reasons, have "locked in" to a particular way of dealing with one another. A concept from both chaos and complexity theories (Arthur, 1990; Briggs & Peat, 1989), "lock in" basically means that systems often tend to become "hardened" into certain patterns or structures. These patterns may or may not be maximally beneficial to the organism or system. It is also possible that a particular lock in has worked well in the past but is no longer functional. Gottman's work (1993, 1994) indicates that most couples, troubled or not, tend to form certain fixed patterns of interaction. Couples whose patterns are functional and satisfying and who tend to do well with one another over time are "stable couples;" couples with tenuous, unsatisfying, and troubled patterns he calls "unstable couples." For most couples, their patterns of interaction are probably a complex product of the histories of each of the partners, the partners' personalities, emotional and physical vulnerabilities and styles of interaction, the history of the marriage, and the current environment. It is unlikely that one or another of these factors would be the only component of the couple's interactional style. It is important that the couple therapist think broadly and flexibly and not make the assumption that any one of these factors represents the only relevant variable to be assessed or addressed. Since lock in is such a key concept in TECT, the therapist must always be thinking of strategies to help the couple make even the most minimal changes leading to a modified style of interaction. There are a variety of ways in which this can be done, and strategies applied to "unlocking" the couple's fixed interactions vary.

ASSESSMENT

First we consider how to assess the couple for treatment.

Level of Motivation for Change

The first question to be assessed in working with a couple is determining whether the individuals are motivated to make changes in their ways of interacting with one another. The model that I use in understanding each partner's motivation is the Prochaska Stages of Change Model (Prochaska, Norcross, & DiClemente, 1994; Prochaska & DiClemente, 1986). Although originally developed to examine how smokers went about the process of stopping nicotine use, it has been applied to many different life-change processes and appears to be a useful generic model.

The model can be viewed as follows: Although the pattern shown in Figure 8.1 is the most likely course of change, a couple may begin the process of change at any point and move to any other point on the model. An individual may make a particular type of change by moving from any given point on the change process to any other point on the model. The process shown in the graphic, however, is the most likely course of change. Once someone begins a particular course of change, that person may have "slips" and move back and forth between the stages until he or she is able to achieve the desired change. The individual may also "get stuck" in a particular stage. My discussion shows examples of these various stages from couple treatment. Each partner

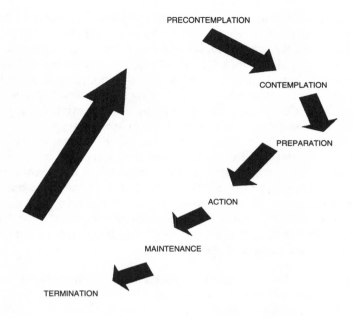

FIGURE 8.1. Prochaska and DiClemente change model.

may be in a different place on the change process; this disparity in motivation is quite common in those coming for couple treatment.

The steps along the change process are considered below.

Precontemplation

In Prochaska's model, an individual in this stage has little motivation to make changes in a given area. The precontemplative alcoholic individual has no interest in stopping drinking and views his or her drinking as nonproblematic. If someone is coming to couple treatment in precontemplation regarding possibilities for change in the marriage, he or she is often doing so because they are being pressured by the spouse. The precontemplative ("dragged in") spouse either does not see a problem, feels that the other partner is "making a mountain out of molehill," or feels that the marriage is beyond repair and cannot be changed. (There is relatively little likelihood that a couple would come for couple therapy if both were in precontemplation. By definition such a couple would be without motivation to change or get treatment. The only circumstance under which such an unmotivated couple would appear for therapy together might be if ordered to do so by the courts.)

I have seen the precontemplative partner "pushing" for couple therapy when he or she is looking for the opportunity to make "one last try" to work things out (all the while actually intending to leave his or her spouse); in this case, the "last try" is for public consumption. In the future, when talking about the dissolution of the marriage, the partner can say, "I'm no quitter. I tried everything to keep us together and nothing worked." Or, "The couple therapist did us no good. She wasn't skilled enough and that led to the end of our marriage." In other cases, a precontemplator might come in to deposit his or her soon-to-be ex-spouse in the hands of a good therapist. "I have to leave her, but she is so depressed and vulnerable that I want her to be getting professional help, which will allow me to feel less guilty about going." The greatest likelihood, however, is that the unmotivated spouse will be very reluctant to engage in couple therapy.

Assessment Implications. It is useful to be clear about a precontemplator's motivation. If he or she has minimal interest in change, this should be recognized as soon as possible. By achieving this clarity, extended periods of time will not be wasted working with a spouse who has "*both* feet out the door." In cases where one spouse is not interested or willing to make changes in the marriage, the therapist should generally move in the direction of individual therapy with the other spouse. Sometimes the motivated spouse becomes convinced that the marriage or relationship will not work if only one person is interested in its survival. The treatment then becomes focused on the process of separation. When the couple therapist is dealing with a "closet" precontemplator, the therapist may quickly sense that the relationship is "hanging by a thread." In addition, the precontemplator is generally *not* eager to work on any issues at all, despite protestations to the contrary. In many of these situations, there is ongoing infidelity or a long-term, hidden affair on the part of the spouse in precontemplation. If the seemingly unmotivated spouse does appear to have some even minimal interest in change, however, he or she can be treated like the contemplators below.

Intervention Implications. In general, the task with precontemplators is to get them to stay in the treatment if they have even some *minimal* willingness to pursue therapy or to clarify that they really don't want to pursue the treatment and are there because of pressure or social desirability. For the relatively unmotivated individuals or couples who are not attending the treatment for ulterior reasons, it is often useful to provide the partners with information regarding couple therapy. For example, "It may be three or four sessions before you see how this treatment can be beneficial." "This therapy will be helpful by assisting the two of you in beginning to talk with one another and listen better to what each has to say." "You can best facilitate the treatment by carrying certain elements of what we are talking about outside of the sessions," and so on.

Contemplation

This stage of change is characterized by ambivalence. The partner or partners who are contemplative "can't live with her/him and can't live without her/him." The majority of couples coming into treatment are in contemplation. They care about one another, but they are hurt, angry, resentful, and isolated. In part, they would like to work out their difficulties; at the same time they may feel that "too much damage has been done," or "this is too little too late," or "we have a love–hate relationship." As was true with precontemplation, it is often the case that the partners are in different places regarding their stage of change. The husband, for example, may be in early contemplation regarding the problem and the wife in preparation, as seen in the following example.

JIM: *She* seems to think that we have a problem in our marriage.

THERAPIST: Do you see a problem?

JIM: Only that she has a problem with it.

MELINDA: I don't even know if I want this anymore. Sometimes I do and sometimes I don't, but he is so dense he's out of touch with reality. I really want things to get better and for us to have a normal marriage. The only time he even talks to me is when he wants to have sex.

JIM: That's just not true. Tell the doctor what really goes on. I try to talk with you and you ignore me.

MELINDA: Of course I ignore you. You're only interested in the things you like. You don't pay any attention to the kids or the house or anything but your work and that damn boat of yours. I'd give anything for you to be interested in Brad's report card or Louie's soccer or my work.

Assessment Implications. Contemplation among couples coming for therapy is ubiquitous. The uncertainty and ambivalence indicate that there is something to work with. The positive side of the ambivalence can be explored and built upon. ("What are the things that you love or care about in your spouse?" "Your ambivalence says to me that there was a time that things were better in the relationship. Are there some things about that time that you still recall? What were they?") In addition, the therapist will be working with the couple to reduce those negatives that inhibit the relationship and lead to uncertainty. The task with couples where one or both partners are in contemplation is to help them move to preparation.

Intervention Implications. The couple or partner in contemplation is dealing with mixed feeling about the marriage. It is useful to be able to explore both sides of the ambivalence and to help the partners remember the more positive aspects of their relationship that may be "forgotten" in the midst of their conflicts with one another.

Preparation

In preparation the partner or partners are committed to the change process in their marriage, are minimally ambivalent, but have not really begun to make attempts at changing their interaction. One or both are clear that there is a problem and that things need to change. The couple in preparation is eager to get expert input from the clinician about what to do in order to "get things going" between them.

Assessment Implications. Couples with one or both partners in preparation are often well motivated for therapy and eager to work with the clinician. Such couples will want strategies that they can practice at home, books and articles to read, movies to watch, and so on. The passive, silent couple therapist approach is anathema to such a couple.

Intervention Implications. For couples in preparation and action, it is important that the therapist be *active enough*.

Action

Individuals or couples in action have often been trying to make changes on their own or have sought help from other treaters. They are very eager to make improvements and to try new strategies to better their marriage.

Assessment Implications. Although such couples seek treatment, they are relatively easy treatment candidates. Minimal input on the part of the therapist will often go a long way toward helping them progress dramatically. These couples may initially "look worse than they are." A crisis or painful betrayal may have adversely impacted the couple, but there remains a strong interest in keeping the relationship together and improving the marriage. In some of these couples, it may be useful to supportively "allow the swelling to go down" before pushing in one direction or another. It has been my experience that, with some of these treatments, the couple, once they emerge from crisis mode, will begin to do very well. Both individuals will be highly receptive to input and be more likely to do homework and actively participate in the treatment.

Possible Combinations

Table 8.1 describes the possible combinations of stages of change in partners and the implications of each combination.

General Considerations

When thinking about a stages of change model with couples, it is important to understand the following:

1. A couple can move no faster than its less motivated (earliest in the change process) partner. Even if one is in contemplation and the other in action, it is the one who is in contemplation who governs this aspect of the process.
   a. A precontemplator can halt the process of couples therapy completely if he or she views the problem or issues in the marriage as nonexistent or has already made the decision to leave the marriage.
2. Interventions must acknowledge both partners' levels of motivation.
3. Intervention must always be stage based. That is, one intervenes differently with a couple in which the "early one" is in precontemplation than a couple in which the "early one" is in contemplation or preparation.
4. Part of the goal of the intervention is to help the members move forward on their levels of change and motivation for the relationship.

When one partner is in precontemplation (for reasons other than having made the decision to leave the marriage), part of the therapist's task is to help that partner look at reasons for continuing the marriage. A central goal is to help this partner become contemplative about the marriage.

TABLE 8.1. Stages of Change Applied to Marital Interaction

	Spouse 1			
Spouse 2	Precontemplation	Contemplation	Preparation	Action
Precontemplation	If both spouses are in precontemplation, it is highly unlikely that they will show up for couple therapy unless they are forced to do so by the courts or for some other exogenous reasons.	If one spouse is in precontemplation and the other is in contemplation, the rate and likelihood of change is determined by the precontemplator. The contemplator may easily become disheartened by the negative or "out of touch" perspective of the precontemplator.	The precontemplator sets the timing again here. The partner in preparation is less likely to become demoralized than the partner in contemplation.	It is unusual for partners to arrive with such disparity. Although possible, the one in action would likely have succeeded in moving the precontemplator by this point, or the precontemplator would have demoralized the spouse in action back toward preparation or contemplation.
Contemplation		A likely state for couples coming for treatment. Both are ambivalent and uncertain regarding the future of the relationship.	One partner is uncertain regarding his or her motivation for change, and the other is clear that he or she would like things to be different.	One partner is clearly committed to change, and the other remains ambivalent.
Preparation			Both spouses are ready to make changes but have not yet begun to do so.	One spouse has begun to make changes and has tried to modify the marriage; the other is positive about change but has not taken any or many steps to do so.
Action				Both partners are working actively on changing the problems in their marriage.

Other Factors in Assessment

Among the other questions to be asked during assessment of a couple are the following: What is the goal of the treatment? What would the partners like to focus upon? Why have they attended this meeting? What would the partners like one another to focus upon? Why now? What made this the point that they came in for treatment? In addition to focus, what are the strengths of this relationship?

CASE EXAMPLE: THE ROTHFORDS

Below, the reader will find Session 3 of my work with Bob and Lisa Rothford. The couple, both in their late 30s, with two young children, had come in for their first visit about a month before the session described. They had been married for 11 years and had dated for 3 years prior to their marriage. Bob had had brief first and second marriages, without children, in his early 20s.

About 6 weeks before their first session with me, the couple's conflict about Lisa's failing business came to a head. Bob, who always had seen Lisa as a spendthrift, was angry about Lisa's decision to buy this franchise business and was now furious that it appeared to be failing. Lisa viewed Bob as unsupportive and angry toward her. She felt that she had purchased this business in order to help Bob out. She saw the business failure as "unfortunate" but "not my fault." Bob was intensely resentful that Lisa's actions were driving them further and further into debt. Another point of great contention between them was Bob's view that during a major medical crisis he had, Lisa had not been supportive of him.

The couple's anger escalated to the point that Bob had moved into a friend's apartment for a week. They sought treatment from a couple therapist but felt that the counselor was "so passive that she just made matters worse." The sessions became "shouting matches" and "nothing positive came out of them." At that point Bob went to his oncologist and asked for another referral. (Bob had been diagnosed with a serious but treatable cancer several years before I began working with the couple. He saw his oncologist on a regular basis, and this physician had become his primary care doctor.)

Prior to the session discussed below, I had tried to help Bob and Lisa start to talk with one another and consider their motivation and readiness for changing the relationship. Both seemed to want to continue the marriage, and Bob moved back home after the first session. I believe that both, although ambivalent, wanted the relationship to work. I perceived them as both in *contemplation* regarding changing and improving the relationship. Although their fighting was intense (as you will see below), they also appeared to share a genuine desire to continue the relationship and keep their family together. I have presented this couple to various training groups as one in which one partner or the other was viewed as being uncommitted to change, and therefore in precontemplation. Although it may be difficult to fully clarify in reading a transcript of one single session, it was clear in working with this couple that both partners, although angry and hurt, also had a strong need and desire to maintain the relationship.

The couple began this session just as they had ended the previous visit, fighting about money and responsibility. They immediately launched into this discussion and were about 5 minutes into the session when the following interchange began.

BOB: I felt and always felt that Lisa's attitude, once we had started absorbing major financial responsibilities . . . short-term credit cards and things like that started happening, my feeling was that she continued to act like she was employed.

LISA: You don't think you have an attitude?

BOB: I'm here because I have all sorts of screwed up attitudes about this, Lisa!

LISA: The only reason I would lie and sneak, which I am known to do, is because I can't stand being told that I cannot have this, and he can have what he wants. Maybe it is a problem that I have, when he says "You are not allowed to buy a chair," but then he goes out and buys me a new $1,500 brooch for a Christmas present when I have a 1-week-old infant. It's like, wait a minute, I want a chair to sit on, but I have been accused, I swear to you, of driving this marriage down the tubes.

THERAPIST: It sounds like these are major monumental issues for both of you. I'd like you to proceed with this discussion with you, Bob, playing Lisa. Just switch roles and do it as best you can. I want to continue this, but just do it from the other person's perspective.

This couple begins the session with intense arguing and recriminations. They have done something similar in their earlier session. There is little to be gained from a continued exchange like this. Couples in this type of intense conflict can fill whatever time is available to them. Therefore, I make the decision to *change things* behaviorally and have them continue the argument from one another's perspective. In these types of locked-in situations, it is most important to help the couple make some type of change. The specifics of that change are much less important than the change itself. *The reader should keep in mind that, once they switch roles, they will be speaking for the other person.* It is important to note that this exercise would not be appropriate for couples where one or both are in precontemplation. In such a situation the partner or partners who are uncertain about being in treatment at all would balk and see such an exercise as "infantile" or "game-playing." A couple in action might enjoy and productively use such role playing as well.

The reason that this exercise is particularly useful for those in contemplation is that it allows them to explore their own ambivalence *and that of their partner.*

BOB: It's hard for me to feel what the point is behind what she feels because I disagree with her reservation.

THERAPIST: And I'm sure she disagrees with yours as well. But what I'd like for you to do for a brief period here is just get into her perspective, even if that means sort of setting aside your own for a brief period. And I'd like you [Lisa] to do the same. I'd like you both to continue this discussion from the other's perspective.

LISA: Who starts?

THERAPIST: Let's just continue talking about the chair.

LISA: I'd rather make it a discussion about a sofa. (*laughing and putting on a deep, manly voice*) I don't think we are ready to buy a sofa yet, Lisa.

BOB: Every nice home I go to there are things, beautiful, matching, seven couches in a house, and we have just this old one you refuse to replace.

LISA: Well, you can't always have what you want and until you learn to stop spending money that is sending us to the poorhouse, you can't have that sofa. You will just have to wait, that's all. We are going to have to wait and determine together what is the appropriate time.

BOB: Well, I'm just going to go out and buy it, and you'll have to deal with the charge. I'll just go out to Stafford Furniture. I'll just go out and spend money, it doesn't matter.

LISA: (*shifting out of character*) I would never say anything like that!

[Don't allow the couple to comment on one another's performance, as this can become an argument.]

THERAPIST: Just keep it going.

LISA: Okay, dear, if you want, why don't you look in the papers for an inexpensive sofa, and next week sometime we can go look for one.

BOB: I don't want to buy a used sofa. I want to buy a new one.

LISA: I thought we had an agreement this fall that no money would be spent on that front room. We had an agreement.

BOB: I never made any agreement.

LISA: We sat there, and we had an agreement. You're *always* breaking these agreements.

BOB: I didn't make any agreements. You said something about my having to help out part time with the new financial structure in buying this new condo. I didn't make any agreements. You pushed me. Yeah, I said something you said and I said yeah, but you pushed me into it, and I never said I would. Those were *your* agreements, not mine. They were yours.

LISA: Well, as usual, you've just gone and done what you're not supposed to do and you have created all this extra debt in this condo, so from now on, I am not going to say another word to you until December.

THERAPIST: (*to Lisa*) Don't come out of role yet. Just tell me what "Bob" is feeling emotionally.

LISA: I am feeling a total lack of control over my life. She's just spending, and I'm so stressed out. I have just assumed this huge gigantic mortgage, and she's just spending us into the poorhouse.

THERAPIST: So you feel scared?

LISA: I feel angry.

THERAPIST: You don't feel any fear?

LISA: I don't think so, just really angry.

THERAPIST: (*to Bob*) What do you feel "Lisa?"

BOB: (*sadly, almost tearful*) I am feeling controlled, that I am not equal to him, that there isn't enough money, enough material things for me to put the kind of life I want around me materially and to put that together. This is not enough, it is important to me, very important to me, what I physically have around me, furniture and the way it looks, and household, and I want all that together, and I want all that together now, and I can't get it and I feel unfulfilled.

THERAPIST: Deprived?

BOB: Somewhat, maybe too strong a word, but uh . . . yeah, I guess, deprived.

THERAPIST: Anything else?

[The interaction above was becoming very intense. Lisa's intervention below breaks the intimacy and "pulls" the couple back to an argument. Other times, it is Bob who does so. Do such couples have a self-destructive wish? Are they trying to sabotage their interactions? Are they playing something out from their histories? It is unclear. What is clear, however, is that the "call of the lock-in" is very powerful and pervasive. Couples with severe marital difficulties will "snap back" to their typical patterns of interaction until they begin to learn and practice new modes of participating in the marriage.]

LISA: (*huffy and angry*) Well, during the fall my wife had several yard sales to finance her . . . purchases which I absolutely hate. I hate yard sales, and find them so embarrassing, and she just added all of this extra stress onto our lives to do this.

BOB: Well, it is the one opportunity I have to turn over what I don't like and doesn't fit into the house in terms of the decorating that I want to do. It's an opportunity to clear out a lot of junk that we've accumulated and make some money. I don't know why you have such a problem selling junk.

LISA: Nothing ever stays the same in my house. Do you know we have had *five* dining room table sets since I've been married?

BOB: Not five, not five that are dining room tables. Eat on, maybe, but not dining room tables.

THERAPIST: I'd like to have a discussion. Again, staying in these roles, I'd like you to have a discussion about the cancer. Talk about your feelings about it and her feelings about it.

[Bob had had a bout with cancer 2 years before. He felt that Lisa had not been supportive or caring and had resented him for getting sick. Although he seemed in fine health, Bob's resentment about the cancer and Lisa's lack of support came up often in their arguments. I switch to this issue, because I feel that while they are in role this may be a valuable area to cover. It appears to be at the heart of Bob's frequent complaints that Lisa doesn't really take his perspective on things.]

LISA: Well, I feel very frightened, and I feel angry and resentful against Lisa because I have to spend the rest of my life working, and I don't know how much longer that will be, so I'm just going to work until I die, while she just lies around and does nothing and spends my money.

THERAPIST: You feel like you are going to die sooner?

LISA: Well, I feel like I don't know how much longer I have. I feel like maybe I don't know how much longer I'm going to live. I don't want to spend that amount of time going nowhere, just working myself to ... ah ... death, basically.

THERAPIST: Do you like what you are doing?

LISA: No, I don't like what I'm doing.

THERAPIST: And you feel like you are *having* to do it?

LISA: (*nods*) Mmm-hmm. And I feel that I am in this position because of my wife's material needs.

THERAPIST: In terms of your feelings of vulnerability, do you feel like this cancer is going to kill you? That you are dying from this or that. This is something that is making you very vulnerable?

LISA: Yeah, I feel like I probably will die from this, and I don't know when but probably sooner than if I didn't have it. I'll probably be facing more treatment which I just recovered from so I hate to think about that.

THERAPIST: When do you think that will happen?

LISA: Well, maybe within a decade. And ... I just feel like life is too short, and I don't want to necessarily be spending it like this.

THERAPIST: So you feel scared and resentful and angry that Lisa is putting you through this position of having to do things you don't want to do?

LISA: Yup, exactly. It was her decision to buy this condo, and she pushed me into this, and it is nothing but a financial mess, and, you know, it's just all her fault. If we could have just rented another 6 months to a year, we wouldn't have had to be in this financial situation.

THERAPIST: And what do *you* feel about the cancer?

BOB: (*long pause*) I think I feel some resentment that it's happened. I have two babies, and I need to be with them and want to be with them and to do what I expect him to do in terms of that. This issue of immortality, mortality, is very scary to me and not part of what I planned this script of how our life would go. It is very scary stuff to me. I still haven't dealt with my dad's death. What that loss has meant to me, and I'd rather not think about it, I'd just rather not deal with it. I'd rather just push on and deal with happy things, and it's too scary for me.

THERAPIST: Do you think you are pushing it away?

BOB: No. I think I push away his issues and his concerns because I can't deal with it. I've got kids to deal with, and I need him to provide, and they need him to provide. And I can't deal with the fact that he might die or is upset about the fact that he is vulnerable.

THERAPIST: Do you feel scared for him?

BOB: (*switching back to own role*) I don't know . . . I just don't know if Lisa feels that way.

THERAPIST: (*turns to Lisa*) Do you feel scared for yourself, Lisa?

LISA: Very much so.

THERAPIST: So you feel scared that you'll be left with the two kids.

[The reader should note that despite the clear anger in their interactions, this couple has great perceptiveness about one another's feelings and an ability to empathize with one another. This empathy and perception of the other is often submerged by their anger and struggles. It is, however, in my experience a very significant factor in predicting improvement. Most worrisome are those couples in which both partners are without a clue about one another's feelings.]

BOB: I've left you with this huge insurance policy, why do you have to feel afraid for that?

THERAPIST: Try not to come out of role just yet.

BOB: (*back in Lisa's role*) Well, you always say that, but I don't want to have to collect that insurance policy. I don't think we should be paying the monthly premium for it.

LISA: (*back in Bob's role*) That is ridiculous. Don't you realize I can never get that insurance policy again?

BOB: It's still a lot of money, and we don't have enough money for other things that I want to get. To me it just seems like an awful lot of amount of money. James and Mimi don't have it.

LISA: (*very gruff voice*) The discussion is closed! I am never changing the insurance policy that I have. Forget it, Lisa. Not even up for discussion.

THERAPIST: (*to Bob*) But you looked very sad before when you were talking about your fears about death. You were very upset.

BOB: Well, it's just very upsetting, the fact that he had this brush with a very serious problem and his oncologist had said that it either could never reappear, or it could reappear within a year, so he should try to live a normal life. It does worry me when I think about it, but I don't like to dwell on the fact that he might die, and I just want to push it aside and move on.

THERAPIST: Lisa (*to Bob*), do you feel like pushing it aside has any impact for Bob?

BOB: He says that it does. I'm not sure it does, but he says it does.

THERAPIST: (*to Lisa*) What is the impact for you? Stay in Bob's role this time.

LISA: . . . well, it makes me angry, and it's just such a serious issue, and it seems to be nonexistent, so . . .

THERAPIST: You feel like Lisa won't talk to you about it?

LISA: Yes, that's correct.

BOB: I feel I talk to him about it. I mean, I went to the hospital every day that he had chemo and . . .

LISA: She bugs me.

THERAPIST: In what way?

LISA: It just seems like she could never do anything right at the hospital. You know, I mean, whether it was getting me a cold cloth or trying to feed me, I mean it, just . . .

THERAPIST: You felt pissed off?

LISA: Yeah, you never got the food in right. I'm sure glad my mother and father were there.

THERAPIST: So you felt like she wasn't a help at all to you?

LISA: Not really. I think she was thinking more about herself.

THERAPIST: How do you feel that Lisa could be more helpful to you around this issue?

LISA: By taking a little bit of the financial pressure off.

THERAPIST: What could she do emotionally, just emotionally?

LISA: Just be a little bit more sensitive, maybe discuss, you know, be more willing to discuss this issue and maybe become a little bit more intimate.

THERAPIST: Are you talking about physical intimacy?

LISA: Well, a lot more, in that regard.

THERAPIST: But you are talking about that she would listen to you more?

LISA: Well, it's just that we *never* discuss it [the illness] at all, so . . .

THERAPIST: Do you initiate it?

LISA: No, I never discuss it either.

THERAPIST: What about you, Lisa. Do you bring it up? Do you like to talk about it?

BOB: No, I don't tend to bring it up, and I also don't find Bob particularly perceptive to me.

THERAPIST: You've felt you've tried?

BOB: No, I don't feel like I've tried very much or very hard but my sense is that . . . he doesn't tend to want to seek me out to discuss it anyway. That he holds these things in and either he talks to other people about them, or he thinks about it while he's running or spending time alone, and he never really opens himself up except when we are having arguments and lists the things that are stressing him. He doesn't make it a point of being a topic that he wants to constructively talk about or obtain my emotional support for.

THERAPIST: Do you feel like if you brought this up, Lisa would turn you off, or that she would listen, or . . .

LISA: No, I think she would listen, it's just, ah, I don't know, it's such a personal thing, that . . .

THERAPIST: What is a personal thing?

LISA: Well, this whole issue of my health, and there is nothing she can do about it, so, we have just not been getting along at all. So I just feel like . . . and she won't go to bed with me, she won't sleep with me—so I'm . . . I'm not going to get intimate with her on that sort of level.

THERAPIST: You find you are punishing her by not talking about it?

LISA: No.

THERAPIST: What about yourself? Are you punishing yourself?

LISA: Uh, well, I have always been a kind of quiet person, so it's not like . . . I don't think I'm really punishing myself.

THERAPIST: Is it hard for you to keep it inside?

LISA: No. It's harder for me to talk about it.

THERAPIST: It's harder for you to talk about it? Let me stop the role play. Let me just ask, because it was a cross conversation, what it has felt like for you to play one another's role, what it has been like the last 15–20 minutes to take Lisa's role and vice versa?

LISA: Well, for a split second I had to think more about his feelings, how he perceives things, and so, instead of being me, me, me, it shows the other side. I think it is a little more constructive ... so ... but ... I mean, I'm not sure it was that accurate, but ... (*takes a deep breath*)

[This is an important perception on Lisa's part. Her tone is what I often think about as a "softening" which must occur if progress is to take place. If one fails to get a softening between the partners the likelihood of change is quite minimal. Similarly, if a couple does this role reversal exercise and shows little or no empathy for the partner's position, prospects for change are poor. It is significant that this softening has occurred, but it will not be unexpected for them to start to fight again later in the session. Progress with couples can often be a repeated cycle of improvement followed by backsliding.]

THERAPIST: You don't have to be accurate.

LISA: Yeah.

THERAPIST: What was it like to be Lisa?

BOB: Well, in so many areas, so many questions seemed perplexing, because I didn't know how to really explain what Lisa might be feeling. I don't mean to say this to press any buttons, but, so much of what I see with Lisa is a level of rage. I don't understand.

[Bob is attempting to shift back to an argument. If not handled correctly, this type of provocation will bring Lisa back into fighting mode very quickly. For a couple therapist, such an interaction can feel frustrating and make the therapy seem fruitless. It is important to retain an optimistic stance and assume that this type of "snap back" will happen many times before the couple retains the skills and trust in one another needed to change.]

THERAPIST: I think both of you show the rage at this situation.

BOB: Well, we show the rage differently.

THERAPIST: Right, right. I think you both show it very differently, but I think that it's this fury and rage that prevents you from moving in a constructive fashion. I think that both of you are reasonable people. Other people like each of you and can relate generally well to you. I think what happens between the two of you is that in a split second, the barriers go up, and they fly up, and, and . . . you are in a fight with one another and there is very little constructive that happens, and I think that both of you have your own sort of way of blocking . . . your wall. I think you [Bob] do it in a quieter way, in a different sort of way, in a more intellectualized way, but I think it is there. It really must be dreadful, for both of you, to feel so shut off in the relationship. To be lonely with another person is almost worse than being lonely, alone.

BOB: (*nods yes*)

[There is some continued discussion for about 10 minutes about how hard it is not to become disappointed with one another.]

THERAPIST: Let's stop there. There are a few things that I just want you both to think about. I think the situation between the two of you is *very* difficult. But the one thing I think is that both of you know what the triggers and what the buttons are and what gets things going in these fights, and I think pushing the buttons serves you absolutely no purpose. Zero. This approach does absolutely nothing to change the situation, to improve the situation. All it does is allow you to vent your steam about the situation. And I think that what it also does is ruins the marriage, it ruins the possibility for a relationship because you keep on pushing the button, pushing the button, pushing the button, and the marriage will clearly go down the tubes under those circumstances. I said to you before: I think there is a basis for a relationship between the two of you. I think that both of you, while doing that role playing exercise, which I will do with you again, which was a success in these sessions, could get some of the perspective of the other. I think that both of you, when you stop and try, can stand in the other's shoes, and get some sense of what is going on. But it is so easy to light the match and throw it on the floor and get the flammable mixture going. And I think sometimes that what both of you have to do, if you have an interest in saving this marriage, is bite your tongue more about things. I think there are some discussions that are going to have to take place about the condo. I think there are some discussions that are going to have to take place about your health difficulty. I think there are going to have to be some discussions about vulnerability, mortality, the future. I think there are going to have to be some discussions about the responsibilities that you [Bob] feel about money and about your [Lisa's] feelings in terms of Bob's illness. But I think there are also some things that are going to have to be left unsaid for the time being. Not that you will never be able to talk about them, but they serve absolutely no purpose at this point in the marriage except for knowing that it's terribly hard for both of you, gets you going in opposite directions, gets you in a fury with one another, and breaks down any possibility of communication. You have to think about where it is you need to bite your tongue, and not talk about a topic like that. It's just not being constructive, not useful to you.

[According to Gottman one of the most difficult things for unstable couples to do is end the argument. Much like the Energizer Bunny, their arguments just keep going and going. A skill often needed by these couples is how *not to talk about something*.]

BOB: Can I just ask one question because I think both of us go through different periods of strength on this. If the other person breaks down and starts a fight, and in the last 2 weeks breaking twice in a 3 to 4 day period, what should the other person do? Just literally bite your tongue and walk out of the room, or . . .

THERAPIST: Not taking the bait. Not go after it because you both know how to do it extremely well; it is a dance both of you do with great agility at this point. Both of you can do it, and you are pros at it. You could join the Master's circuit and be able to win the couple's conflict competition. But maybe, you don't need to do that. It serves no purpose at all. You know how to get her going, she knows how to get you going, and both of you know the parts to play. You *are* *experts* at it; you don't need to demonstrate that you are experts at it. You need to stop, and figure out ways to stop. The thing I would be very interested in hearing about from both of you next time are places where you could have gotten into conflict with one another, but didn't do that. Were able to halt that. Think about that each day until we meet. "Where did I prevent an argument?" "How did I jump in and stop the pattern?" Just think about that, we probably won't talk about it much here, just give it thought. The other thing I would like you to do, and let's be sure to talk about it next time, is [think about] your reactions to this session and what went on today here. I would prefer if you did not discuss your reactions with one another, but note them down so that we can talk about them here. I really want to go into some detail with that if that is okay.

[For this couple where anything can be a provocation, I would rather save the discussion of the session to our next visit, rather than have them do it at home, as I might with other couples.]

LISA: Sounds fine.

THERAPIST: So we'll get together in 2 weeks. Okay?

BOB: Okay with me.

[I almost always end the session with a homework assignment or assignments that the couple can work on between visits. The type of assignment is closely tied to the content and process of the couple's relationship and to their stage of change. For this contemplative couple, the important task is to help them build skills to stop the argument.]

Follow-Up

I saw this couple for 13 visits over a 10-month period. Over this time they felt themselves to be significantly improved and communicating "much better" with one another. Bob was able to let go of his anger regarding Lisa's business, and Lisa became more supportive of Bob and his concerns over his illness. Their sexual relationship, which had been virtually nil, became much better and was satisfying to both of them. They left treatment with the knowledge that they could return as needed.

Is it surprising that the couple was able to make so much progress over this period? I think not. Even with the high level of visible conflict, there is an intensity and strong feeling of emotional involvement. In general, when couples only have hate and disdain left for one another and have lost the interest in maintaining even the anger, they are closer to dissolution than this couple. The ambivalence (contemplation) gives the therapist something to work with. If the partners are so tired of the conflict that they have even "lost the energy to fight," and if they are so pessimistic about change that there is little intensity available for trying, the prognosis is grim.

About 18 months later I received a call from Lisa that things were very difficult again. Bob's company had moved out of the state after a hostile takeover by one of their competitors. Bob and Lisa did not want to move to the new location, and Bob had been unemployed for the past 3 months. Lisa had gotten a job to try and help out, but Bob's concerns regarding his lack of a job and the poor financial situation were taking their toll. Bob had begun to drink heavily and was arrested for driving while under the influence. (He and Lisa claimed that before the unemployment, drinking was not a problem.) The couple had started arguing again. Lisa, however, felt (and Bob agreed when he came in) that the arguments were much less severe and vicious than they had been prior to treatment. The skills that the couple had learned were useful to them in being able to end fights and helping them move in a more constructive direction.

They reentered treatment with me and were seen for eight visits in this second course of treatment over a 7-month period. Much of the focus in this treatment was about their both being able to deal with the stress of Bob's unemployment and support one another through this stress. About 4 months into this second course of treatment, Bob got an excellent (but demanding) position.

A little over 2 years after the second course of treatment, I saw the couple for one last course of therapy. Bob's mother had died suddenly and this had sent him into a severe depression. Lisa again called to initiate the treatment. This therapy lasted three sessions over two months and was again useful to them. They were very clearly functioning much better than during either of the two earlier courses of treatment.

I have not seen the Rothfords for about 4 years but expect that I may again have contact with them in the future. There are many couples I see in courses of treatment that have interludes of 10, 15, or even 20 years.

ENDING TREATMENT

As is the case in much of the treatment I do (Budman & Gurman, 1992), I do not view myself as "ending" treatment with most of the couples with whom I work. Instead, I perceive of myself as being similar to a primary care doctor. Couples like the Rothfords often return for additional therapy months or years later. When they come back, many of these couples have used the input from an earlier course of treatment and are ready to make some additional changes. For others, there is a sense that they have "slipped a bit" since the end of the prior treatment and are coming back for a "tune up." For some of these couples, I have seen their children (now grown) in couple therapy, and I am able to have a multigenerational perspective on the family and their relationships.

I will almost always end a treatment with the statement to the couple that "the door is always open." They need not view return to treatment as a failure, or an indication that the prior treatment did not work. Instead, just as the primary care patient returns to his or her family physician when new problems occur or old ones reassert themselves, my couples came back periodically as needed.

My estimate is that the average number of visits that I see a couple is about six to eight over a 5- or 6-month period in a given episode of treatment. I have seen some couples for years in sessions that are spread apart by 3 to 6 months. Others I see very frequently (every other week or so) for 3 months or more and then begin to spread the sessions further apart. There are probably several hundred couples who view themselves as being in treatment with me, even years after their last visit. I feel privileged to have had the opportunity to have worked with these people and have been allowed into their lives.

REFERENCES

Arthur, W. B. (1990). Positive feedbacks in the economy. *Scientific American, 262,* 92–99.

Baucom, D. H., Epstein, N., & Carels, R. (1992). A cognitive-behavioral model of marital dysfunction and marital therapy. In S. H. Budman, M. F. Hoyt, & S. Friedman (Eds.), *The first session in brief therapy* (pp. 225–254). New York: Guilford Press.

Briggs, J., & Peat, F. D. (1989). *Turbulent mirror: An illustrated guide to chaos theory and the science of wholeness.* New York: Harper & Row.

Budman, S. H., & Gurman, A. S. (1988). *Theory and practice of brief therapy.* New York: Guilford Press.

Budman, S. H., & Gurman, A. S. (1992). A time-sensitive model of brief therapy: The I-D-E approach. In S. H. Budman, M. F. Hoyt, & S. Friedman (Eds.), *The first session in brief therapy* (pp. 111–134). New York: Guilford Press.

Gottman, J. M. (1993). The roles of conflict engagement, escalation, and avoidance in marital interaction: A longitudinal view of five types of couples. *Journal of Consulting and Clinical Psychology, 61,* 6–15.

Gottman, J. (1994). *Why marriages succeed or fail.* New York: Simon & Schuster.

Gottman, J. M., & Krokoff, L. (1989). Marital interaction and marital satisfaction: A longitudinal view. *Journal of Consulting and Clinical Psychology, 57,* 47–52.

Jacobson, N. S. (1981). Behavioral marital therapy. In A. S. Gurman & D. P. Kniskern (Eds.), *Handbook of family therapy* (pp. 556–591). New York: Brunner/Mazel.

Prochaska, J. O., & DiClemente, C. C. (1986). Toward a comprehensive model of change. In W. R. Miller & N. Healther (Eds.), *Treating addictive behaviors: Processes of change* (pp. 3–27). New York: Plenum Press.

Prochaska, J. O., Norcross, J. C., & DiClemente, C. C. (1994). *Changing for good.* New York: William Morrow.

Wallerstein, J. S. (1994). The early psychological tasks of marriage: Part 1. *American Journal of Orthopsychiatry, 64,* 640–650.

Wallerstein, J. S. (1996). The psychological tasks of marriage: Part 2. *American Journal of Orthopsychiatry, 66,* 217–227.

PART III

◄◦►

COLLABORATIVE
MODELS

The Wile and Lawrence, Eldridge, Christensen, and Jacobson approaches, although quite different from each other in method, both represent collaborative models. As the basic building block of the intervention, the therapists help each patient to shift a behavior that promotes a change in feeling so that the couple can move away from an embattled position to a cooperative one.

Both systems have been with us for some time. Wile originally published his unique perspective on marital conflict in 1981. He observes that the partners will naturally feel slighted, angry, and competitive; everyone does sometimes. The problem comes when they feel unentitled to their feelings and bottle them up. According to Wile, couples fight when they try like mad to avoid a fight. He teaches his couple partners, through his own script writing, to give voice to their natural dissatisfactions and to help their spouse, but most importantly themselves, to *accept* how they are really feeling. He coaches each member to acknowledge his or her true thoughts, which then leads the pair away from an alienated or adversarial stance and toward collaboration.

The Lawrence, Eldridge, Christensen, and Jacobson model is of particular interest as an evolving, research-based approach. Jacobson began with a traditional, behavioral-learning model of couple work. Then he exhaustively studied the efficacy of his approach and found the long-term outcome statistics unsatisfactory. Lawrence, Eldridge, Christensen, and Jacobson, influenced by Wile, added acceptance training to their approach before introducing the behavioral exercises, thus creating their new, integrative couple therapy model, which they offer us here. How-

ever the Christensen–Jacobson group introduce acceptance very differently from Wile. They teach it in structured fashion according to the
social learning principles that they know so well, not through the creative script-writing approach mastered by Wile. In the two models we
see illustrated, then, two different methods of working toward the same
goal, greater emotional acceptance and collaboration in the couple.

JAMES M. DONOVAN

9

◄O►

COLLABORATIVE
COUPLE THERAPY

DANIEL B. WILE

I present a vignette to describe the theory of relationships from which this couple therapy approach emerges. Let us say I am at a party with my wife, Joanne. I look across the room and see her talking in what seems to me too animated and intimate a way with a good-looking man. Let us say that I feel a jealous twinge. It lasts just a moment, but it changes everything. Why? Because I see my jealousy as inappropriate, a sign of immaturity, an indication of being hung up. In a word, I feel *unentitled* to that jealous twinge. That is a key idea in collaborative couple therapy: The degree of entitlement a person feels to the experience he or she is having at the moment.

I hear the rush of my positive self-opinion escaping into space and the clank of my negative self-image wheeling into place. I've lost my safety net: My good will toward myself, my ability to give myself the benefit of the doubt, the positive inner voices that had been cheering me on. I'm at a *crossroads moment,* by which I mean that I have in front of me three paths—attack, avoid, or confide—each of which leads to its own distinctive couple system: adversarial, alienated, or collaborative.

AN ADVERSARIAL COUPLE SYSTEM

I attack—or, rather, I *think* of attacking. I make the adversarial shift of everyday life: from "I shouldn't be jealous—there isn't any reason" to

201

"But does she have to stand so close to him?" That is, I come up with a reason. As soon as Joanne is alone, I head toward her to tell her off. But like a grandmaster anticipating the next several chess moves, I know what will happen:

DAN: How can you flirt like that, and right in front of me!

JOANNE: What are you talking about? I wasn't doing anything, and you weren't anywhere near me.

DAN: You know exactly what you were doing. Don't pretend you don't.

JOANNE: I'm *not* pretending—and I don't particularly care for your tone.

DAN: I don't have a tone.

JOANNE: Are you kidding? You rush over here, you accuse me of doing things I'm not doing. You're trying to control me like I'm some child!

DAN: Oh, I'm trying to control you, huh? You're waltzing around the room flirting with every man you see trying to make me jealous. You're trying to control *me*.

I don't want to get into that fight. I don't want to hear "You're trying to control me." I don't want to say "You're waltzing around the room flirting with every man you see trying to make me jealous"—since I know that's not true. I'm saying it in the heat of the moment. That's the problem: all that *heat*. By attacking Joanne, I would be shifting us into an adversarial couple system, a fast-moving fire that, once ignited, is self-fueling. I don't want to ignite that fire and start that exchange in which each responds to the other's last stinging comment by stinging back. Not that I mind doing a little stinging, but I don't want to get stung back.

Also, it would be humiliating. Let us suppose that Joanne and I really *were* at such a party and that I really *were* to make such a scene. I'm a couple therapist. After spending the whole day dealing with partners caught in adversarial couple systems, I'd feel ashamed of getting into one myself.

AN ALIENATED COUPLE SYSTEM

So, halfway to Joanne, I shift gears. I hear the rumble of a new mental state sliding into place: From "attack" to "avoid." When I reach Joanne, I *don't* say, "How can you flirt like that!" Instead, I say:

DAN: This is a dull party, don't you think? What do you say we leave?

I'm trying to get us out of there. But Joanne wants to stay. *Of course* she wants to stay. She's got that guy to flirt with, doesn't she?

I head for the bar, on the way bumping into a beautiful woman— which gives me an idea. I'd feel better if I had my own attractive person to talk to. But there's a problem. When, as now, I feel demoralized, I lose the ability to talk to beautiful women. In fact, I lose the ability to mingle at all. I end up in the corner leafing through art books.

JOANNE: (*coming over to me*) You're over here by yourself. Is something wrong?

DAN: No, I'm just tired. That's all.

JOANNE: Are you sure that's all?

DAN: Yes.

JOANNE: Maybe we *should* go home.

I want to go home, but I don't want to be seen as unable to cope.

DAN: No, really, I'm okay. I'm enjoying this book.

When we eventually do leave, things don't get any better. In the car, our conversation is strained. My evasiveness exerts a dragging effect on Joanne; it infects her. Arriving home, I try to be chatty in an effort to generate spontaneity, but it rings hollow. My withdrawal has snapped us into an alienated couple system, a self-reinforcing exchange in which each person's carefulness, inhibition, and overpoliteness stimulates the same in the other much as whispering stimulates whispering.

DAN: (*giving up on the evening*) I'm tired; I think I'll go to bed early.

JOANNE: I'm not sleepy. I think I'll stay up and read.

DAN: (*trying to head off* total *disconnection*) You can read in bed.

JOANNE: But the light disturbs you.

DAN: No, it'll be okay.

JOANNE: Are you sure?

DAN: Yes, really.

JOANNE: But I don't want to disturb you.

DAN: You wouldn't.

JOANNE: I don't know. Maybe I'll come up a little later.

What an excruciating exchange. It would sap all the energy I had left. When Joanne and I are an alienated couple system, our conversation is reduced to polite, ritualized, careful, socially acceptable comments. I feel trapped in my thoughts and feelings without a way to reach through to her. It's like feeling lonely in a crowd.

A COLLABORATIVE COUPLE SYSTEM

I don't want to feel lonely in a crowd. But I don't want to get into a fight either. I'm not in the mood. (I'm *never* in the mood.) I need a scriptwriter, an expert who can come up with the perfect dialogue. With a scriptwriter's help, I wouldn't have to choose between starting a fight ("How can you flirt like that!") and tiptoeing around ("This is a dull party, don't you think? What do you say we leave?"). With a scriptwriter acting like a kind of Cyrano de Bergerac, feeding me lines, whispering in my ear, I could have told Joanne:

DAN: I'm afraid to tell you this but—okay, I'll tell you. I got a little jealous when you were talking to that guy.

That's brilliant! It's *confiding* in Joanne rather than criticizing her. It's bringing her in on what I was struggling with in a way that might get her empathizing. Of course, it might not.

JOANNE: Well, that's ridiculous!

Immediately, I would want to shoot back, "What's ridiculous about it? You were trying to *make* me jealous." I'd be reacting to Joanne's attack by attacking back, propelling us into an adversarial couple system. It'd be a crossroads moment, and I'd be taking the attack path. But quickly my scriptwriter whispers an alternative, which I immediately recognize as more satisfying to say:

DAN: (*to Joanne, following the scriptwriter's recommendation*) Yes, my jealousy *is* ridiculous. That's what I think about it, too—I feel ashamed—which is why it's so hard to bear your agreeing with me.

Again brilliant! Instead of attacking, I would again be confiding. Who could resist such a charming admission?

JOANNE: (*smiling*) Well, I guess I did rub it in a little.

Joanne is softening (see Johnson, Chapter 2, this volume), which helps me do the same.

DAN: I know it's not the greatest thing to have to worry about your husband's jealousy every time you talk to a guy at a party.

Is it safe to say this? Aren't I handing Joanne a weapon she can use against me? Can I be sure she won't say "You can say that again!"?

I know she won't! I heard the grinding of the collaborative couple system shifting into place. When Joanne and I are in such a system, it would never occur to her to turn what I say into a weapon against me. (Later, when we are again in an adversarial couple system, it might.)

JOANNE: Actually, I can see how it might look—you know, how I was talking to that man.

In response to my looking at things from Joanne's point of view, she is looking at things from mine, which makes me want even *more* to look at things from hers.

DAN: But I shouldn't jump to conclusions.

This comment just popped out of my mouth. I couldn't have stopped it. Suddenly—I don't have to think about it—I'm admitting, confiding, and appreciating Joanne's dilemma. I don't need a scriptwriter. I can come up with my own lines, and they come out easily and naturally. My eloquence returns. I become capable of talking to the most beautiful woman at the party, and I am doing so right now.

JOANNE: But I can see how you might.
DAN: Oh?
JOANNE: Things were pretty quiet in the car; then we walked in here, and suddenly I became this total extrovert.

When Joanne and I are in a collaborative couple system, we are able to figure out what neither of us could singly (see Johnson, Chapter 2, this volume, Step 6 of therapy).

DAN: You just went into the "party mode." I shouldn't have taken it so personally.

Earlier, when Joanne and I were in an adversarial couple system, we automatically looked for ways to disagree with and tear down what the other had just said. Now, in a collaborative couple system, we automatically look for ways to agree with and build on what the other says.

DAN: It *was* quiet in the car. I guess I was reacting to that.

JOANNE: I was worried about the party. That's probably why I was quiet.

DAN: You were?

JOANNE: I didn't know anyone who was going to be there.

Joanne and I are engaged in a collaborative couple system, which, like the other two (alienated and adversarial) is self-reinforcing. But whereas these other two are *negative* self-reinforcing cycles (stinging in response to being stung, withdrawing in response to withdrawal), the collaborative couple system is a *positive* self-reinforcing cycle. Each of us is confiding, admitting, reaching out, and giving the other the benefit of the doubt in response to the other doing the same.

THE FRAGILITY OF A COLLABORATIVE COUPLE SYSTEM

A collaborative couple system, however, is fragile. Its continuation requires that each partner feel that the other is doing enough confiding, admitting, and reaching out in return. It requires the maintenance of an atmosphere of warm acceptance, a holding environment. Were I to remain in a collaborative couple system—that is, to accept and build upon Joanne's comment that she was worried about the party—I would say, "Yes, I know. It was my office party; you were coming as a favor to me. I feel bad about dragging you along." But what I *do* say is:

DAN: You knew the Jacksons.

That's not accepting and building upon what Joanne just said. That's looking for weaknesses in it, for ways to poke holes in it. Instead of appreciating what Joanne is trying to say, which is that she didn't know enough people at the party to feel comfortable, I am focusing on a minor inaccuracy in her statement—an overstatement, a bit of poetic license, an exaggeration for emphasis. I am ignoring the spirit of what she is saying and holding to the letter of it. I am arguing with her. We are at a crossroads moment, and I have taken the attack path.

Why am I doing that? Because I feel *bad* about dragging Joanne to the party (even if she ended up having a better time than I did). I need to convince her that she *did* know people at the party, and, as a result, she had no reason to dread it, and, as a result, I *wasn't* really dragging her to it.

JOANNE: Yes, I knew them and I knew you—but those were the *only* people I knew.

Frustrated by the ease with which she is answering my objection, I bring out the big guns.

DAN: Well, if you didn't want to go, why didn't you *tell* me?

I don't think of this as bringing out the big guns but simply as telling Joanne what is true. I don't realize that what I'm really saying is: "Joanne, if you're so inhibited and immature that you can't say what you want, then don't blame me"—which, of course, is the heart of the matter: I'm trying to get the blame off me by putting it onto Joanne. I've made the adversarial shift of everyday life. I took a feeling I was having ("I feel bad about dragging you to parties") and turned it into something that Joanne was doing wrong ("It's your own fault for not telling me you didn't want to go").

JOANNE: I *did* tell you.
DAN: No, you didn't.
JOANNE: Remember, I said . . . ?

There is a therapist I know who would say at this point: "You're acting like a couple of 3-year-olds in a sandbox fighting over a pail and shovel." I don't say that to my clients. I spend too much time in this sandbox myself. Of course, Joanne *is* primarily at fault here. It doesn't seem fair. My therapy approach is based on the idea that no matter how irrational a partner's position may seem, there is always a way to show it to make sense. That's what I do all day—find the hidden reasonableness in what partners say—just to come home to find the one person in the world who truly *is* unreasonable.

SHIFTING AMONG THREE COUPLE SYSTEMS

At any moment, partners are confiding what is on their minds, which means that they are in a collaborative couple system; or they are not confiding, which means that they are in an alienated couple system. Unless there is blaming going on, in which case they are in an adversarial couple system. That is what a couple relationship is. Every couple is going to spend time in each of these three systems, much as everyone entering a triathalon is going to spend time running, biking, and swimming. Couples differ primarily in which of these three predominates and the manner in which each of them expresses itself. For some couples, being in an adversarial system means an out-and-out battle; for others, it may be an exchange of looks.

As couple therapists, we deal with couples who are caught in adversarial or alienated relating; that is, they're fighting or withdrawing. Every couple therapy approach has its own characteristic way of trying to shift partners *out* of these two states. Communication skills trainers give partners rules to shift them from fighting or withdrawing (e.g., "Make 'I-statements' not 'you-statements' "; "Repeat what your partner just said in your own words and check to see if you have it right"). Marital behavior therapists try to get partners to behave in loving and caring ways—to compliment one another, do thoughtful things, say "I love you"—in an effort to jump-start a self-perpetuating exchange of positive reinforcers. Cognitive therapists bring out and refute the unrealistic expectations and the automatic thoughts (the negative self-talk) that lead partners to fight and withdraw. Psychodynamically oriented therapists confront the leftover influences from childhood that lead to fighting and withdrawing and that prevent partners from developing a mature relationship. Object relations theorists try to get partners to rein in their projections and to create a holding environment for one another. Social constructionists use positive reframing to create a more positive spirit.

My way of dealing with fighting and withdrawing is to function as each partner's scriptwriter. I try to get some confiding going in an effort to jump-start a collaborative couple system. I show partners the dramatic shift that takes place when they confide the thoughts and feelings they're having *about* their partner or *about* the relationship. I was confiding such a feeling when I told Joanne "I'm afraid to tell you this, but—okay, I'll tell you. I got a little jealous when you were talking to that guy."

In saying this, I was appealing to her as a resource and confidant in dealing with this problem I was having with her. I was turning this problem in our relationship into a moment of intimacy.

There is a map in my mind that enables me to track partners through their sequence of crossroads moments so that I can then show them how to confide. Using this map, I see things in threes. When a partner attacks, I mentally label it as such, and I imagine the avoiding and confiding comment that he or she could have made instead. Then I

watch to see how the other partner, in response, attacks, avoids or confides—and, in response to that, how the first partner attacks, avoids, or
confides. All the while, I look for opportunities to introduce confiding.

BECOMING EACH PARTNER'S SCRIPTWRITER

I will use this made-up fight between Joanne and me to demonstrate.
But let us now say that I'm not Dan, but their therapist, Daniel B. Wile,
PhD. (I made myself one of the partners because I wanted to talk from
the inside about what it is like to be a partner; *now* I want to talk from
the inside about what it is like to be a therapist.) At our next session,
Joanne and Dan tell me about this incident at the party. Thinking in
terms of threes, I recognize how Dan considered "attacking" but ended
up "avoiding."

THERAPIST: (*looking for feelings that Dan might have "confided"*) Okay,
    Dan, there you were at the party. You looked across the room and
    saw Joanne talking to that man. What did you feel?

I'm searching for a soft, vulnerable feeling, such as "When I saw
you talking in that way, I felt lost, forgotten, and unloved."

DAN: I don't see why she had to stand so close to him!

That's not a soft, vulnerable feeling. Dan is using my question to
attack Joanne—which isn't surprising, since they are presently in an
adversarial couple system. I feel like telling him: "That's not a feeling; I
asked you what you were feeling." But that would be attacking Dan for
attacking Joanne. I would be engaging in an adversarial way with him,
when what I want to do is to engage in a collaborative way. I want to
create an atmosphere of safety and acceptance that might enable him to
reach out toward Joanne.

In collaborative couple therapy, the therapist relates to partners in a
collaborative way and has the goal of enabling them to relate that way
to one another.

THERAPIST: (*relating to Dan in a collaborative way, which, in this case,
    means accepting what he has just said and building from there*) Yes,
    and what did you *make* of her standing so close to him?

Since Dan is in an adversarial relation with Joanne, he is likely to
answer "She's a flirt!", or "She's always doing things like that," or "I

don't know; ask her!" That is, he's likely to turn my question into ammunition to use against her. If I am to wrest him away from his adversarial interaction with Joanne and into a collaborative one with me, I need to say something with more impact.

THERAPIST: (*to Dan, laying out possible things he could be feeling in the form of a multiple-choice question*) Did you feel hurt—thinking she might have forgotten you were even there? Did you feel abandoned—thinking that she only cared about him and she didn't care about you at all? Did you feel angry—seeing her as crossing the line of appropriate behavior and, perhaps, even trying to make you jealous? Did you think that she didn't mean anything by it but just didn't realize how it might look?

Why do I think this has impact? Dan has been arguing his case to a person (Joanne) who automatically dismisses what he says. It can be a shock to him, therefore, to find someone (me) who is seriously considering what he is saying and, moreover, helping him elaborate it. It can be a relief to no longer be the only one arguing his case.

But isn't Joanne going to think I'm taking his side? I don't think so. She knows, from seeing me operate in previous sessions, that I will devote equal effort to developing her side.

But should I really ask Dan, "Do you think she was trying to make you jealous?" Won't that feed his suspicions? Do I want to give him ammunition he can use in his fight against Joanne? It was a surprise when I first discovered it, but developing a person's argument (complaints, case, position, reality), rather than trying to talk him or her out of it, can provide a way out of the stinging-in-response-to-being-stung adversarial system.

It shouldn't have been a surprise. What keeps a fight going, after all—what makes an adversarial system self-sustaining and unresolvable—is that neither partner gets a chance to make his or her point, air his or her grievances, fears, doubts, suspicions, and longings, and feel that the other has heard. I'm trying to provide such an airing for Dan. The person Dan really needs to hear him is, of course, Joanne. But it can mean something to him that at least I have heard.

DAN: (*softening*) It's not exactly that she forgot I was there. It's more that . . . that . . . that . . .

Dan is deescalating. He is adopting a more conciliatory stance as a result of finally feeling heard. (People don't always respond to finally feeling heard by deescalating. At times they react by taking the opportunity to express all their pent-up rage about the matter; that is, they escalate.)

DAN: It's more that ... I don't know ... I suddenly felt so ... well, left out and unimportant.

There is the soft, vulnerable feeling. Dan's whole body relaxes. All he needed was to get that out—which required first, of course, that he figure it out. A wave of relief sweeps through him. I hear the kaplunk of the collaborative state shifting into place.

DAN: (to Joanne) You weren't even doing anything wrong. It was just a party. A person is supposed to be friendly at a party. I was just being overly ... overly ...

I know what Dan is about to say: That he was being overly "sensitive" or "jealous" or "possessive." I'm sitting there congratulating myself for being a wonderful therapist, for engaging Dan in a manner that's bringing forth this admission. I feel jolted, therefore, when Joanne interrupts to say:

JOANNE: *(indignantly)* Of *course* I wasn't doing anything wrong!

I say to myself: *Why did she have to say that—and in that tone? And at this delicate moment when Dan was reaching out. It's going to completely derail him. He certainly isn't going to admit now that he was overly sensitive, jealous, or possessive. She's made sure of that! He's probably going to take back what he has already said. What's wrong with her? Can't she see that Dan was being conciliatory? If she is immediately going to thwart every positive move he makes, what hope is there? Maybe she is unreasonable, just as Dan says.*

THERAPIST DISAPPROVAL

Couple therapists continually find themselves privately siding with one or the other partner—and they can change sides quickly. A moment ago I was siding with Joanne; now I'm siding with Dan. *What's her problem?* I ask myself. *Is she trying to sabotage the therapy? Dan makes a positive step and she punishes him. Could she be acting out some unresolved issue from childhood? Is she competitive? Is that her problem? Is she narcissistic? Is she trying to reassert control? Does she have a prob-*

*lem with intimacy—or with men? Maybe that's it. Dan reaches out, and
she gets nervous. Is she simply spiteful?*

These thoughts coursing through my mind indicate that I have
shifted to an adversarial mode. When I make such a shift, I immediately
lose the ability to:

- Listen
- Identify with the client—here, Joanne
- Empathize with her
- Appreciate her point of view
- Remember that she *has* a point of view
- Point to the confiding path
- Remember that there *is* such a path
- Look for the hidden rationality and appropriateness in what on
  the surface appears to be her irrational and inappropriate behavior
- Function as her scriptwriter

In a word, I lose my ability to do collaborative couple therapy. I
need a mental adjustment to restore my psychotherapeutic capabilities. I
see the specter of my mentor rising up in my mind telling me:

THE MENTOR: *Well, let's recognize that you've made the adversarial
shift of everyday life. Therapists do it too, you know. You're seeing
her as competitive, narcissistic, and spiteful. But don't worry, that's
bound to happen. You're disapproving of Joanne because she's
doing a poor job of representing herself. She isn't pulling you into
her experience. She isn't confiding. She isn't talking about her
thoughts and feelings in a way that would get you to empathize and
to identify with her. She isn't charming you, warming your heart,
winning you over.*

*Of course, that's also her problem with Dan: She isn't winning him
over. And that's Dan's problem with her: He isn't winning her over.*

*But look! Your disapproval toward Joanne puts you in contact
with the relationship problem of the moment: The poor job she is
doing of representing herself. That's the therapy right there! Your
job is to become spokesperson for Joanne—the partner whom, at
the moment, you are siding against—and then for Dan as well.*

The specter of my mentor, with all that she represents, readjusts my
mind. I hear the *whoosh* of my adversarial feelings rushing out the window and my collaborative feelings kaplunking back into place. My therapeutic capabilities have been restored. My feeling of disapproval, which
had brought about the loss of these capabilities, has been transformed

into a therapeutic instrument pointing me to the relationship problem of the moment: The particular way in which Joanne is doing a poor job of representing herself.

BECOMING SPOKESPERSON FOR THE PARTNER WHOM YOU ARE SIDING AGAINST

My way to help Joanne do a better job of representing herself is to figure out how what she's doing makes sense.

THERAPIST: (*to Joanne*) It looked like Dan was being conciliatory, but either it didn't seem conciliatory to you, or it was too little too late, or you've heard it all before, or you know something that I don't know, or it seemed like I was taking Dan's side, or it touched on something we haven't talked about yet—or *something*.

I'm telling Joanne "I know there must be a reason for your not being won over by what Dan just said, and I'm just trying to figure out what it is." In listing these possible reasons, I'm trying to prime the pump of her own thinking about the matter.

JOANNE: None of those things, really. It's more that . . . (*to Dan, softly*) it scares me how quickly things can go bad between us.

A moment ago Joanne was attacking: "I wasn't doing anything wrong!" Now she is confiding: "It scares me. . . . " My comment has shifted her from an adversarial into a collaborative state. She is winning me over, and my guess is that she is winning Dan over, too. I sit there congratulating myself for being a wonderful therapist—for so deftly bringing about this shift.

But uh-oh! Dan has a big frown on his face.

DAN: (*to Joanne*) You don't think standing two inches away from him was doing something wrong? Everyone was looking at you! You were making a complete fool of yourself!

Dan obviously hasn't heard a word of what Joanne and I just said. He's still back there fuming over Joanne's earlier "I wasn't doing anything wrong!" He felt stung by it and was simply waiting for us to finish so he could sting back. Feeling frustrated by Dan's so quickly destroying the collaborative spirit I had worked so hard to establish, I have the following 10-second mental tantrum: *Why does Dan have to be so thin-skinned? That's not going to help. He's so defensive—and narcissistic; he gets wounded so easily. And he's immature; he gets upset when things don't exactly go his way. And he always has to be in control. I don't understand what Joanne sees in him.*

I have again made the adversarial shift of everyday life, but now with respect to *Dan*. Again I have lost my therapeutic capabilities: My ability to listen to him, to empathize with him, to identify with him, and to look for ways in which his reactions might make sense. Again I hear the voice of my mentor telling me: "Your job is to become spokesperson for the partner who at the moment you are siding against."

Well, I know who *that* is.

THERAPIST: (*moving his chair next to Dan, facing Joanne, speaking for Dan, and thus* literally *becoming his spokesperson*) Okay, Dan, what you're saying in effect is: "Joanne, I'm still back on what you said a moment ago—I haven't heard anything since. Because it really stung!"

As Dan's spokesperson, I am having him confide that he felt stung—in contrast to what he did, which was simply to sting back. I am showing him how, at that crossroads moment, he could have confided rather than attacked.

But should I be speaking for Dan? Shouldn't he be speaking for himself? I think not, because I'm speaking for him in a way that he *can't* speak for himself. I'm having him confide. When you are in an adversarial state, as Dan is right now, you can't confide—you can only attack or defend. I'm demonstrating something that in the natural course of events couldn't and wouldn't occur.

DAN: It didn't just sting. I felt totally pissed!

Dan is telling me that I am misstating and minimizing what he felt.

THERAPIST: (*still speaking for Dan, welcoming his correction and incorporating it into the statement*) Right, "I felt totally pissed! And what pissed me was, well, to start with, I was trying to be conciliatory. Okay, I'm not proud of how I behaved at the party. I feel really bad about it. I was feeling left out and unimportant . . . "

As Dan's spokesperson, I'm having him do what people never do when they're in an adversarial state: admit things; and confide things. Being in an adversarial state means that you can't admit anything (except as a vehicle for proving the other person wrong, as in "I'm willing to admit that I was partly at fault here; that's the problem: You never admit anything!").

THERAPIST: (*continuing to speak for Dan*) " . . . But I was hoping that you'd like my admitting that you weren't doing anything wrong at the party. And I was hoping that you'd *really* like what I was about to say—what I was getting up my *courage* to say—that I know I was being . . . well, overly sensitive."

I'm trying to present Dan's position in a way that will be more satisfying to him than the way he put it and, at the same time, easier for Joanne to hear.

JOANNE: (*to Dan*) You were going to say that?

Joanne likes it. It *is* easier for her to hear.

DAN: (*snidely*) Of course! What do you think?

In response to which I tell myself: *Why does Dan have to be so vindictive? Joanne was coming around. She was softening. But no! Dan has to ruin it by making this totally gratuitous attack. I give up!* (I have shifted into an adversarial mode.)

DAN: (*to Joanne*) But then you had to get on your high horse!

Oh, so that's it! (I have shifted back into a collaborative mode, which enables me to resume as Dan's spokesperson and scriptwriter.)

THERAPIST: Okay, Dan, so you're saying to Joanne: "Yes, I was about to admit that I was oversensitive. But no, you had to get on your high horse. So *forget it!* I take it all back. I feel totally exposed and demolished and enraged and like never admitting anything to you ever again!"

I'm trying to express the outrage that, because Dan has been unable to do so, has kept him in an adversarial state.

DAN: (*hiding a smile*) Well, I don't take it *all* back.

Dan's smile reveals that he has shifted from an adversarial to a collaborative state—as a consequence of my having provided sufficient expression for his outrage. You can't smile when you're in an adversarial state; you can only smirk or snicker. You *can* smile when you're in an alienated state, but it is a forced, awkward, polite, social smile. Dan's collaborative response immediately elicits one from Joanne.

JOANNE: (*hiding her own smile*) I hope you don't take back the part about being "oversensitive." I really liked that part—although I don't think you really were so oversensitive. I *was* acting a little strange at the party.

Joanne's immediate response, now that Dan has become collaborative, is to jump over to his side and start looking for evidence to support what he has been saying. That's what happens when partners shift into a collaborative couple system; they automatically start looking for ways to go along with, agree with, and build on what the other person has been saying.

DAN: (*surprised and pleased*) Oh?

JOANNE: I was so glad to find someone I could talk to that I may have overdone it a little. I wasn't in the mood for a party. I didn't know anyone who was going to be there. I was afraid it wouldn't be any fun.

REVEALING THE CONVERSATION
HIDDEN IN THE FIGHT

This excerpt demonstrates three elements in the collaborative couples therapy effort to develop each partner's position:

1. Interviewing partners in search of the thoughts or feelings they might confide
2. Suggesting possibilities to grease the gears of their own thinking about the matter, at times making it a multiple-choice question
3. Speaking for them (in a method reminiscent of *doubling* in psychodrama)

At times, I conduct a conversation. I go back and forth between the partners, reshaping what each says to make it more satisfying to that person and easier for the other to hear. At times, I *have* the conversation for them. Taking my role as scriptwriter seriously, I create the entire script. Here is how I do that later in the session with Joanne and Dan:

THERAPIST: (*to Joanne and Dan*) There's a conversation you've been having that you might have missed because of the fight that you were also having. So let me exclude the fight so that we can clearly see the conversation. In this conversation, Dan, you began by saying, in essence: "Joanne, I was about to admit that maybe I was being overly sensitive—until you jumped on me, at which point I no longer felt like admitting anything." Then, Joanne, you said: "Well, yes, I *did* jump on you. I was upset about how fast things can get bad between us—how fast we jump on one another."

Joanne and Dan are intrigued by my finding this thread in what had seemed to them at the time a jumble of confusing and contradictory comments. I am revealing the conversation buried in the fight.

THERAPIST (*continuing*) Then, Dan, you said: "Well, okay, I'm not proud of what I did at the party. Why mince words? I was jealous." Then, Joanne, you said: "Well, I appreciate your admitting that, which immediately makes me want to admit that I *was* acting a little strange at the party, so you were on to something. You asked why I was so quiet in the car on the way over. I was worried that I wouldn't know anyone. I was so happy to find someone to talk to that I might have overdone it a little."

I'm describing the conversation Joanne and Dan might have been able to have were they in a collaborative couple system. I'm taking what they said in a blaming way that made it hard for the other to hear and am putting it in a form that makes it easy to hear—which, interestingly, is also a more satisfying form than what the partner originally said for him or herself.

THERAPIST: (*continuing*) Then, Dan, you said: "It's a relief to know that I wasn't *entirely* crazy. But now I'm upset about something else, for dragging you to the party." And, Joanne, you said: "It's no big deal. Don't worry about it. I drag *you* to parties. I'll tell you what I *want* you to worry about. I want you to worry about what I just said: How quickly things go bad between us and how awful it is when they do."

Why am I telling Joanne and Dan what they said? Weren't they there? Yes they were, but they were shifting in and out of an adversarial couple system, which means that they were unable to notice the conversation they were having.

THERAPIST: (*continuing*) Then, Dan, you said: "Yes, things *can* go bad between us quickly. You talk to some guy at a party and suddenly I feel left out and unimportant. It's like——." Well, actually, Dan, you didn't say what it *is* like, so let me suggest some possibilities and you can say if any of my guesses are close. Here, I'm you, talking to Joanne and you'd say: "Joanne, it's like I suddenly feel unlovable and unimportant and that maybe you should leave me out." Or, "It's like suddenly I don't exist anymore, it's just you and that guy." Or, "Our relationship goes *poof,* and I feel all alone." Or, "I feel humiliated and that everyone *is* watching." Or, "I feel I shouldn't be jealous and something is wrong with me that I am." Or, "I feel helpless; I need to get us out of there, and I can't figure out how to do it."

Should I be speculating about Dan's feelings? Isn't there a rule against such mind-reading? Shouldn't it apply to therapists also? I don't think so. I'm mind-reading to grease the gears of Dan's own speculations. I'm pointing him in the direction of soft underbelly feelings. Dan tears up slightly—which happens to people when someone brings to the surface thoughts and feelings that they have been struggling with alone. Something in my comment has touched him. And Joanne is touched by his being touched. I have taken the argument that he had been having with Joanne and have turned it into a moment of intimacy.

CAPTURING A THERAPEUTIC APPROACH IN A MOMENT

Why have I devoted so much space to describing just a few minutes of a single therapy session? Because collaborative couple therapy can best be understood by taking such a microscopic look. In this look, we saw how the therapist:

> Looks for opportunities to show partners how, by confiding thoughts and feelings about the partner or about the relationship, they can turn the relationship into a curative force for dealing with problems arising in the relationship.
>
> Uses his or her moment-to-moment feelings of disapproval to locate the relationship problem of the moment, namely, the particular ways the partners are doing a poor job of representing themselves.

Expresses the sense of rage, fear, helplessness, or hopelessness that, because the partner has been unable to express it adequately, has blocked his or her shift out of an adversarial or alienated state into a collaborative one.

Models a way of talking that doesn't occur in reality: Confiding in your partner when you're in a state in which you can only attack, defend, or avoid; appreciating the validity of your partner's position when your automatic response is to impeach it.

DEVELOPING A JOINT PLATFORM

If I'm modeling a way of talking that couldn't occur in reality (given the state of mind of the partners at the moment), what do they take away with them? What do they get out of it? The answer is, an increased potential to have such conversations when they *are* in a position to do so—for example, *after* a fight. Ordinarily couples don't want to talk about their fights afterwards. They're afraid of rekindling them—which they probably would. People are often emboldened to attempt such conversations, however, after hearing the ones I construct for them.

When partners attempt such conversations, they rarely talk in the ways I model for them. They come up with their own modified, personalized versions. Jasmine and Kevin, a couple I had been seeing, came in one session reporting success in short-circuiting fights that ordinarily would have spiraled out of control. One of them would turn to the other and say something like:

"Do we really want to be doing this?"
"What I'm saying is coming out a lot harsher than I wanted it to."
"I'm doing what I vowed never to do: Act like my father."
"I guess I'm being a little defensive here."
"You're probably right, but I'm too angry at the moment to want to admit it."
"Should we stop now or go on and ruin Sunday also?"
"This is the moment in the fight that I usually storm out and refuse to talk for the rest of the afternoon. But I don't feel up to it today."

These are potential turning-point statements. Made at the right moment (at a let-up in the fight when neither partner feels stung and needs to sting back and when both are weary of the fight)—and if not too much water has flowed over the dam—such comments can snap partners out of their adversarial couple system and into a collaborative one. The speaker is inviting the other partner to join him or her on a joint platform to look at the adversarial exchange they have been in.

None of these comments is one that I modeled for Jasmine and Kevin. They aren't parroting me. These comments emerged out of their improved ability to create a joint platform—something I *did* have something to do with. My therapeutic effort is devoted to showing partners how, at any moment, they can become resources and confidants to one another in dealing with the problems they are having with one another. I take whatever is on their minds—what they are talking about, the problems they report from the week—and I create the conversation they'd be able to have were they looking at it from a joint platform.

Although partners say things in fights that they don't mean, it is often only in fights that they say what they do mean. Partners can use what one of them blurts out in the course of a fight as an access-point into a conversation they may need to have. Joanne and Dan used his blurted out accusation about her flirting at the party to start a later conversation in which Joanne expressed how upset she is about how quickly things go bad between them, and Dan expressed how upset he is about how quickly he can feel forgotten and discarded.

The problem isn't so much these feelings in themselves as it is the lonely, isolated manner in which Joanne and Dan had been struggling with them. Confiding in one another about them, they no longer feel so alone. They are building (incorporating) their problem into the relationship in a way that makes it much less a problem. Creating a joint platform from which to look at the difficulties that you are having with your partner is in itself often a solution to them.

RELATION OF COLLABORATIVE COUPLE THERAPY TO OTHER APPROACHES

For more on collaborative couple therapy see my previous writings (Wile, 1981, 1988, 1993, 1994, 1995). I apply to couples a general form of psychodynamic thinking, ego analysis, developed by Bernard Apfelbaum (1966, 1977, 1982, 1983, 1988; Apfelbaum & Apfelbaum, 1985; Apfelbaum & Gill, 1989; Wile, 1984, 1985), which he built upon ideas from Freud (1926/1959) and Fenichel (1941).

At the core of Apfelbaum's thinking is the idea of entitlement. People feel unentitled to many of the thoughts and feelings coursing through their minds. Dan felt unentitled to his jealous twinge; he felt humiliated by it. The question then became: Did he feel entitled to the *next* feeling coursing through his mind: his *humiliation* about being jealous? If he did, he might have been able to tell Joanne: "I'm afraid to tell you this but—okay, I'll tell you. I got a little jealous a moment ago when you were talking to that guy." He'd be taking her into his confidence, something that he could do only were he to feel sufficiently entitled to this feeling to be able to take himself into his confidence.

What we deal with in therapy is the result of feeling threatened by and unentitled to thoughts and feelings. At such moments, people try to talk themselves out of the unacceptable thought or feeling, maneuver around it, or put the blame on someone else. They try to distract, justify, soothe, or numb themselves. Dan thought of getting a drink, finding a beautiful woman to talk to, getting out of there, and putting the blame on Joanne. The terms that Freud used to describe such events are *repression* and *defense*. But it is a repression and defense in the fine-grain of the moment and in reaction to the person's sense of unentitlement to the thought or feeling of that moment.

Although developed from psychodynamic roots, collaborative couple therapy often appears to have more in common with family systems theory, cognitive therapy, and social constructivism. Collaborative couple therapy can be thought of as an application of family systems thinking to couples. A couple relationship is defined as shifting among three couple systems. The therapeutic task is to harness the power of the collaborative couple system to deal with the alienated and adversarial couple systems.

The goal of collaborative couple therapy is a *cognitive* one: To put partners in a position in which they can think, reason, talk, and see the big picture; that is, to shift into a collaborative couple system. The first task, however, is for therapists to put their own cognitive houses in order: to get *themselves* in position to think, reason, talk, and see the big picture.

Part of getting ourselves in such a position requires reexamining some of our traditional forms of psychotherapeutic thinking. There is a developing awareness in psychotherapy that many of our standard terms, concepts, and interventions are pejorative and pathologizing. Kohut (1984) drew attention to what he saw as a hidden moralism in classic psychoanalytic thinking. Wachtel (1993), Josephs (1995), and Stolorow, Atwood, and Brandchaft (1994) have written particularly incisively about pejorative interpretations. Behaviorists have been aware of this problem for some time (see Wachtel, 1982; and Jacobson & Christensen, 1996). Johnson (1996) has eloquently described the pejorative tone of and the distortions implicit in the concept of dependency. The cutting edge of contemporary family therapy—social constructivism, as represented in particular by narrative therapy and solution-focused therapy—starts from the recognition that many of the traditional ways we think about and talk to clients reinforce the self-critical thinking (stories, narratives, discourses) that lies at the root of their problems (see Eron & Lund, Chapter 12, this volume).

In collaborative couple therapy, the shift from pejorative to non-pejorative thinking occurs within the session and in the fine-grain of the moment. The therapist's awareness that he or she has just adopted a pejorative, accusatory, pathologizing stance cues him or her to the relationship problem of the moment: the particular way that this partner, feeling unentitled to his or her thoughts and feelings, is unable to confide them and, instead, attacks or avoids (eliciting the therapist's negative response).

SELECTING ISSUES AND COUPLES

In adopting a short-term approach, therapists typically think that they have to limit therapy to the number and type of issues that can be dealt with in the time available. Such limiting is unnecessary in collaborative couple therapy, since there is only one issue: to increase the partners' ability to create a joint platform from which to talk about *whatever* is at issue. Each session is the next lesson in this effort. Like bowling lessons, each new one can help, and you can stop at any point.

Also like bowling lessons, the sessions may be weekly, biweekly, intermittently, on demand, or whatever. Partners are provided with audiotapes of their sessions so that they can listen back—now from a more observing position—and catch what they might have missed the first time. The decision when to terminate therapy is made by the partners; they may resume at any time.

Couple treatment is sometimes viewed as consisting of phases such as (1) creating a therapeutic alliance, (2) dealing with resistance and control issues, (3) the emergence of core interpersonal fears, and (4) producing a therapeutic effect. In collaborative couple therapy, all of these occur concurrently; the single therapeutic task (developing each partner's perspective and creating moments of intimacy) simultaneously creates a therapeutic alliance, deals with resistance and control issues, brings forth core interpersonal fears, and produces whatever therapeutic effect is to occur.

There is no need for the therapist to preselect which couples might benefit most from collaborative couple therapy. Since partners get an immediate taste of what the therapy is going to be like—that is, there are no preliminary phases such as creating a therapeutic alliance—the partners are quickly in position (after just 15 minutes, one session, two sessions, or whatever) to judge for themselves whether therapy shows promise of helping—or at least enough so to try another session or two.

Couple therapy is essentially an experiment. It's an experiment to see whether, in the presence of the therapist, the couple can talk more usefully than they can on their own and whether the positive effects generalize to their lives outside the session. (In the case of spousal battering, therapy is conducted only if the battering has stopped.)

Every person has his or her set of underlying issues and unresolvable personal problems. Every relationship has its set of unresolvable problems. When you start a relationship, you are in essence choosing a particular set of unresolvable problems. There are always going to be disagreements—ways in which, and issues over which, the partners rub one another the wrong way. There are always going to be incompatibilities—conflicts over which the partners have not yet arrived at (and may never arrive at) a fully satisfactory compromise or accommodation. What's crucial is how the partners relate about the moment-to-moment manifestations of these incompatibilities. The goal is to increase the partners' abilities to confide in one another about these manifestations and, by so doing, to build the problem into the relationship. This includes, for Dan and Joanne, their becoming increasingly familiar with (i.e., creating a joint platform from which to discuss) Dan's humiliation about feeling left out and unimportant and Joanne's dread about how quickly things go bad between them.

In collaborative couple therapy, we take whoever the partners are and whatever is happening between them and try to build the relationship out of that.

Is this kind of couple therapy appropriate for nonpsychologically minded clients, for example, those who wouldn't sit still for the kind of detailed, back-and-forth conversations that I just constructed for Joanne and Dan? People *will* sit still, no matter how nonpsychologically minded, as long as the therapist is making sense of an exchange that had left them confused and disheartened.

Let us say that my conversation for Dan and Joanne *didn't* make much sense to him. He gives a dismissive shrug. My task then is to find words for that shrug; that is, to relate to him collaboratively about it. After asking about his reaction, I would put together the following statement for him:

THERAPIST: (*as Dan's spokesperson*) Okay, Dan, so you're saying that the long, involved statement I just made a moment ago didn't make much sense to you. It was just a bunch of words. All you know is that when Joanne is upset with you, as she seems now, you get confused, blank out, and don't know *what* to do.

I'd expect Dan to nod his head to *that*.

THE HUMAN CONDITION

Collaborative couple therapy is based on a view of human beings as scurrying after thoughts and feelings that elude their grasp. A relationship provides a way of catching up with some of them. In the session, Joanne caught up with her distress about how quickly things turn bad, and Dan caught up with his distress about how quickly he feels left out and unimportant.

For a few moments, Joanne and Dan had a intimate relationship from which to observe the nonintimate (alienated, adversarial) relationship they had been having. They got together in the act of talking about how they had been at odds. The goal of therapy is to provide partners with an increasingly more usable joint platform from which to recover from their inevitable adversarial and alienated exchanges and to scan their fights for the useful information contained in them.

REFERENCES

Apfelbaum, B. (1966). On ego psychology: A critique of the structural approach to psychoanalysis. *International Journal of Psycho-Analysis, 47,* 451–475.

Apfelbaum, B. (1977). A contribution to the development of the behavioral-analytic sex therapy model. *Journal of Sex and Marital Therapy, 3,* 128–138.

Apfelbaum, B. (1982). The clinical necessity for Kohut's self theory. *Voices, 18,* 43–49.

Apfelbaum, B. (1983, August). *Introduction to the symposium "Ego Analysis and Ego Psychology."* Paper presented at the Annual Convention of the American Psychological Association, Anaheim, CA.

Apfelbaum, B. (1988). An ego-analytic perspective on desire disorders. In S. R. Leiblum & R. C. Rosen (Eds.), *Sexual desire disorders* (pp. 75–104). New York: Guilford Press.

Apfelbaum, B., & Apfelbaum, C. (1985). The ego-analytic approach to sexual apathy. In D. C. Goldberg (Ed.), *Contemporary marriage: Special issues in couples therapy* (pp. 439–481). Homewood, IL: Dorsey.

Apfelbaum, B., & Gill, M. M. (1989). Ego analysis and the relativity of defense: Technical implications of the structural theory. *Journal of the American Psychoanalytic Association, 37,* 1071–1096.

Fenichel, O. (1941). *Problems of psychoanalytic technique.* New York: Psychoanalytic Quarterly.

Freud, S. (1959). Inhibitions, symptoms and anxiety. In J. Strachey (Ed. and Trans.), *Standard edition of the complete psychological works of Sigmund Freud* (Vol. 20, pp. 77–174). London: Hogarth Press. (Original work published 1926)

Jacobson, N. S., & Christensen, A. (1996). *Integrative couple therapy: Promoting acceptance and change*. New York: Norton.

Johnson, S. (1996). *The practice of emotionally focused marital therapy: Creating connection*. New York: Brunner/Mazel.

Josephs, L. (1995). *Balancing empathy and interpretation: Relational character analysis*. Northvale, NJ: Jason Aronson.

Kohut, H. (1984). *How does analysis cure?* (P. E. Stepansky & A. Goldberg, Eds.). Chicago: University of Chicago Press.

Stolorow, R., Atwood, G., & Brandchaft, B. (Eds.). (1994). *The intersubjective perspective*. New York: Jason Aronson.

Wachtel, P. L. (Ed.), (1982). *Resistance: Psychodynamic and behavioral approaches*. New York: Plenum Press.

Wachtel, P. L. (1993). *Therapeutic communication: Knowing what to say when*. New York: Guilford Press.

Wile, D. B. (1981). *Couples therapy: A nontraditional approach*. New York: Wiley.

Wile, D. B. (1984). Kohut, Kernberg, and accusatory interpretations. *Psychotherapy: Theory, Research, Practice, and Training, 21*, 353–364.

Wile, D. B. (1985). Psychotherapy by precedent: Unexamined legacies from pre-1920 psychoanalysis. *Psychotherapy: Theory, Research, Practice, and Training, 22*, 793–802.

Wile, D. B. (1988). *After the honeymoon: How conflict can improve your relationship*. New York: Wiley.

Wile, D. B. (1993). *After the fight: Using your disagreements to build a stronger relationship*. New York: Guilford Press.

Wile, D. B. (1994). The ego-analytic approach to emotion in couples therapy. In S. M. Johnson & L. S. Greenberg (Eds.), *The heart of the matter: Perspective on emotion in marital therapy* (pp. 27–45). New York: Brunner/Mazel.

Wile, D. B. (1995). The ego-analytic approach to couple therapy. In N. S. Jacobson & A. S. Gurman (Eds.), *Clinical handbook of couple therapy* (pp. 91–120). New York: Guilford Press.

10

◄o►

INTEGRATIVE COUPLE THERAPY

The Dyadic Relationship
of Acceptance and Change

ERIKA LAWRENCE
KATHLEEN ELDRIDGE
ANDREW CHRISTENSEN
NEIL S. JACOBSON

Any form of couple therapy may sound promising in theory. However, therapy is only useful if couples improve. We as clinicians have developed numerous forms of couple therapy without testing them to see if they are truly effective. Yet there are a number of couple therapies that do have empirical support. Greenberg and Johnson cite empirical evidence supporting their emotionally focused marital therapy (e.g., Johnson & Greenberg, 1987; see Johnson, Chapter 2, this volume). Snyder presents data in support of insight-oriented marital therapy (Snyder & Wills, 1989). Of all of the interventions that couple therapists have tested and supported empirically, however, traditional behavioral couples therapy[1] (Christensen, Jacobson, & Babcock, 1995) is by far the most widely tested. It is also the only form of couple therapy the clinical psychology division of the American Psychological Association lists as meeting the criteria of an "empirically validated treatment" (Crits-Christoph, Frank, Chambless, Brody, & Karp, 1995). Yet only half of all couples who are treated with this therapy experience long-term improvement (Jacobson, Schmaling, & Holtzworth-Monroe, 1987).

Traditional behavioral couple therapists view relationship distress as arising from a decrease in interaction that is reinforcing and an increase in interaction that is aversive. Partners also experience "reinforcement erosion" (Jacobson & Margolin, 1979), in which they become accustomed to once pleasing behavior and no longer find it as rewarding. In addition, many couples do not have the communication and problem-solving skills to handle the inevitable conflicts that arise in any long-term relationship. Their inability to manage these conflicts leads to tension, anger, and distress.

Based on this model of relationship distress, traditional couple therapists try to restore relationship satisfaction and reduce conflict by getting partners to change their actions toward one another. In a strategy called "behavior exchange," therapists help partners generate lists of positive acts and encourage them to increase and reinforce demonstrations of that behavior. In the strategies of communication training and problem-solving training, therapists teach couples to communicate more effectively and solve their conflicts more amicably. Further, they often assign homework to encourage partners to practice the skills they've learned in therapy at home.

Couple researchers have conducted two dozen studies on traditional couple therapy in five different countries (Baucom & Hoffman, 1986; Hahlweg & Markman, 1988; Jacobson, 1978, 1984). In controlled outcome studies, researchers have shown that this type of behavioral therapy is superior to no treatment control conditions and leads to decreased verbal aggression such as insults, increased relationship satisfaction, and increased positive behavior (Baucom & Epstein, 1990). In a longitudinal study, Jacobson (1984) found that 72% of treated couples improved after treatment, with 58% scoring in the maritally satisfied range. Most of these couples maintained their gains through 6 months. However, approximately 30% relapsed to a distressed level after 2 years, the majority declining between years 1 and 2 (Jacobson et al., 1987). Thus, only 50% of all couples treated with traditional behavioral therapy achieve and maintain gains in marital satisfaction (Jacobson et al., 1987). The couples who typically improve are younger and less distressed, more emotionally engaged, and less polarized in their disagreements (Baucom & Hoffman, 1986; Hahlweg, Schindler, Revenstorf, & Brengelmann, 1984; Jacobson, Follette, & Pagel, 1986).

Because of the limited effectiveness of behavioral couple therapy, many professionals have tried to modify it and test new protocols against the existing strategies. For example, several researchers have compared cognitive marital therapy (i.e., cognitive restructuring techniques) to the behavioral techniques and have not achieved superior results (e.g., Baucom, Sayers, & Sher, 1990). Other researchers have *added* cognitive strategies to the traditional interventions and have also not achieved superior outcomes (e.g., Emmelkamp et al., 1988). Fincham, Bradbury, and Beach (1990) argue that cognitive techniques have not yet received an effective trial when combined with traditional couple therapy. Nevertheless, researchers' attempts to enhance traditional behavioral treatment with cognitive techniques so far have not been empirically successful.

Andrew Christensen and Neil Jacobson have also attempted to enhance behavioral couple therapy. They have added strategies to help couples emotionally accept each other *before* trying to implement the changes in communication and problem solving stressed in traditional behavioral therapy. Christensen and Jacobson call their new intervention integrative couple therapy[2] (ICT; Christensen et al., 1995; Jacobson & Christensen, 1996). They include the three existing behavioral change techniques mentioned earlier: behavior exchange, communication skills training, and problem-solving training. However, they have added four new strategies to promote acceptance: (1) empathic joining around the problem, (2) unified detachment from the conflict, (3) tolerance building, and (4) self-care. Christensen and Jacobson have conducted a pilot study with 21 couples, comparing ICT to behavioral couple therapy. The couples who received their new treatment did better than the couples who received traditional couple therapy alone (Jacobson, Christensen, Prince, Cordova, & Eldridge, 1999).

In sum, behavioral couple therapy has limitations but is the first couple therapy to be declared empirically valid. Further, based on initial evidence from the pilot study, Christensen and Jacobson's therapy is the first modified version of behavioral couple therapy to *outperform* it. Christensen and Jacobson are currently conducting a large-scale clinical trial to compare ICT and traditional couple therapy and are writing a manual for couples (Christensen & Jacobson, 1999).

INTEGRATIVE COUPLE THERAPY: SESSION BY SESSION

ICT consists of 20 to 25 sessions: 3 to 4 for assessment, when we gather information; 1 devoted to feedback, when we present the couple's dynamic and relationship themes; and 15 to 20 for treatment and termination, when we implement the emotional acceptance and change strategies. Because Christensen and Jacobson are still conducting clinical trials to determine the efficacy of ICT, we recommend that therapists use it in its existing format and length. Pending further empirical support, we will begin experimenting with comparable short-term versions.

Assessment Phase

During the assessment phase, we give couples several questionnaires to fill out and meet with them together for two or three sessions and with each partner individually for one session. We evaluate five areas of the marriage and then determine how best to help the couple. The five marital areas we assess are (1) level of distress, (2) level of relationship commitment, (3) what issues are causing conflict, (4) why these issues are so problematic for this couple, and (5) what individual and relationship strengths are holding the couple together. As we assess each area, we make decisions about which treatment strategies would be most beneficial for each couple and the order in which we should implement those techniques.

Distress

To determine a couple's level of distress, we give the partners questionnaires and discuss their discord during both the conjoint and individual sessions. First, we administer self-report questionnaires that measure relationship satisfaction. The standard questionnaires we use are the Dyadic Adjustment Scale (Spanier, 1976) and the Marital Satisfaction Inventory (Snyder, 1979). Second, we assess their distress during the two to three conjoint sessions. For example, a very distressed couple might discuss separation, have tremendous difficulty listening to each other, or only discuss their problems with an enormous amount of anger. Third, we assess each partner's distress level during the individual session. Often, partners will enter therapy but won't feel comfortable expressing how unhappy they are with their marriage in front of their partner. In these cases, we can usually get a better sense of how distressed they are when we speak to them individually. For example, a husband may not divulge that he wants to separate in front of his wife but will tell us privately.

Commitment

We evaluate a couple's level of commitment through questionnaires and individual sessions. First, we administer self-report questionnaires such as the Marital Status Inventory (Weiss & Cerreto, 1980), which assesses the specific steps each partner has taken toward divorce (e.g., consulting a lawyer), and the Dyadic Adjustment Scale, which has an item that measures level of commitment. Second, we discuss each partner's commitment to the relationship during the individual sessions. Although some couples may be willing to discuss a lack of commitment during the conjoint sessions, we find that partners are more willing to admit that their commitment to the relationship is low privately.

Before we conduct separate interviews, we let both partners know that our role in therapy is to be the *couple's* therapist, not either partner's individual therapist. Because of this role, we are in a difficult position if one partner shares a secret during an individual session. We are obligated to maintain confidentiality but keeping secrets would prevent us from forming an alliance with the couple as a unit. Therefore, if either partner divulges something important during the individual interview, we encourage him or her to disclose the secret. In the extreme, we may insist that the partner divulge the information to his or her partner in order for us to proceed with therapy.

There are several examples of issues that we believe need to be disclosed before we can continue couple therapy. For example, one partner may confide that couple therapy is a last ditch effort before filing for divorce. In this case, we would encourage the individual to share this. Further, if the couple decided to separate, we would do separation counseling instead of couple therapy.

Another relevant example is when one partner reveals an affair. We have three ways of responding to this situation. First, we encourage the partner to end the affair. Second, if he or she will not end the affair, we encourage disclosure to the partner. Third, if the partner will not disclose or end the affair, we refuse to do couple therapy. We believe it is fruitless to begin couple therapy when one partner is keeping a secret that makes it difficult, if not impossible, to improve the relationship.

Divisive Issues and Why They Are Problematic

In conjoint and individual sessions, we assess the third and fourth domains, issues that divide the couple and reasons why these issues cause such problems with relationship satisfaction and intimacy. We try to understand why couples are in conflict by examining how they have developed incompatibilities and how they have attempted to cope with them. Conflicts, as conceptualized in ICT, derive from normal differences between partners. These differences develop because of partners' personal histories, their genetic make-up, their current stressors, and their gender and cultural socialization. As partners cope with their differences, they often engage in self-defeating behavior that leaves them feeling even more polarized.

For example, Dave and Liza, a couple in their mid-20s, married 4 years ago. Early in their relationship, they agreed upon and were happy with the amount of time they spent at work and at home. Last year, Dave's company promoted him, and since then he has spent less time with Liza. Liza became angry with Dave about their increased time apart, and Dave withdrew further from her. He spent even more time at work and was less connected to Liza when he was home. In sum, the amount of time Dave and Liza spend together, a topic they initially agreed on, became an area of disagreement, led to an increase in anger and withdrawal, and resulted in an increase in incompatibility.

We call our analysis of a couple's incompatibilities and their efforts to cope with them our "formulation" of their problems. This formulation provides the conceptual framework for our treatment.

Individual and Relationship Strengths

Partners' strengths include individual qualities that originally attracted them to each other and aspects of the relationship that are keeping the couple together. Identifying the healthy, functional aspects of the relationship is important for several reasons. First, by closely examining a couple's dyadic strengths, we gain information about how they have successfully resolved conflict in the past. For example, a couple may exhibit an admirable tenacity to stay with a problem until it is solved. Second, individual strengths are often key to helping partners achieve emotional acceptance, one of our main goals. The qualities that each partner initially found attractive in the other may have become the source of their incompatibilities over time. Reminding partners of the positive aspects of the now-aversive behavior may help them become more accepting of it. For instance, Amy is a 37-year-old lawyer who married Michael, a 35-year-old journalist, 12 years ago. When they first married, Amy was attracted to Michael's ability to "live life to the fullest." She now views these qualities as irresponsible and financially risky. During treatment, we reminded Amy of the positive features she originally saw in Michael's behavior to help her begin to accept their differences.

We also look at the extent to which couples approach their problems collaboratively. The degree to which couples see themselves as a unit guides the order of our strategies. If partners see their problems as stemming from joint contributions, they are more willing to change; therefore, we can begin treatment with a greater focus on the traditional behavioral techniques. In contrast, if partners see each other as adversaries, they will be less willing to change. We would then begin treatment with the emotional acceptance strategies to help each partner better understand the other's feelings and thoughts. After the acceptance strategies have softened couples so that they feel less antagonistic and more empathic, we would introduce the change strategies.

Feedback Phase

In the feedback session, we discuss with the couple the five areas of assessment and our plan for treatment. We try to model effective communication skills by reflecting each partner's side of the conflict in a sympathetic light and emphasizing the cyclical nature of their arguments. Most of the feedback session is devoted to our formulation of the couple's problems. The following excerpts are from a feedback session for Don and Linda, an Asian-American couple in their 30s who frequently argue about demonstrations of affection. The therapist describes Don's and Linda's different levels of emotional expressiveness as arising from their very different childhood experiences.

THERAPIST: (*to Linda*) Both your [mother] and your father were quite up front with criticism, judgment, and anger. And you grew up with what you would consider a normal amount of anger, rejection, criticism. A pretty high level perhaps by other people's standards. And it seems like if there was one theme that you might have taken from your family background it is perhaps a special sensitivity to being rejected.

THERAPIST: (*to Linda about Don*) He has a very even temper, not a lot of highs or lows and doesn't show those. And, in fact, he was rewarded and shaped in his family and culture not to show a lot of emotion and not to be very expressive. And at work he even gets rewarded for that—he gets into less conflict, and things go better. So for family reasons and for work-related reasons, this certain pattern was effective for him, but he acknowledges and agrees that it comes out being flat with you, that he might feel very cozy and connected with you and Linda, you're feeling, "Where is he, what is he thinking, what is he doing? If he's thinking anything, he's not sharing it with me."

LINDA: (*Looks at Don and nods in agreement.*)

THERAPIST: And so rather than seeing an even-tempered person pursuing the middle way, you look at him and think he's "romance-dead." So Linda, you're having a lot of feelings of disappointment and frustration and abandonment, and prior to now it built up and built up, and then the volcano erupts. And then you would say, "Approach me more!" and he's (*therapist shrinks back and looks fearful*).

That's the bind; that there's so much anger coming from your hurt spot because your expectations are so different from [one another].

The therapist frames Don and Linda's dynamic as caused by a basic difference in styles of expressing affection. Although both partners already recognize that they differ in this domain, and that their opposing styles lead to conflict, they are at an impasse. Linda feels she needs more warmth and is considering abandoning the relationship if Don does not provide more affection. Although Don is trying to change, his ingrained style of communicating is undemonstrative. Further, it is hard for him to respond to Linda's demands with more kisses, hugs, and loving statements, because he fears her anger and withdraws from it. It is exactly when she demands affection that he is least able to show it. Consequently, Don is frustrated that Linda believes his lack of affection represents a lack of love for her and that his attempts to be loving have gone unnoticed and unacknowledged.

We work to help couples see their differences as common and understandable. In the above excerpt, the therapist points out the reasons Don and Linda have opposite styles to encourage them to perceive each other's behavior as the natural consequence of each one's particular background, rather than as demanding, blameworthy, unloving, or intentionally hurtful behavior. This explanation for the way they relate to each other also highlights how challenging it is for them to change, because it describes their styles as lifelong traits, thus validating their struggle to meet each other's expectations. For example, the therapist sympathizes with Don's struggle to be more expressive and with how difficult it is for Linda to withhold her demands for more affection. This allows them to view each other more empathically and to be less blaming. Further, the therapist describes Linda's demands in ways that highlight Linda's feelings of disappointment, frustration, and abandonment. This description enables Don to see Linda's reactions as understandable responses to unmet expectations rather than as unreasonable demands for more affection.

We first present the formulation in the feedback session, then subsequently throughout treatment in the context of discussing ongoing conflicts. For Don and Linda, one primary goal of treatment was for them to understand the reasons for their own and their partner's reactions and to understand that their problems with expressiveness stem from a basic difference between them that leads to polarization. Once partners embrace this perspective and become more sympathetic to one another, aversive behavior may spontaneously decrease and/or reactions to negative actions may become less intense. Specifically, Linda might appreciate Don's difficulty showing affection, given his upbringing and her angry demands, and Don might understand Linda's need for more affection given her family background and his unresponsiveness. Such understanding would increase emotional acceptance of Linda's needs and Don's lack of demonstrativeness, leading to a reduction in Don's frustration with Linda's demands and in Linda's anger about Don's inexpressiveness.

Treatment Phase Overview:
Four Types of Discussions during Therapy

During the treatment phase, we choose the content of each session based on the issue that is most emotionally salient to the couple. The four types of discussions we usually have during therapy sessions are (1) a discussion of a recent positive incident (e.g., a conversation that went well); (2) a discussion of a recent conflictual incident (e.g., a conversation that went poorly); (3) a general discussion of a difference between partners and the way each partner's behavior affects the other; and (4) a discussion of an upcoming event where the couple anticipates that they will have a conflict. The most common discussion targets a recent incident, either positive or negative. Recent positive incidents are important because we can help the couple understand what they did well and reinforce any constructive behavior they used.

However, we typically wind up focusing on the second type of discussion, conflicts that the couple was *not* able to resolve. This is especially common during the early stages of therapy, when partners have more arguments than constructive conversations. When we discuss a recent conflict, we focus on the thoughts and feelings that triggered each partner's behavior during the initial stages of the disagreement. This is far more productive in therapy than rehashing a heated conflict. The middle or later stages of an argument often consist of criticisms, insults, and accusations. It is more difficult for partners to accept hurtful behavior like this in each other. Therefore, we try to help partners understand and articulate the thoughts and feelings that led up to their hurtful words and actions. When partners hear these emotions, it is easier for them to understand and accept how their partner behaved. For example, it is easier for a wife to understand and accept her husband's fear about bringing up the controversial topic of buying a new car than it is for her to understand and accept the angry accusations he ends up making about her in the heat of an argument about this purchase. Further, focusing on thoughts and feelings, rather than on what each partner did, helps couples get past their anger and facilitates their recovery from the incident.

General discussions, the third type, often follow descriptions of recent incidents. We use general discussions to reiterate our formulation of the couple's problems or to modify that formulation. Our goal is to keep our nonblaming conceptualization of their relationship constantly in their awareness.

We discuss upcoming incidents, the fourth type of discussion, when a couple anticipates a conflict. For example, Mark and Angela were in their early 20s and had lived together for 2 years when they came in for couple therapy. They frequently argued about Angela's parents, who disapproved of Mark. As Thanksgiving drew closer, and they prepared to go to Angela's parents' home for the holiday, Mark became irritable and withdrawn. Both Mark and Angela expected that they would argue when they returned home after Thanksgiving, because they typically argued after seeing her parents. To combat this, during the last session before Thanksgiving, the therapist focused on Mark's fears about seeing Angela's parents and on Angela's anxiety and frustration as she tried to appease both Mark and her parents. Next, the therapist explored the thoughts and feelings that triggered Mark and Angela's typical conflict after they came home. Once Thanksgiving came around, because they had discussed the visit in advance, Mark felt more comfortable talking to and participating in activities with his in-laws. Further, Angela made more of an effort to facilitate conversations between her parents and Mark.

Treatment Phase 1: Emotional Acceptance Strategies

As we mentioned earlier, we choose whether to start with emotional acceptance or behavioral change strategies based on the immediate needs of the couple. Occasionally, we will begin with the behavioral techniques. For example, a highly collaborative couple in which both partners are motivated to change their own behavior would be ripe for traditional couple therapy strategies. However, in most cases, we start with the emotional acceptance interventions and follow these with the change techniques.

We use four strategies to help couples achieve emotional acceptance: (1) empathic joining around the problem, (2) unified detachment from the conflict, (3) tolerance building, and (4) self-care. Our goal is to get partners to see each other's behavior in a more sympathetic light and to work as a team to solve their conflicts. We want partners to be more "emotionally accepting" of each other, so that each will be more open and responsive to the behavioral change techniques during the latter part of treatment.

Emotional Acceptance through Empathic Joining around the Problem

Most couples who enter therapy are focused on blaming their anger and frustration on their partner. Others are withdrawn and emotionally disengaged from each other. With both types of couples, any expression of positive emotions often appears superficial and forced. Therefore, our first strategy is to help partners feel closer. The first step in restoring intimacy is helping them talk and listen to each other without accusations. We do this by encouraging couples to talk about their experiences rather than discussing what they believe their mate thinks or feels. If speakers focus on their own feelings and stop blaming their partners, then listeners are freed from coming up with defenses, contrary examples, and counterattacks; they can just listen and understand. When partners are angry or defensive, it is difficult for them to understand or empathize with each other's behavior.

Once couples are communicating more effectively, our overriding goal is to restore intimacy by encouraging partners to express feelings that will elicit compassionate or empathic responses from their mates. We differentiate between two types of emotions to accomplish this goal. One type are the "hard" emotions, such as frustration, resentment, blame, and disgust. The other type are the "soft" or vulnerable emotions, such as fear, sadness, and disappointment. For angry couples, eliciting a compassionate response from a partner typically requires a disclosure of soft feelings from his or her mate. In emotionally disengaged couples, fostering empathic responses may require that partners voice their hard emotions. In short, we take a functional approach to this task by considering the characteristics of each couple to determine which type of disclosure, such as angry or sad, would serve to foster "empathic joining" around the problem, which then may restore intimacy in the relationship.

Johnson and Greenberg (1987), who developed emotionally focused marital therapy, use similar strategies to encourage partners to express feelings related to attachment needs (see Johnson, Chapter 2, this volume). Although our approach is not based on attachment, we believe that when partners express anger, they also feel hurt; when they voice resentment, they feel disappointment; and when they make accusations, they feel insecure about their partners' feelings toward them. Further, although we believe partners feel afraid, sad, and disappointed, they may be only dimly aware of these emotions or may be uncomfortable voicing them for fear of feeling too vulnerable. Once therapists create an atmosphere in which partners can stop blaming each other, express softer emotions, and receive compassion and support from each other, they will feel closer in their relationship.

When Matt and Sheri, a married couple in their 50s, entered therapy, they were extremely angry. In their formulation, the therapist described Sheri as filling the "domestic" role in the relationship because she was the oldest of her family and had shouldered many of the caretaking responsibilities of raising her younger siblings. She enjoyed being in control at home and was comfortable taking care of her husband and the household duties. In contrast, Matt was an only child and wasn't as comfortable as Sheri in the role of caregiver. This difference had never been a problem during their marriage until financial trouble forced them to take in boarders for income, a responsibility Sheri could not handle on her own. Eventually, Sheri began voicing her frustrations to Matt, who became defensive and withdrawn. A pattern of attack and withdrawal was apparent by the time they entered therapy. In the excerpts below, Matt and Sheri discuss a recent argument that highlights this typical pattern.

SHERI: And then when I came out there and saw the socks I felt anger again in myself.

THERAPIST: Okay, so now it's the second time. You feel . . . ?

SHERI: I felt anger.

THERAPIST: Because, you're feeling . . . ?

SHERI: We talked about it. I said, "What are your socks doing there?" and he said "Oh, I can put them away," so then I figured, "Okay, he won't do that again."

THERAPIST: But the second time, then you feel anger?

SHERI: Yeah, I was angry.

In this excerpt, the therapist tried to elicit feelings such as hurt from Sheri by saying, "Because you're feeling . . . ?" but Sheri continued to focus on the specific incident and her anger. Sometimes partners will spontaneously share their vulnerable feelings, but frequently the therapist needs to suggest emotions they might be experiencing, such as fear or sadness, to get them to elaborate on the soft instead of the hard feelings.

THERAPIST: And that anger comes from feeling . . . ? (*pause*) My guess is it's similar to some feelings you talked about before.

SHERI: Well, a feeling of being ignored, ignored completely because obviously he picked up those, and then he just ignored me and went right on about his business dropping his socks again.

THERAPIST: So, you weren't important?

SHERI: No, no. And when I holler he does it, and otherwise [the socks] pile up on the floor.

THERAPIST: So, you felt ignored. So, if we were to make a general principle about when you've expressed a feeling or request to Matt and it seems to you that he's not honoring it, not respecting it, not responding to it, because it's not visible to you that he is, you feel ignored. And I'm thinking of what you've said before, that you also feel sort of alone in this or kind of like you don't have a partner. Is that right?

SHERI: (*Nods in agreement.*)

THERAPIST: So try and say that in your own words to Matt because I think this is something that happens over and over again in your relationship. Let's try to make it a general principle. Say what I said: "When this happens, I feel this."

SHERI: When I do make a request or express my feelings and you answer me with, "I'll do it later," or go on about what you're doing, it makes me feel like I'm on my own—I'm doing this alone. It makes me feel like I don't have a partner. It makes me feel I've got to do all this myself. I don't want to be that way. It's hard for me to feel good about myself.

In this excerpt, the therapist hoped to encourage Sheri to elaborate on vulnerable emotions by suggesting that she might have felt the same way she described feeling in previous arguments with Matt, such as feeling unimportant and alone. By making this suggestion, the therapist related this particular argument to other incidents and to a general pattern or theme for Matt and Sheri. Eventually, Sheri moved away from the angry, blaming stance and disclosed two soft emotions that are evoked in this pattern: feeling alone and without a partner and not feeling good about herself.

Ideally, once disclosures go from hard to soft, the listening partner changes from defensive to compassionate. Sometimes the listener responds empathically without therapist intervention, and the effect can be a dramatic increase in intimacy. However, at times the therapist needs to prompt the listener to reflect the feelings just expressed.

THERAPIST: Just sticking to that first part, Matt, of what she said, what did you hear her say? When this happens, how does it feel to Sheri?

MATT: That she's not feeling honored, not feeling, what's the word? She's feeling alone and not respected.

THERAPIST: What happens to trigger that? What is it that causes her to feel alone, in her eyes?

MATT: (*defensively*) When she doesn't feel she's getting attention, doesn't feel that I'm hearing her.

THERAPIST: Because of what?

MATT: Because of the way I'm responding, I suppose.

THERAPIST: (*excitedly*) Yes, exactly, Matt, there's something about the way that you respond to her. It's probably just who you are and the way that you're used to being in the world, which is not really very verbal and not really very responsive that, for whatever reason, ends up leaving her feeling that she doesn't have your attention, or that you're not honoring or respecting her. And she is then left feeling alone, and that you're not a team or a partnership. When she gets a response from you that feels to her like a nonresponse that you may know inside yourself means "I'll get to it. That's fine, that's no problem, I understand," she feels like she hasn't been able to completely let go of it and say, "It's yours now. I feel relieved; we're in this together."

The therapist attempted to describe the sequence of events without blaming either partner, pointing out each one's understandable reactions. Matt's reaction was explicated as an internal, unobservable process of considering Sheri's words rather than a dismissal of them. So far, Sheri has been unaware of Matt's internal consideration and has reacted based on the belief that he has not responded.

Although the therapist eventually elucidated Matt's perspective in the situation, that he knows he is responding to his wife so her anger seems unjustified, it would have been preferable to address his feelings sooner, before describing the sequence of behavior, to prevent him from becoming defensive and disregarding what the therapist said subsequently. The less defensive the listener is, the more likely it is that he or she will respond with compassion to vulnerable disclosures.

Emotional Acceptance through Unified Detachment from the Problem

Our second treatment strategy is to help couples approach their problems in a detached, objective, intellectual way rather than in an emotional way. By distancing from a conflict, partners can work as a unit to resolve their arguments more constructively. Christensen and Jacobson's goal of "unified detachment" is similar to Daniel Wile's objective of encouraging couples to develop a "shared platform" (Wile, 1995). Both approaches seek a vantage point from which couples can discuss their problems without blame or defensiveness. However, Wile's emphasis is on using the "shared platform" as a place from which couples can discuss primarily the feelings they are unable to get across, particularly those to which they feel "unentitled." In contrast, Christensen and Jacobson seek a position where couples can analyze any important aspect of their conflict.

To encourage partners to achieve "unified detachment," we discuss their sequence of behavior during a recent conflict. We coach partners to delineate their actions objectively rather than blaming each other. We may also look at similarities between this recent conflict and arguments they have had in the past. Seemingly unrelated issues (sex, time spent with friends vs. time at home, whether to buy a house or continue renting) often stem from the same few relationship themes (one partner wanting more intimacy and the other wanting more autonomy). By focusing on the concrete behavior and the associations between conflicts, we help partners to discuss their problems as an "it" that they share rather than seeing each other as adversaries. A unified detachment intervention is demonstrated with another example from Matt and Sheri's therapy.

THERAPIST: There is a lot that's invisible inside Matt. A lot of things that go on in your mind that are not immediately apparent to Sheri. And, sometimes she thinks there's more going on, like maybe she thought you were upset or something, and she makes assumptions about what's inside your head for lack of information. And before she even met you she was probably good at that. [And] when you're good at responding to people's needs, you've got really big antennae. That's how I always think about it, [Sheri] you've got these big antennae sticking out there and you're always looking for some data. (*The therapist demonstrates antennae by putting her fingers pointing up from her head.*)

SHERI: That's a good description. (*Sheri and Matt laugh.*)

THERAPIST: So in the absence of any information you're kind of searching even further, and you'll start creating something inside yourself.

MATT: That makes sense.

THERAPIST: So there's a lot of good things that come with having those kind of antennae. It makes you very sensitive to other people, and aware of what they need when they need it. But it can also get you into trouble sometimes, and that's part of what we've realized that occurs sometimes between you and Matt. She takes your neutral and turns it into a negative. If you're very sensitive you always look for the possibility of a negative, because then that means you have to do something to tend to it.

The therapist's primary goal in this intervention is to move partners away from a blaming stance by allowing them to detach from the emotion of the conflict and see it as an objectively understandable sequence of reactions. In this excerpt, the therapist highlighted the understandable reasons why Sheri makes assumptions about Matt's emotions, which moved Matt away from accusing her and toward a nonblaming explanation for Sheri's reactions to him. Additionally, the therapist used the techniques of humor and metaphor to create unified detachment by describing Sheri as having "big antennae that stick out there," at which the couple laughed. Such techniques allowed Sheri and Matt to distance themselves from the problem and examine it dispassionately.

Next, the therapist focuses on Matt's experience, highlighting the understandable reasons for his negative reactions to Sheri's anger:

THERAPIST: [I]t's also important for you [both] to understand where Matt gets stuck. The dynamic of what occurs between the two of you leaves you [Matt] unable to be very sympathetic to what Sheri is feeling. I think this pattern happens over and over, and even in these incidents you're describing. It's all a circle, but we'll start with [Sheri]. There's something she needs, or wants, or feels, so she'll say a little something. So you see him, in your eyes ignoring it or not responding, so you say it strongly. It's understandable as we've learned about the differences between the two of you that Matt's not a verbal person. But it doesn't mean that he's not thinking about it, and that's where you get stuck. Sheri thinks you're still ignoring it; she still feels ignored.

The therapist used nonblaming and descriptive language throughout, and emphasized the dyadic cycle between Sheri and Matt: Sheri expresses herself and Matt responds with internal consideration; Sheri doesn't realize he's responded and becomes angry; Matt sees her reaction as unjustified and extreme because he knows he really has responded, just internally. Ideally, Matt and Sheri will eventually begin to describe their conflicts using this nonblaming language and obtain some detachment from the hurt and frustration associated with these arguments. Further, they will be able to recognize that this argument is consistent with the specific theme—responsibility and caretaking—that runs through many of their conflicts. This detached, nonblaming, intellectual view will then decrease the hurtful reactions, prevent further escalation, and reduce recovery time after the conflict.

Emotional Acceptance through Tolerance Building

Our third goal is to help partners become more tolerant of each other's actions. In contrast to the first two strategies, which are designed to promote intimacy, tolerance simply reduces the pain associated with negative behavior. To accomplish this goal, we use three strategies. First, we present the positive aspects of the partner's aversive behavior. Second, we have partners "fake" hurtful behavior to desensitize their mates and to help the "fakers" see the emotional effects of their actions. Third, we have the two role play conflicts that include the aversive behavior in order to desensitize the "receiving" partner to the behavior.

Our first strategy to promote tolerance is to present the positive aspects of partners' actions. We acknowledge the pain the partner "receiving" the behavior feels. However, we also highlight the positive features of the behavior. Depending on the function of this act in the couple's life, we may frame it as a quality that originally attracted the partner. Alternatively, we may emphasize how differences in partners' actions complement each other. For example, Sarah is a 31-year-old lawyer who married Bob, a 37-year-old social worker, 9 years ago. When Sarah and Bob entered therapy, one of Sarah's complaints was that Bob wanted to have sex more frequently than she did. After discussing this issue over several sessions, Sarah came to realize that Bob's sexual overtures also made her feel desirable. Further, she remembered that, when they first married, she was uncomfortable being sexually assertive, and so Bob's expressiveness complemented her behavior. Finally, Bob came to understand why his sexual overtures made Sarah uncomfortable.

Our second strategy to increase partners' tolerance is to have them "fake" aversive acts. One partner identifies an action that angers or hurts him or her. We tell the partner who does the behavior to fake it several times during the coming week, but only when he or she is not feeling like doing the behavior. We say this in front of the partner "receiving" the action. We accomplish two goals by having couples fake conflict. First, the person faking the behavior usually does not react emotionally in response, because the action is feigned. Therefore, he or she can better observe the receiving partner's pain and prevent the incident from escalating. Second, the receiving partner knows that his or her partner will fake this behavior in the coming week. Therefore, the receiving partner is less likely to react as strongly as he or she usually does and thus is less affected during the interaction. Over time, the association of the aversive behavior with a reduced emotional reaction desensitizes the receiving partner to the faker's hurtful actions. Further, the therapist concludes this intervention by asking the receiving partner how he or she normally feels and reacts during this type of interaction. Therefore, even if the reaction were mild during the exercise, the faker has another chance to hear how his or her behavior typically affects the partner.

At times, couples have difficulty role playing a conflict and find themselves laughing during the exercise. This can also be effective— although we will not have promoted desensitization, the laughter will have diffused what is normally an extremely stressful interaction. The couple will have achieved unified detachment through the use of humor.

For example, Mick and Jimmy are a gay couple who have been together for 4 years. When they started couple therapy, Jimmy complained that Mick was frequently angry with him. The therapist told Mick, *in front of Jimmy,* to fake being angry with Jimmy twice in the coming week and to observe how it affected Jimmy. During that week when Mick faked being angry at Jimmy, he was able to see Jimmy begin to get hurt and defensive, because Mick's perceptions of Jimmy's behavior were not clouded by his own anger. This exercise changed Jimmy's reactions as well. Whenever Mick expressed anger that week, Jimmy wondered if he were faking the anger. Therefore, he did not always react with hurt or defensiveness and was better able to tolerate it. The normally aversive behavior had less significance and a softer impact on Jimmy.

Our technique of asking couples to fake behavior is similar to the paradoxical techniques of strategic family therapy (e.g., Sluzki, 1978). Strategic therapists will often "prescribe the symptom" as a way of paradoxically decreasing the symptom's frequency. They will instruct a couple to engage in the aversive behavior and will invent a rationale to disguise the true reason. In contrast, we have couples fake hurtful actions in order to desensitize partners and to give the fakers insight into the pain they may create. We give an appropriate rationale to the couple and are open about the technique.

Our third strategy to build partners' tolerance is to have couples role play an argument during a therapy session. The couple acts out a typical conflict, and then the partners discuss the feelings and thoughts that arose or would normally arise for them during this argument. We accomplish two goals through role playing. First, we help couples understand that, no matter how much progress they make in therapy, future conflicts, or "slip-ups," are inevitable. If partners know that they will revert to their old patterns at times, they are more likely to "tolerate" the lapses and recover from them faster, because they will consider them isolated incidents rather than irreparable relapses. Second, we use role playing to desensitize couples to future arguments because the pair act the conflicts out without the anger that typically accompanies them.

We follow the role play with a discussion about why each partner acted as he or she did. Because the couple reacted calmly during the enacted conflict, the partners can discuss their behavior without feeling defensive. They can also respond to each other's pain with compassion rather than with anger and blame. Role playing conflict helps partners to understand how their behavior affects each other. Further, each partner can begin to understand why the other exhibits aversive behavior and becomes less affected by it.

The following excerpt demonstrates a therapist using this intervention with Jack and Ellen, a businessman and a housewife having problems with their sexual relationship.

THERAPIST: It only makes sense that you will go back at some point to what you've done habitually for years, but how you handle it when it happens is most important. You had a minor incident of it last night I think, which is what I'm talking about. Essentially, it sounds like you, Jack, pulled away a little bit at the suggestion of "No" to sex. And that's sort of the old pattern, that if you were turned down you might feel like you needed to really withdraw in a significant way to get into your own head and distance yourself, and that would be the old way. And then you [Ellen] would feel horribly abandoned. That's going to happen again. Last night you kept it from becoming a big deal because [Jack] you didn't retreat, you stayed with her and [Ellen] you didn't ascribe all sorts of malice to him about dumping you because you weren't going to have sex. So it was really a twofold thing. Now what I'd like to have you do is imagine a situation where essentially [Jack] you're feeling somewhat aroused and you [Ellen] are not really in the mood. Talk to each other and do it the bad way. Do it how it would go wrong.

JACK: (role playing, puts his hand on Ellen's thigh)

ELLEN: (role playing, pushes Jack's hand away) That's enough. I'm not really feeling sexy.

JACK: You're not?

ELLEN: No.

JACK: Okay.

ELLEN: Are you mad?

JACK: No. (long pause)

ELLEN: You are.

JACK: No, I'm not.

ELLEN: You're disappointed.

JACK: (*strongly*) Yes.

ELLEN: You're mad.

JACK: No I'm not mad; I'm just disappointed. (*pause*)

ELLEN: So you're not going to talk to me.

JACK: Sure, I'll talk to you. (*pause*)

ELLEN: Can I touch you?

JACK: Sure. (*pause*)

ELLEN: (*not role playing*) You would say "No."

JACK: (*matter-of-factly*) Yeah, I probably would.

THERAPIST: So you would probably say "No." And would you be getting up and leaving the room?

JACK: I would probably scoot over in bed and just stay away from her, if she doesn't want to be touched.

THERAPIST: Okay, give a really bad way you would handle it.

JACK: I would get up and leave, but I don't do that too often.

THERAPIST: Pretend to do that.

JACK: Well, I would get up and go in the other room, but I would lay there for a long time. I would lay there as long as I felt comfortable, and then I would get up and excuse myself and go to the other room.

ELLEN: (*gently*) You wouldn't excuse yourself; you would just leave.

THERAPIST: So he just got up and left. What do you do?

ELLEN: I feel horrible. I stay in bed, but I don't sleep; I toss and turn. And I just get a sick feeling like he's mad at me, doesn't want to be by me, because I don't want to have sex. And I sort of dread the new day coming, and I dread that it's not here quick enough because of the restless sleep, and I just feel sick.

THERAPIST: And what are you feeling, [Jack]?

JACK: I'm feeling sick, too. Because I feel like it's a misunderstanding more than anything.

Jack goes on to describe the misunderstanding. Although Ellen believes he is angry with her, he leaves the room simply because he cannot sleep when he is aroused and needs to distract himself by watching TV in the other room. The following excerpt concludes this role play:

THERAPIST: So, is this how you feel?

JACK: Yeah. (*Jack and Ellen nod in agreement.*)

THERAPIST: All right. Now, what in fact can you do differently?

JACK: (*jokingly*) Have sex! (*Jack and Ellen laugh.*)

THERAPIST: (*laughing*) That's one option.

ELLEN: I think what happened last night that was different is that we treated it more lightly.

The therapist's first intervention was to acknowledge that slip-ups will occur. We point out this possibility when couples feel optimistic about the relationship, for it is at precisely this time that they can hear and accept that future hurtful behavior is inevitable. Subsequently, when a slip-up does occur, partners are more likely to view it as an expected occurrence. This results in less blame and increased tolerance of the aversive behavior than if they viewed it as a total regression of the relationship. In turn, the conflict will not escalate to previous high levels, and recovery will be faster.

The therapist's second intervention was to encourage Jack and Ellen to role play conflictual behavior, to help them learn to tolerate these interactions. If partners role play an argument when they are devoid of the strong emotions that typically accompany it, they can observe their own and their partner's responses to the interaction more objectively. They can see their own behavior as potentially hurtful, and therefore perceive their partner's reactions as more understandable. In this excerpt, Ellen eventually understands Jack's need to leave the room when she says no to sex, and Jack understands Ellen's distress when he leaves without saying anything. Previously, Jack blamed Ellen because he thought her distress was irrational, and Ellen blamed Jack for being cold and unloving. In future arguments about sex, Ellen is more likely to understand why Jack leaves, and Jack will likely understand why Ellen gets upset when he leaves.

Emotional Acceptance through Greater Self-Care

Our fourth goal is to help partners learn to take care of themselves when they are feeling needy and vulnerable rather than depending on their partner exclusively to take care of them. This intervention is more relevant to couples in which one or both partners are fairly dependent on the other. The more dependent individuals are, the more distressed they will be when their mates are not able to meet their needs. Increasing each partner's ability to care for him- or herself decreases the responsibility of the other to fulfill these needs and allows the couple to spend more time focusing on improving the relationship. For example, increasing a wife's ability to care for herself when she is feeling sad or anxious allows her to manage these feelings better when her husband cannot care for her. Further, because the wife's needs are being met more effectively, she is more likely to understand what makes it difficult for her husband to console her emotionally.

Couples typically feel most vulnerable during arguments. Therefore, we focus on helping individuals learn how to care for themselves during these times. We encourage partners to generate ways to protect themselves and to minimize escalation of conflicts. For example, we may suggest leaving the situation, seeking comfort from friends, or assertively setting boundaries. However, we encourage partners to come up with strategies to protect themselves without alienating their partner or worsening the situation. We would not condone a self-care strategy that might upset the other partner. For example, if a husband tends to withdraw when his wife gets angry, we would not encourage him to withdraw. In contrast, if he has difficulty controlling his anger when a conflict arises, removing himself from the situation until he is calmer and can discuss the issue more constructively would be an effective tool.

This technique is only used in terms of how it fits into our case formulation. For example, if a husband attacks his wife for being too dependent on him, we would not use this technique to collude with the husband against the wife and focus on helping her become more independent. Instead, we would use this specific conflict about the wife's dependence as one example of an overall theme in their relationship, such as a struggle over the amount of closeness versus distance each partner desires. We would use our strategies of "empathic joining" and "unified detachment" to help them deal with this problem.

The strategy of encouraging self-care behavior can be tricky when a couple is caught in a demand–withdraw cycle of conflict. If a wife's chief complaint is that her husband is not supportive enough, she may demand more from, him and he may withdraw further from her. In this case, we would help the wife become more independent, so her need decreases, rather than pushing the husband to do more for her. Importantly, we have found in clinical practice that if the wife is more independent, and consequently less demanding, the husband is more likely to be motivated to move closer to her, and intimacy is actually enhanced. This would be more effective than directing the husband to be more intimate. Indeed, one of the chief limitations of traditional behavioral couple therapy is that couples were taught specific behavior techniques to improve intimacy rather than creating a context where it could happen spontaneously. Additionally, as we coach the wife to be more independent and able to care for herself, we would use the emotional acceptance techniques to try to create intimacy within the relationship, which was her initial request.

Sometimes couples do not use the self-care strategies they generate in therapy. However, even bringing up the topic accomplishes our overall goal of helping partners be more emotionally accepting of each other. Simply suggesting to partners that they can do things (e.g., go out with friends, write in a journal) to make *themselves* feel better is useful. Couples then feel less dependent on and less angry with their partners when they feel depressed, disappointed, or anxious and their mates are unable to care for them. The following excerpt illustrates this strategy with Don and Linda, the Asian-American couple we presented earlier. In this session, the therapist helps Don find an outlet to use when he and Linda begin to argue.

THERAPIST: (*to Don*) What can you do when things aren't going well to protect yourself and tap into your own resiliency?

DON: Sports. It's always been sports, and sleep. I play team sports or ski or that kind of stuff.

THERAPIST: Now, how do you do a team sport with your busy schedule?

DON: Well, I have a basketball league I'm part of.

THERAPIST: And then you can shoot hoops on your own.

DON: I've been trying to think of different things I can do, just as an individual at home. Skipping rope or something.

THERAPIST: It has to be nourishing. When [you're] feeling [yourself] getting into old patterns that [you] know are just going to end up making [Linda] more angry and making [you] want to withdraw more, it's finding things that you can fit into the lifestyle. And sports is one. Some kind of activity, so even like jump-roping, or something you could spontaneously just pick up and do.

DON: Right, jump-roping could be. But the other side is sleep. In the past if I was upset, I'd always give myself one day to go ahead and feel upset or feel crummy. And then sleep and rest sort of took that away and allowed me to pick it up and deal with it again first thing in the morning. And that's become more difficult. Partly because Linda has different needs in relation to problem resolution. She wants to resolve it now, and if I feel stressed or stretched it's harder for me to resolve it now.

THERAPIST: It's hard to say to Linda, "I really need to sleep on this one." The odds are against you escaping to sleep. You'll need to talk to her about it so she knows you're not in silent withdrawal, but you're trying to figure out how to get some sports time or some sleep time.

The therapist aided Don in finding helpful outlets, or ways to care for himself when faced with Linda's anger. To increase the likelihood that self-care strategies will be utilized by partners, they should be relatively convenient. The therapist helped Don find a strategy—jumproping—that was readily available to him and could be engaged in easily. Additionally, the therapist needs to ensure that self-care strategies are innocuous. The therapist suggested that Don's use of sleep as a self-care strategy will likely trigger Linda's sensitivity to his withdrawal and therefore may not be an appropriate self-care outlet for him to use. Self-care interventions provide an outlet for partners when they cannot cope with the other's aversive behavior. If partners can seek solace in their outlets, they are less likely to demand changes from their partner, leading to less conflict escalation and quicker recovery.

Shifting from Emotional Acceptance Strategies to Behavioral Change Strategies

So far we have discussed four techniques developed by Christensen and Jacobson to help couples increase their emotional acceptance of each other's differences and behavior. Often, when couples come in for therapy, each partner's agenda is to get the *other* to change. By using the emotional acceptance strategies, we shift the partners' focus from pressuring each other to change to *accepting* each other's differences and behavior. After we have implemented the emotional acceptance techniques, partners sometimes make two types of spontaneous changes. First, partners usually experience fewer demands to change and feel that their mates understand their thoughts and feelings. They feel less defensive about their actions and begin to appreciate how their behavior affects their partner. This shift often leads partners to change their own actions before we even introduce any of the change techniques. Second, partners feel more like a team and less like adversaries. Therefore, they stop behaving the way they used to during conflict. Because most couples come in for therapy because of problems with communication and conflict, this change improves their ways of solving problems. Again, this often happens before we incorporate communication and problem-solving training.

We believe these two types of "spontaneous change" are preferable compared to deliberate, structured change. Because these shifts in behavior come about in response to natural contingencies, such as by being reinforced for disclosing vulnerable feelings to each other, we believe the changes will be more durable. Unfortunately, however, our acceptance strategies are not sufficient for many couples; they need additional, directive interventions. Therefore, we switch to traditional couple therapy interventions when we believe the acceptance techniques have generated as much improvement as they can. We believe couples will be more receptive to change because we have started by promoting acceptance. Further, during the implementation of change strategies, we often come back to acceptance techniques when clients have difficulty with directed change interventions.

Treatment Phase 2: Behavioral Change Strategies

Behavior Exchange

Our goal when we implement behavior exchange strategies is to increase a couple's happiness with their relationship by having partners do more positive things for each other. Coming on the heels of acceptance work, the increase in positive actions has more powerful results than if we implemented the behavior exchange strategies at the beginning of therapy. First, the partner increasing the behavior is more willing to make this change, and the partner receiving the action sees the change as more genuine and is more likely to reinforce it by responding positively. Second, because partners are more willing to make this change, they are more likely to continue doing this behavior, even if the therapist is not present to suggest it or to praise and reinforce them for doing it. Therefore, any changes in relationship satisfaction at this point are likely to continue after therapy.

There are three steps to the behavior exchange techniques. First, we help partners identify specific actions they could do that would please their mates. Second, we have partners increase that behavior in the coming week, to make them and their mates happier with the relationship. Third, we prompt partners to recognize and acknowledge the acts done for them so they will reinforce their mates' relationship-enhancing behavior.

The acts chosen should provide maximum gratification for the receiver with little cost to the giver, such as actions that are not controversial and do not require new skills. Examples may include helping do the dishes, putting the children to bed, or kissing your partner good morning. The identified behavior is typically positive, because it is easier for partners to increase positive actions than to decrease aversive ones.

Also, performing an act is more noticeable to the receiver than suppressing one, so the receiver is more likely to be positively affected by it.

In this excerpt, the therapist introduces the behavior exchange task to Matt and Sheri toward the end of their treatment.

THERAPIST: What are those things that could contribute to you feeling more connected with each other, closer to each other, more affectionate? From gentle little things like a little touch on the shoulder, or a smile, or bringing you a cup of coffee, the little things that happen during the day as well as some of the bigger things. We want to try to build some ways for the two of you to be more connected and close. And we can't expect that we're suddenly going to create closeness at every moment, but we want to know what those ingredients are that lead to that, so that when you can, you can be trying to build those in. Okay?

The therapist often instructs couples to put their ideas in writing and encourages them to define very specific actions. Such recorded specificity prevents ambiguity, confusion, and forgetting, which increases the probability that partners will exhibit the pleasing behavior and notice when their mates exhibit the actions. Often, however, identifying target behaviors that are positive, innocuous, and specific is a difficult step for couples.

THERAPIST: Matt, you just said to talk more consistently with each other, and there are probably a lot of little examples. It could be just chatting, and you can write out as many of those things as you can think of that are the kinds of things that you'd like to be able to share. So, what's something that you can think of, Sheri? Something that would make you feel connected and close.

SHERI: Something that would be connected and close to him? (*pause*) It's just, we have been so unconnected for so long. It's going to be a whole new—I mean, I can't even explain.

MATT: It's like a new start, fresh, if it works. They haven't always worked.

THERAPIST: I know. It seems sort of intimidating when you look at closeness and connection as these big things that we're going to suddenly have together, and we haven't had for so long. But what I want you to start with is just little tiny things, because, actually, closeness is developed out of really little things that can build up to bigger things. Start by thinking small. If you woke up in the morning, what are some of the things that could be happening and that Matt could do, you could do together, that would make you feel close to him?

SHERI: It would make me feel close to you when we're driving in the car if you didn't back-seat drive when I'm driving. I would feel—that would make me feel good.

THERAPIST: Is there something he'd be doing instead?

SHERI: Well, we could be talking, chit-chatting about the beautiful day, the mountaineers out.

THERAPIST: Okay, Matt, another thought that comes to mind of something you'd like more of, or that would help you feel more connected? Something Sheri could do, something you could both do?

MATT: It would be nice if we could—just recently we haven't had much time to get out, just together.

THERAPIST: Go out together as a couple?

MATT: Yeah, or to go to a play with some of our friends.

THERAPIST: Okay. And I want you when you're writing these down to get really specific because when you bring them back next time and we start talking about them, I'm going to ask you to really fine tune them as to how could we make that happen. Not just to say I want to go out together, but to think about what kinds of things would I want to do, what would be the activities that I'd want to share. And [the] same thing with talking together—what are the kinds of things that I'd want to talk about?

The therapist encouraged Matt and Sheri to generate positive actions each would like the partner to increase instead of specific behaviors each could increase in him- or herself. However, it is often more productive for the therapist to allow the giver as much choice as possible in which acts to increase and when to do so. Couples are more likely to view changes positively when the partners believe the actions are done because the partner chose to do them rather than because the therapist or receiver told the partner to do so.

Communication Skills Training

Our goal for communication skills training is to teach couples basic skills to more effectively solve their conflicts. Once a couple is able to implement these new techniques, we add the more involved strategies of problem-solving training.

We teach couples two types of skills to improve their communication. First, we teach them skills to use when they are speaking or expressing their feelings about a conflict. Second, we teach them specific techniques to use when they are listening to their partners. When speaking, couples are taught to express their own feelings and reactions to their partners' behavior, such as by using "I" statements. We do this to prevent partners from focusing on what they believe to be their mates' feelings and intentions or from making accusations against their partners. When in the listener role, couples are taught to summarize the speaker's experience in such a way that the speaker agrees with the summary. Once the summary is deemed accurate, the partners switch roles. The listening partner becomes the speaker and is allowed to express his or her own feelings, which will then be summarized by the new listener.

Often, the listening partner will have difficulty expressing his or her partner's experience in a sympathetic way. Alternatively, he or she may capture part of the speaker's feelings but not the whole picture. When either of these difficulties occurs, we encourage the speaker to positively reinforce the listener for the pieces that are accurate. We will often model this positive feedback if the speaker does not readily provide it. We then encourage the speaker to clarify the missing or inaccurate portions of the summary.

In the following excerpt, Henry, a 40-year-old electrician, and Charlotte, a 32-year-old housewife, are guided in communication training by the therapist.

THERAPIST: [Henry,] what I'd like you to do is practice a listening skill right now. First, tell her what you've heard her say. Then, [Charlotte,] I'm going to ask him to share his feelings, and I want you to just listen, feed it back, and validate the feeling. So we aren't trying to problem-solve this now. We're just trying to listen to each other's feelings. So, [Henry,] what have you heard her say so far about the sister? Tell her.

HENRY: You want us to get along again. You'd like the relationship to be mended so that you can feel comfortable having your sister over.

THERAPIST: What is a change that she feels has happened in the relationship that she would like her sister to see? This is one thing she said that you missed (*pause*) . . . Something she said about working more as a team now and being more united, that she would like her sister to see the two of you doing.

In the example, the therapist assisted Henry in his active listening skills, specifically to reflect Charlotte's entire message. Ideally, the therapist would have first reinforced Henry for the part he did correctly.

Once Charlotte completely expressed her feelings and was comfortable that Henry understood those feelings, the therapist instructed Henry to express his feelings about the conflict.

THERAPIST: Now switching roles, [Henry,] what is your hope that might come out of this, and what's your worst fear? And tell her, and she's going to listen and then feed it back to you.

HENRY: The best case is your sister would say she was sorry and that she was out of line, to apologize and leave it at that. My worst fear is that I'll have to apologize to her for something, when I didn't do anything. Just to make things right.

CHARLOTTE: I hear you saying that the best case would be that she come and apologize to you, to us, and she'd really understand that she was wrong.

HENRY: That she apologize for advocating divorce as a solution. That she acknowledge that that's wrong, that that's a mistake. That advocating that you leave me, and all that, was way out of line.

Although the therapist is directive, couples are not just taught to speak pleasantly to each other. Instead, they are encouraged to express genuinely both positive and negative emotions in a constructive way. Further, instead of teaching an entirely new way of speaking, we foster communication that is closely aligned with the skills already present. Typically, couples know how to communicate effectively, but haven't used these abilities for some time. We elicit the skills they already have, polish them, and encourage the use of them when they are most needed—in conflict situations. Approaching communication training in this way improves the likelihood that couples will continue to use these skills without therapist intervention.

Problem-Solving Training

Once couples are able to use the general communication skills, we add a series of detailed techniques to help them more effectively solve their conflicts. We have two goals for problem-solving training. First, we want couples to solve their immediate conflicts by using these skills. Once they have resolved these issues, they feel relieved from the burden of them and are more hopeful about the relationship. Second, and more importantly, we want couples to learn the skills they need to solve problems in the future, after they leave therapy. We use the behavior changes couples make in solving their current conflicts as an example of how they can solve problems on their own in the future. To achieve these goals, we distinguish between the two stages of problem-solving: problem definition and problem solution. During the problem definition stage, couples generate a specific statement describing the issue. During the problem solution phase, they use specific skills to help them solve their conflicts.

The first stage, the problem definition phase, consists of five steps. First, we encourage couples to come up with a positive aspect of each other's aversive behavior. (This is the same strategy used to promote tolerance of the aversive behavior, as discussed earlier.) Second, we help the couple state their conflict in descriptive, behavioral terms rather than with personality descriptions and generalities. Third, we encourage each partner to express his or her feelings about the issue and listen to each other using the communication skills each has already learned. We define the problem in terms of the couple's specific actions *and* in terms of how each partner feels and reacts to the other's behavior. Fourth, we help each partner acknowledge his or her role in perpetuating the conflict. We believe both partners cause and maintain their relationship problems, and we want couples to see their difficulties this way. Fifth, we help the couple create a summary of the overall issue, known as their "problem definition."

The second stage is the problem solution phase. During this phase, we use five techniques: brainstorming, weighing pros and cons, negotiating a solution, implementing the solution, and revising the solution. First, we have couples brainstorm all possible solutions to their problem and write each idea down without evaluation of its merits. We try to use humor and may even encourage couples to come up with "silly" solutions to promote a nonjudgmental atmosphere. Second, we have couples weigh the pros and cons of each solution. Third, we have partners jointly negotiate a solution, which may be a combination of more than one idea on the list. Fourth, they implement this solution during a trial period. Finally, based on how the trial period goes, they revise the solution and implement it again.

During the problem definition and problem solution phases, we use four techniques to promote the couple's autonomy: instruction, behavior rehearsal, feedback, and "fading." First, we instruct couples how to communicate when discussing their conflicts. We explain each skill and the reason for its implementation. We encourage the couple to practice these skills in therapy and at home. Second, we have couples "rehearse" the skills by attempting to solve a current problem during a therapy session. Third, we provide feedback about their actions. We point out the skills that are helping them to solve their conflicts and suggest ways to change the unproductive behavior. Fourth, over time, we "fade" from the process. After couples practice a few times during therapy and receive feedback, we have them practice at home on their own and thus we become less active in their discussions. At this point, couples often want to work on resolving their own issues rather than waiting until their next therapy session. As the partners practice their new communication and problem-solving skills, they are able to solve many of their conflicts without the therapist's input.

Termination Phase, Booster Sessions, and the Therapist–Couple Relationship

From the onset of therapy, we explicitly inform couples that the protocol calls for 20 to 25 sessions; we believe this preparation outright makes termination easier for the couple. Within these parameters, we determine when couples seem ready to terminate. We believe that couples are ready when they come in with less conflictual material and are able to talk about their issues more productively. At this point, we usually space the sessions farther apart, which we believe makes termination easier for the couple as the pair gradually become less dependent on the therapist. We may include booster sessions, should a problem arise that partners are having difficulty solving or should they want to review the skills they have already learned. For example, toward the end of therapy, a couple may schedule a session only after an angry conflict, because then they know that they can make productive use of a therapy session. By spacing out the sessions at the end, couples have time between sessions to practice the skills they have learned in therapy.

When couples terminate, we collect outcome data to determine whether partners' marital quality has improved. For example, we administer the Dyadic Adjustment Scale (DAS; Spanier, 1976) at the last session. Partners' scores on the DAS can also inform us whether a couple is indeed ready for termination based on the pair's levels of marital quality.

For instance, Matt and Sheri were ready for termination when they began to have fewer conflicts and were able to discuss the ones they had without blaming each other. They identified these arguments as consistent with the themes running through most of their conflicts. They were even able to laugh about some of their arguments in retrospect. These gains were reflected in their DAS scores at the last therapy session, which indicated increased relationship satisfaction from pretreatment to posttreatment. Prior to treatment, Sheri's DAS score was 105, and Matt's was 87. (Lower scores indicate more distress, and a score of 97 or lower is considered indicative of clinically significant marital distress.) Matt was clearly much more distressed than Sheri at the start of therapy. Interestingly, at termination, Matt was more satisfied than Sheri, although both were out of the significantly distressed range. At posttreatment, Sheri's DAS score rose to 110 and Matt's rose to 120. In answering an open-ended question about what they liked about therapy, Matt and Sheri both indicated that increased understanding of their partner was crucial.

SHERI: It opened up Matt. He could see where I was coming from and vice versa. We were talking more, understanding each other's feelings. He understands he has to be more communicative.

MATT: The therapist did a good job. She helped us to understand each other better, to be more patient. Understanding why helped clarify a lot of things.

When couples offer statements such as these, we can see the importance of increased understanding in relationship improvement. In ICT we strive to extend a couple's awareness about each other and their conflicts by consistently illuminating the basic differences between partners, the reasons for those differences, how arguments are caused by those differences, and the emotions elicited by conflict. When couples understand more about each other and their disagreements, they are more likely to accept or tolerate aversive behavior. Consequently, conflicts arise less frequently, do not escalate the high levels reached previously, and are resolved more quickly.

INCLUSION AND EXCLUSION OF COUPLES

We have used ICT with a range of couples: heterosexual, homosexual, married, not married and living together, and couples who are only dating. We treat couples even when one or both members has an Axis I or Axis II disorder. However, there are four reasons why we would exclude a couple from treatment. First, for obvious reasons, we do not treat individuals who are actively psychotic (e.g., from a current episode of schizophrenia, a current episode of bipolar disorder, or an organic brain syndrome). Second, we do not offer therapy to individuals who meet criteria for borderline, schizotypal, or antisocial personality disorders. These individual problems often prohibit constructive work on the relationship. Third, we do not treat individuals who meet criteria for a current episode of alcohol or other substance dependence. We believe the substance problem needs to be treated prior to beginning couple therapy. Fourth, we exclude couples from treatment who report moderate to severe violence. Like many clinicians, we believe that partners in moderately to severely violent relationships are better suited to individual rather than conjoint therapy. We have specific criteria, based on the Conflict Tactics Scale (Straus, 1979) for excluding couples from conjoint treatment. In general, these criteria focus on injury and intimidation. When violence or the threat of violence has or could lead to injury and/ or intimidation, we believe that couple therapy could compromise the victim's safety (usually the woman).

PRELIMINARY DATA:
EVIDENCE THAT ICT WORKS

We have had positive outcomes in clinical settings with ICT. However, the best test of whether a therapy works is empirical data. Jacobson et al. (1999) have preliminary data from a pilot study comparing couples treated with ICT ($n = 9$) to couples treated with traditional behavioral couples therapy (TBCT) ($n = 11$)[3]. They measured relationship satisfaction with the Global Distress Scale of the Marital Satisfaction Inventory (Snyder, 1979). Statistically, ICT couples reported nonsignificantly higher levels of relationship satisfaction after treatment. This was true for husbands [$F(1, 19) = 1.93$, ns; effect size = .62] and wives [$F(1, 19) = 2.20$, ns; effect size = .78].

Jacobson et al. (1999) also computed partners' improvements in marital quality based on clinical significance—whether partners' marital quality scores improved reliably (not based on chance) and whether partners' marital quality scores improved to the point that they were in the range of maritally satisfied couples. (See Jacobson & Truax, 1991, for a detailed explanation of how this is computed.) Based on these criteria for clinical significance, 55% ($n = 6$) of couples treated with traditional behavioral therapy were maritally satisfied after treatment; 9% ($n = 1$) improved but were still in the maritally distressed range; and 36% ($n = 4$) either did not change or worsened. In contrast, 78% ($n = 7$) of ICT couples were maritally satisfied after treatment; 11% ($n = 1$) improved but were still distressed; and 11% ($n = 1$) either did not change or worsened. In sum, 64% of traditional therapy couples either improved or recovered by the end of therapy, compared to 89% of the ICT couples, in which only one couple reported marital distress after therapy.

The 6-month and 1-year follow-up data suggest that for both ICT and traditional couple therapy, couples maintain these differences. Of the traditionally treated couples, neither husbands [$t(6) = 1.23$, ns] nor wives [$t(7) = 0.54$, ns] reported significant improvement in relationship satisfaction from pretest to 6-month follow-up. However, for ICT couples, both husbands [$t(5) = 4.50$, $p < .01$] and wives [$t(5) = 4.01$, $p < .05$] reported increased relationship satisfaction from pretest to 6-month follow-up. Similarly, at a 1-year follow-up, 3 of the 11 traditional behavioral therapy couples had separated, compared to 0 of the nine ICT couples.

Obviously, such a small sample does not allow us to generalize our findings at this point. However, the results are encouraging and have prompted Christensen and Jacobson to begin a large-scale study of ICT.

CONCLUSION

Traditional behavioral couple therapists seek to bring about behavior change in couples through strategies such as behavior exchange, communication training, and problem-solving training. Traditional behavioral therapy is the most widely tested couple intervention. Further, it is the first couple therapy judged to be empirically valid. However, it still has its limits. Only half of all couples who receive this treatment experience long-term improvements in marital quality.

Christensen and Jacobson have attempted to enhance traditional couple therapy. They retained the behavioral change techniques and developed four novel strategies to bring about emotional acceptance in couples: empathic joining around the problem, unified detachment from the problem, tolerance building, and self-care. Based on preliminary data, ICT *outperforms* TBCT. Christensen and Jacobson have now launched a full-scale clinical trial in Los Angeles and Seattle to examine empirically whether ICT is truly more effective. Although our clinical experience with ICT leads us to believe it is indeed effective, empirical data are our only evidence that our theories and interventions truly help couples.

ACKNOWLEDGMENTS

Preparation of this chapter was supported by a National Research Service Award and by Grant No. MH56223 from the National Institute of Mental Health. We thank James Donovan and Michael Nichols for their valuable feedback.

NOTES

1. Traditional behavioral couple therapy was originally named behavioral marital therapy (Weiss, 1978). The name was recently changed to be more inclusive, because couple therapy need not be limited to heterosexual or married couples, as the original name implies. Further, referring to this therapy as "traditional" couple therapy allows it to be more clearly contrasted with recent attempts to enhance it.
2. Christensen and Jacobson originally named their intervention integrative behavioral couple therapy (IBCT; Christensen et al., 1995; Jacobson & Christensen, 1996). However, this name seemed to imply that the therapy focused exclusively on getting couples to change their behavior rather than focusing on change *and* emotional acceptance. Consequently, they renamed their treatment integrative couple therapy to be more inclusive.
3. One additional ICT couple dropped out of treatment and was not included in the analyses.

REFERENCES

Baucom, D. H., & Epstein, N. (1990). *Cognitive-behavioral marital therapy.* New York: Brunner/Mazel.

Baucom, D. H., & Hoffman, J. A. (1986). The effectiveness of marital therapy: Current status and applications to the clinical setting. In N. S. Jacobson & A. S. Gurman (Eds.), *Clinical handbook of marital therapy* (pp. 597–620). New York: Guilford Press.

Baucom, D. H., Sayers, S. L., & Sher, T. G. (1990). Supplementing behavioral marital therapy with cognitive restructuring and emotional expressiveness training: An outcome investigation. *Journal of Consulting and Clinical Psychology, 58,* 636–645.

Christensen, A., & Jacobson, N. S. (1999). *When lovers make war: How acceptance and change can solve conflict and create greater intimacy.* Book in preparation for Guilford Press.

Christensen, A., Jacobson, N. S., & Babcock, J. C. (1995). Integrative behavioral couple therapy. In N. S. Jacobson & A. S. Gurman (Eds.), *Clinical handbook of couples therapy* (pp. 31–64). New York: Sage.

Crits-Christoph, P., Frank, E., Chambless, D. L., Brody, C., & Karp, J. F. (1995). Training in empirically validated treatments: What are clinical psychology students learning? *Professional Psychology: Research and Practice, 26,* 514–522.

Emmelkamp, P. N. G., van den Heuvell, C., Ruphan, M., Sanderman, R., Scholing, A., & Stroink, F. (1988). Cognitive and behavioral interventions: A comparative evaluation with clinically distressed couples. *Journal of Family Psychology, 1,* 365–367.

Fincham, F. D., Bradbury, T. N., & Beach, S. R. (1990). To arrive where we began: A reappraisal of cognition in marriage and in marital therapy. *Journal of Family Psychology, 4*(2), 167–184.

Hahlweg, K., & Markman, H. J. (1988). Effectiveness of behavioral marital therapy: Empirical status of behavioral techniques in preventing and alleviating marital distress. *Journal of Consulting and Clinical Psychology, 56,* 440–447.

Hahlweg, K., Schindler, L., Revenstorf, D., & Brengelmann, J. C. (1984). The Munich marital therapy study. In K. Hahlweg & N. S. Jacobson (Eds.), *Marital interaction: Analysis and modification* (pp. 3–26). New York: Guilford Press.

Jacobson, N. S. (1978). Specific and nonspecific factors in the effectiveness of a behavioral approach to the treatment of marital discord. *Journal of Consulting and Clinical Psychology, 46,* 442–452.

Jacobson, N. S. (1984). A component analysis of behavioral marital therapy: The relative effectiveness of behavior exchange and communication/problem solving training. *Journal of Consulting and Clinical Psychology, 52,* 295–305.

Jacobson, N. S., & Christensen, A. (1996). *Integrative couples therapy.* New York: Norton.

Jacobson, N. S., Christensen, A., Prince, S., Cordova, J. A., & Eldridge, K. (1999). *Integrative behavioral couples therapy: An acceptance-based, promising new treatment for couple discord.* Manuscript in preparation.

Jacobson, N. S., Follette, W. C., & Pagel, M. (1986). Predicting who will benefit from behavioral marital therapy. *Journal of Consulting and Clinical Psychology, 54,* 518–522.

Jacobson, N. S., & Margolin, G. (1979). *Marital therapy: Strategies based on social learning and behavior exchange principles.* New York: Brunner/Mazel.

Jacobson, N. S., Schmaling, K. B., & Holtzworth-Munroe, A. (1987). Component analysis of behavioral marital therapy: Two-year follow-up and prediction of relapse. *Journal of Marital and Family Therapy, 13,* 187–195.

Jacobson, N. S., & Truax, P. (1991). Clinical significance: A statistical approach to defining meaningful change in psychotherapy research. *Journal of Consulting and Clinical Psychology, 59*(1), 12–19.

Johnson, S. M., & Greenberg, L. S. (1987). Emotionally focused marital therapy: An overview. *Psychotherapy, 24,* 552–560.

Sluzki, C. E. (1978). Marital therapy from a systems theory perspective. In T. J. Paolino & B. S. McCrady (Eds.), *Marriage and marital therapy: Psychoanalytic, behavioral and systems theory perspectives* (pp. 366–394). New York: Brunner/Mazel.

Snyder, D. K. (1979). Multidimensional assessment of marital satisfaction. *Journal of Marriage and the Family, 41,* 813–823.

Snyder, D. K., & Wills, R. M. (1989). Behavioral versus insight-oriented marital therapy: Effects on individual and interspousal functioning. *Journal of Consulting and Clinical Psychology, 57,* 39–46.

Spanier, G. B. (1976). Measuring dyadic adjustment: New scales for assessing the quality of marriage and similar dyads. *Journal of Marriage and the Family, 38,* 15–28.

Straus, M. A. (1979). Measuring intrafamily conflict and violence: The Conflict Tactics (CT) Scales. *Journal of Marriage and the Family, 41,* 75–88.

Weiss, R. L., & Cerreto, M. C. (1980). The Marital Status Inventory: Development of a measure of dissolution potential. *American Journal of Family Therapy, 8,* 80–85.

Wile, D. B. (1995). The ego-analytic approach to couple therapy. In N. S. Jacobson & A. S. Gurman (Eds.), *Clinical handbook of couple therapy* (pp. 91–120). New York: Guilford Press.

PART IV

◄◦►

THE POSTMODERN SCHOOLS

The postmodern approaches to couple therapy have a short but exciting and productive history well summarized by several of our authors at the beginnings of their chapters. Building on the work of Jay Haley, Milton Erickson, and particularly Michael White and David Epston, our postmodernists eschew history taking and co-create a new view of the problem with their clients. Our postmodern writers bypass the problem-laden story and begin to seek constructive solutions building on the *already existing* capabilities and world views of their clients. This work dramatically breaks with traditional psychotherapy which emphasized the opposite, unraveling the patients assumptions about self and other by reentering and reinterpreting the past.

We include strategic therapy here because it is so clearly the parent of the later solution-focused approach. The discussions James Keim initiates with his couples do not concentrate on the past nor on conflicted affect. Keim wishes to understand which strategies have not worked before and to introduce a behavioral prescription, in this case the art of negotiation, which, with his coaching, will carry a far greater chance of success.

When we reach the work of Joseph Eron and Thomas Lund and Steven Friedman and Eve Lipchik, we can clearly see the influence of the earlier strategic approach. These four writers, for the most part, avoid history taking and steer around troubled feeling to quickly restore morale and begin working right away toward *positive solutions*. Eron and Lund and Friedman and Lipchik present the two most similar approaches in this book. However the former seem to work more with the individual members of the couple to resurrect the preferred view of self, and the latter, in more systemic fashion, focus on optimistic outcomes for the couple as a pair.

Neal, Zimmerman, and Dickerson, also postmodernists, likewise title their approach narrative but move into the work very differently from Eron and Lund or Friedman and Lipchik or Keim. They concentrate on the restraints, particularly the power differential, introduced by our cultural assumptions. They help the man and the woman to explore their relationship in terms of these restraints and to reauthor a new narrative more free of cultural images. Of all our writers Neal, Zimmerman, and Dickerson are the most sociological and political.

It seems to me whether or not you follow the postmodern bent is a question of training, clinical experience, and personal temperament. These chapters will appeal to the experimenters among us no doubt, but the postmodern emphasis on flexibility, alliance building, externalizing the problem, and establishing personal agency all hold powerful, specific lessons that can be adapted to any model of couple therapy.

JAMES M. DONOVAN

11

◄○►

BRIEF STRATEGIC
MARITAL THERAPY

James Keim

This chapter describes the version of strategic therapy taught in the 1990s at the Family Therapy Institute of Washington, DC, which was founded in 1974 by Jay Haley and Cloé Madanes. Referred to as the "Washington School" of strategic therapy, this approach is rooted in the work of Milton Erickson, the Mental Research Institute (MRI; especially the work of Don Jackson), and of structural therapists such as Salvador Minuchin and Braulio Montalvo. After a description of the theory and tenets of the Washington School, the application of these ideas are demonstrated with case examples.

The goal of strategic therapy is to facilitate the solution of the presenting problem and to do so in the most efficient and ethical way possible. Toward this end, diagnosis and directives are used as needed. Diagnosis is achieved through describing problems in terms of protection, unit, sequence, and hierarchy. Directives tend to fall into two major categories: urging clients to try ideas that the clients have introduced, and urging the clients to try ideas that the therapist has introduced. The first section of this chapter is dedicated to these issues of diagnosis and directive.

The terms "spouses" and "marriage therapy" are used to generically describe the therapy of two adults in a romantic relationship whether or not the partners are actually married or living together. The terms "therapist" and "clinician" imply Washington School therapists and are not meant to be generic descriptions of how professionals practice. This chapter's description of therapy applies only to the Washington School of strategic therapy and is not a general description of the field.

WASHINGTON SCHOOL DIAGNOSIS

Haley noted that, in the hands of a practical therapist, a "diagnosis indicates ways of bringing about change . . . and by the third session an experienced therapist would have begun change rather than dwell on diagnosis" (Haley, 1971, p. 233). This encapsulates the strategic view of problem description; it is a way of directing the therapist to the best way to facilitate change. Diagnosis should be worded in a way that immediately indicates what needs to change.

The Washington School description of problems is informed by a constructivist view, a focus on client strengths, and a sensitivity to the family life cycle. As is described in detail later in this chapter, diagnosis is achieved through the description of the problem in terms of Protection, Units, Sequence, and Hierarchy (Jay Haley developed the acronym PUSH to describe this method of problem description).

The Constructivist View

This utilitarian view of diagnosis is an example of a strategic therapy's emphasis on maintaining a skeptical, constructivist approach to its own theory. In *Strategies of Psychotherapy*, Haley (1963) quoted Einstein on the tendency to confuse construct and reality. Speaking of scientific discoveries, Einstein wrote: "For to the discoverer . . . the constructions of his imagination appear so necessary and so natural that he is apt to treat them not as the creations of his thoughts but as given realities" (p. i). Clinical theory is better thought of as serving to organize the clinician to be helpful rather than as being empirically descriptive of clients. The belief among constructivists is that one must bend theory to meet the needs of clients or one will end up bending clients to meet the needs of theory.

A Focus on Client Strengths

True to the influence of Milton Erickson and Don Jackson, strategic problem formulation also emphasizes focusing on client strengths. One of Haley's criticisms of psychodynamic thinking was that its orientation "is toward the negative side of people" (Haley, 1980, p. 13). A clinician's view of human potential is regarded as a self-fulfilling prophecy, and focusing on client's strengths rather than on weaknesses is thought to be a key to successful therapy.

There is an emphasis in this approach on avoiding pathologizing language. Such labeling can be damaging to both the client and the therapist to the degree that it limits hopefulness and to the degree that it dehumanizes and oversimplifies clients, problems, and solutions.

Family Life Cycle Theory

Sensitivity to the family life cycle is part of the foundation of this approach. The therapist must have a solid understanding of what is normal at different ages and stages. Family stage sensitivity helps to avoid pathologizing transitions that are better viewed as painful but inevitable growth for the couple and family.

Certain human problems are viewed as being inevitable based on the way a family develops over time (Haley, 1973). The family life cycles stages described in *Uncommon Therapy* include courtship, marriage, childbirth and raising children, middle marriage, weaning parents from children, and retirement and old age (Haley, 1973). Each of these stages influences the nature of marital problem solving.

The goals of marital therapy are often conceptualized as helping clients move from one stage of life to another. Helping couples adapt to a first child or coaching a family through a member's death (Minuchin, 1984) are examples of conceptualizing in terms of the family life cycle. Life-cycle issues inform information collection as well. For example, a therapist dealing with new parents is going to be especially curious as to how the couple finds quality time together.

It is helpful for clients to know that their problems are normal challenges faced by people going through similar life-stage changes. It is perhaps more important for therapists to remember this. As both Erickson (Haley, 1973) and Erikson (1959) pointed out, pain and difficult transition should not necessarily be thought of as necessarily being pathological; they are part of growing. Thus, family life-cycle theory serves to help therapists avoid pathologizing normal but difficult growth.

PUSH: The Washington School's Map

A therapist may believe that there are 50 significant variables involved in the creation, maintenance, or solution of a presenting problem, but that therapist is limited to focusing on just a few in therapy. Clinical theory can thus be thought of as an acknowledged oversimplification. The oversimplification that the Washington School uses is known as the PUSH system for describing problems.

PUSH is an empowering way for clinicians to describe a presenting problem. Its emphasis is not on what creates problems but, rather, on what helps to solve them. Solutions may have nothing to do with causes.

Protection

With the exception of abuse, problem behavior is often viewed as being motivated at some level by a desire to help loved ones. In other words, many problems brought to therapy are thought of as cases of "love gone wrong." They are efforts at *protection* of loved ones that are problematic (Haley, 1976; Madanes, 1981).

This idea that symptoms can have a function is referred to by the Washington school simply as "protection." For example, a clinician might start a therapy by viewing a presenting problem of "nagging" as being an unsuccessful effort on one partner's part to help the other. The term protection is thus used in an interactional sense as opposed to the Freudian concept of individuals protecting themselves through symptoms.

There are two major reasons for viewing problems as being unsuccessful efforts to help. The first reason is that a therapist who believes in the positive motivations of clients tends to intervene in a much more humanistic and empathic manner. A therapist who believes in the negative motivations of clients tends to be more authoritarian and unempathic.

The second major reason for viewing problems as being problematic efforts at protection is that this construct creates lines of inquiry that lead the clinician to explore powerful issues between people. In other words, the concept of protection can lead the therapist to look at issues and relationships that may otherwise have been overlooked.

The concept of protection is viewed as being a construct that is sometimes useful and that is sometimes not. Like all strategic constructs, it is viewed as a tool and not as "reality." One should also note the similarity between the Washington School's concept of protection and MRI's view that symptoms involve problematic efforts to solve difficulties (Watzlawick, Weakland, & Fisch, 1974). Physical or sexual abuse is not viewed as being protective.

Unit

One of the most basic decisions that a therapist must make is whether to focus primarily on the intrapsychic (within an individual's mind) or interactional (Haley, 1976) aspects of a problem. Problems and their solutions are viewed interactionally, and the preferred unit of description is the triangle. In other words, when working with a husband or wife, the therapist would be automatically curious as to possible involvements of third parties such as children, in-laws, or lovers. The therapist would also be sensitive to the ability of third parties to contribute to solutions, and the impact of change upon third parties would be considered.

An important point is for therapists to see themselves as a new point of triangulation for the couple (Haley, 1976). The therapist's ability to help or harm a marital relationship is a further reminder of the influence that other third parties may have.

Sequences of Interaction

As noted above, strategic diagnosis involves a description of the problem that simultaneously suggests what needs to be changed. The description of sequence simultaneously describes the problem and points to what the solution will look like.

Clinicians view problems and their solutions from an interactional perspective. The therapist maps out the clients' stories not only into sequential form (*a* led to *b* led to *c*, for example) but, more specifically, *into an interactional sequence of events*. Problems and solutions are viewed as involving a series of interactions between people. Change is defined in part as the adaptation of new and preferred interactional sequences.

When problems are viewed as interactional sequences, it leads to greater sensitivity to the connectedness of problems within a system. The interactional view inspires a therapist to think that solving one problem sequence may result in a change in other sequences as well. For example, a couple that learns to deal with a problem behavior of a child may apply the same collaboration to handle an in-law problem.

The general tendency is for escalating sequences to be converted into soothing sequences. For example, a discussion between a parent and an adolescent that previously led to an all-out shouting match might convert to the adult's attempting to soothe the angry adolescent instead. Whether or not the adolescent is receptive to the soothing, the attempt by the parent would constitute an important sequence change.

Hierarchy

It is important for the therapist to focus not only on the marital hierarchy but also on the hierarchy of the larger social system. We are interested not only in the balance of influence between the spouses but also in the influence of other levels of hierarchy, such as in-laws, bosses, and children, on the couple.

The "marital hierarchy" is defined as the perceived balance of influence and contribution between spouses. In other words, it is the perceptions of each spouse of whether each is contributing equivalently and whether each is appropriately open to each other's influence. The work of Schwartz (1995) is often used in Washington School training because of its illustrations of what leads couples to perceive balance or imbalance in relationships.

When viewing the hierarchy of the larger system, the Washington School therapist is particularly interested in "cross-generational coalitions" (Haley, 1976). With a couple, a cross-generational coalition occurs when a person (1) seeks to exert influence over a spouse by gaining the active involvement of another generation of the family, such as a child or in-law, or (2) a spouse enters a coalition with a member of another generation of the family to deal with responsibilities that were previously the responsibility of the other spouse.

Cross-generational coalitions are not necessarily pathological; in fact, they may at times be highly adaptive. However, this type of coalition and the situations that produce it are associated with great amounts of stress for all in the family system. Furthermore, recognizing cross-generational coalitions is important because they require greater sensitivity and diplomatic skills on the part of the clinician.

INTERVENTION THEORY

Some clinical theories attempt to explain problem etiology, maintenance, and change. Strategic theory, however, makes no attempt to dictate a theory of problem development and leaves this to each individual therapist. The focus of strategic therapy is on what facilitates change in the context of psychotherapy.

Strategic intervention can appear to be deceptively simple. The problematic interactional sequence of behavior is identified. A preferred sequence is identified. And the clients and therapist work together to make that shift to the preferred sequence. What informs the therapist's advice is a sense of the hierarchy and triangles involved in the problem and its solutions.

One of the defining characteristics of strategic therapy is that each therapy is individually created. For example, the negotiating intervention in Case 2 is used only when it seems individually applicable.

Defining Terms

Three Important Intervention Concepts

Good therapy tends to be (but is not always) characterized by the following:

The Expected Conversation. Good therapy tends to involve conversations that should be happening outside of therapy but, for various reasons, are not. Clinicians zero in on these conversations as they relate to the presenting problem. The Washington School calls these discussions the expected or needed conversations. These are simply discussions of topics that are so "hot" that clients have not felt safe in having them.

Moving from Who's or What's to Blame to What Do We Do about It. Good therapy tends to involve the following change in conversation about the problem: The discussion moves from "Who or what is to blame?" to "What do we do about it?" Miller, Duncan, and Hubble (1997) have described this transition as one of the generic aspects of successful therapy irrespective of the model used. Unsuccessful therapy is characterized by getting stuck in the "Who is to blame" conversation, which blocks problem solving.

Relationship Maintenance. Having fun together and having a time and a place to talk about intimate and important issues are basic requirements of a long-term romantic relationship. This is such a common-sense issue that it is often ignored in clinical literature. But it is difficult for a couple to get past a problem if they or the therapist ignore these maintenance issues. Therapy must respect and reinforce the couple's sense of how much quality time the partners need to spend together. If a couple is not achieving its own standard of relationship maintenance, the therapist should pursue whether or not the couple wants to include the issue in the therapy contract.

The Therapist–Client Relationship

Research on the Washington School therapist–client relationship comes from qualitative study conducted by a third party, Lucy Mabrey. Mabrey's study on qualitative interviews with Institute clients was presented by Thomas and Mabrey at the National Meeting of the American Association for Marriage and Family Therapy in 1995. Mabrey wrote:

Without exception, all clients interviewed felt very accepted by the counselors and affirmed in their individual feelings, whether young children, teens, or adults. A wife commented, "And that made us feel good. She never made us feel like we were failures, or that things weren't irreversible." Many times the warmth of the counselor was given credit for the trust that developed so early into the therapeutic process. (1995, pp. 114–115)

The modern version of strategic therapy emphasizes a trusting, warm relationship with clients and stresses the importance of such a relationship to good clinical outcome (Miller et al., 1997).

The Contract

An essential part of the therapist–client relationship is the clinical contract. The contract establishes that the therapist is doing the client's bidding. Strategic therapists see themselves as being hired by the clients in the same sense that a bricklayer or architect is hired. A student once described the strategic therapist as "an expert servant," and this seems to be an accurate description of what the Washington School aspires to.

Therapy is easiest when there is an equivalence between therapist and client that comes from two balancing roles: The clients are hiring the therapist and are thus the boss; this is hierarchically balanced out by the therapist's having special training, experience, and position (designated by society as being a helper).

Failure in therapy is often viewed as a result of problems related to the contract. Resistance is viewed as a message from the clients that therapists are working on issues other than those contracted for. Therapy is easiest when the contract is for changing the most central issue of irritation in the client's life. Students at the Institute often hear the phrase, "wrap the therapy around that which the client wants most."

The Length of Therapy

The average marital therapy at the Family Therapy Institute of Washington, DC, is about eight sessions (based on our own unpublished research). No time limits are placed on the length of therapy.

Directives

The influence of the therapist can help or harm clients. Ethical practice and awareness of influence are crucial to not doing harm. Helpful use of influence is crucial to facilitating change. The construct that the Washington School uses to describe influence is the directive.

A directive is any sort of encouragement to think or act. Clinical directives are sometimes very mild, such as a therapist's saying "that sounds like a nice idea" or even smiling. At the other end of the scale of influence would be a clinician's statement "you must stop driving while intoxicated." Strategic uses the full range of mild to strong directives.

How Do Directives Facilitate Change?

When conceptualizing the presenting problem, the therapist describes the problem chosen by the clients in terms of sequence and hierarchy. The clients' inputs lead to a description of a preferred sequence and hierarchy. Directives are then used to shift from the problem sequence and hierarchy to the preferred sequence and hierarchy.

Directives need not be focused on the identified patient or even on the identified behavior. Given that the goal is to solve the presenting problem, and the means is a sequence change, one can ask another party involved in the sequence to do something different. One could also ask an identified patient to change a different area of his or her life in the hopes that this will change the presenting problem.

Types of Intervention as Determined by Function

Preparational Interventions. This type of directive is not intended to solve the presenting problem. It is used to facilitate later attempts to directly address the presenting problem. For example, a reframing may make it easier for the client to address the presenting problem. The reframing in such a case would not have facilitated the direct solution of the problem but would have helped to prepare the way. This "preparing the way" gave rise to the term "preparational directive."

Primary Interventions. A primary directive is a direct attempt to solve the presenting problem. For example, a couple may come in for help in negotiating some major life decisions. The therapist might use a structured negotiating technique to help the clients deal with the issues. As this intervention is a direct attempt to solve the presenting problem, the suggestion to use the structured negotiating approach would be considered a primary directive. If the therapist suggested that the couple go out on a date before negotiating a problem, this would be considered a preparatory directive since its intention was to prepare the way for a later direct attempt (negotiating) to address the presenting problem.

Termination Directives. A termination directive is used after the presenting problem is solved, and its function is to help end the therapy. An example of such a directive would be a therapist's asking a couple to discuss and plan how to handle problems that arise after the end of therapy.

Types of Directives as Categorized by Inspiration

Client- and Therapist-Inspired Directives. When a therapist encourages a client to address a problem by trying something that the client has thought of, this is called a "client-inspired" directive. When a therapist encourages a client to address a problem by trying something that the therapist has thought of, this is called a "therapist-inspired" directive.

Although some therapies emphasize one type of directive or the other, the Washington School emphasizes the use of both client- and therapist-inspired directives, and individual style determines which category is used more often. What characterizes the Washington School practice is the mix of both types of directives.

The Range of Directives

Below are 33 of the most commonly used categories of directives (Keim, 1992, 1995). They are explained in detail in the books *Problem Solving Therapy* (Haley, 1976), *Strategic Family Therapy* (Madanes, 1981), and *Behind the One-Way Mirror* (Madanes, 1984).

1. Correcting the hierarchy (Minuchin, 1974; Haley, 1976; Madanes, 1981; Price, 1996)
2. Negotiations and contracts (Jackson, 1965; Minuchin, 1974; Haley, 1976; Madanes, 1981)
3. Changing benefits (Jackson, 1967; Madanes, 1981, 1984; Keim, Lentine, Keim, & Madanes, 1990)
4. Rituals (Haley, 1973; Madanes, 1981; Haley, 1984; Wedge, 1996)
5. Ordeals (Haley, 1973, 1984; Grove & Haley, 1993)
6. Paradoxical restraint from improvement (Haley, 1973, 1976)
7. Paradoxical contracts (Haley, 1963, 1973; Madanes, 1981; Watzlawick, Beavin, & Jackson, 1967)
8. Prescribing the presenting problem with a small modification in context (Haley, 1973; Madanes, 1981, 1984)
9. Changing a parent's involvement (Minuchin, 1974; Haley, 1976, 1980)

10. Changing memories (Haley, 1973; Madanes, 1984, 1990)
11. Prescribing the symptom (Haley, 1973, 1976, 1980)
12. Prescribing the pretending of the symptom (Madanes, 1981)
13. Prescribing a symbolic act (Madanes, 1981)
14. Asking parents to prescribe the presenting problem or the symbolic representation of the presenting problem (Madanes, 1981)
15. Prescribing the pretending of the function of the symptom (Madanes, 1981)
16. Strengthening or weakening relationships (Minuchin, 1974; Haley, 1976; Madanes, 1981)
17. The illusion of being alone in the world (Madanes, 1984)
18. Reuniting family members (Minuchin, 1974; Haley, 1976; Madanes, 1981)
19. Changing who is helpful to whom (Madanes, 1981)
20. Empowering children to be appropriately helpful (Madanes, 1981)
21. Orienting or projection into the future (Haley, 1973, 1976; Madanes, 1981)
22. Prescribing a reversal in the family hierarchy (Madanes, 1981, 1984)
23. Prescribing who will have the presenting problem (Madanes, 1984)
24. Repentance and reparation (Madanes, 1990)
25. Reframing (Satir, 1964; Haley, 1973, 1976; Madanes, 1981)
26. Creating a positive framework (Madanes, 1981, 1984)
27. Finding protectors (Madanes, 1990)
28. Eliciting compassion (Madanes, 1990)
29. The illusion of no alternatives (Haley, 1973; Madanes, 1981, 1984)
30. Asking the client to find a solution (Haley, 1973, 1976; Watzlawick et al., 1974; Fisch, Weakland, & Segal, 1982; de Shazer, 1991)
31. Asking clients to repeat their own previously successful strategies (Fisch et al., 1982; Haley, 1973, 1976; Watzlawick et al., 1974; de Shazer, 1991)
32. Prescribing nonrepetition of unsuccessful efforts to solve the problem (Watzlawick et al., 1974; Fisch et al., 1982)
33. Coaching or providing emotional support to clients to stay on track through difficult transitions (Haley, 1973; Minuchin, 1974).

Application

Strategic diagnosis, as mentioned earlier, uses language that describes what needs to change. The problem is described in terms of protection, unit, sequence, and hierarchy, and the intervention is simply to change the sequence in a way that is hierarchically sensitive, is informed by or changes triangles, and that finds appropriate ways for loved ones to protect and help one another.

A hallmark of strategic therapy is its flexibility. The following cases are examples of different degrees of intervention. Case 1 falls into the category of what Minuchin calls "coaching," or providing emotional support for clients who are basically on track. In addition to the coaching of the sort provided in the first case, the second case requires more active clinical intervention. Case 2 involves structured negotiation, stronger triangulation with the therapist, and ending triangulation with an adult child. In Case 3, the treatment of marital violence requires active participation of third parties in the session as well as the greater use of ritual and consequence.

Case 1: Bob and Mary

Bob and Mary, both age 26, came to therapy with the complaint that their relationship was in trouble. They have two children ages 3 and 1. Bob is a computer repairman, and Mary is a marketing representative. They grew up, met, and married in a small city in the Midwest. Two years ago, the couple moved to a large eastern city after Mary received what she described as a "choice" marketing position that paid 50% more than her previous job.

During the first interview, the therapist met with the couple together first, and began the session with the question "How may I be of help to you?" After chatting with the couple together, the therapist then spoke to each spouse alone and then brought them together again. Both husband and wife complained of constant verbal fighting over child care, house cleaning, and finances. Each reported the fear that they were falling out of love. During the joint and individual interviews, the therapist asked about affairs and other third-party issues, physical abuse, substance abuse, and self-destructive behavior. There was no history of physical abuse or substance abuse or health problems. There had been no deaths or unusual traumas in the extended family in recent years.

After speaking to each of the spouses individually, the therapist once again brought Bob and Mary together. The therapist then asked, "What needs to happen for the two of you to get back on track? If you would, please discuss this with each other here, if you feel comfortable." The spouses began talking to each other and, with only the most minimal prompting by the therapist, were able to get past blaming each other to talking about how to fix things. Bob and Mary, without input from the therapist, began to negotiate more time together and a more organized distribution of labor. Their conversation was so productive that the therapist did not speak for 15 of the last 20 minutes of the session.

Toward the end of the therapy session, the clinician interrupted and said that the hour was coming to a close. The therapist asked if the problem solving that went on in the session was what the clients wanted from therapy, and each spouse emphatically said "yes." The therapist then specifically contracted with the couple to facilitate their problem-solving conversations.

During this first session, the therapist looked into issues involving PUSH (protection, unit, sequence, and hierarchy) but did not need to employ these to inform an intervention; successful problem solving was already going on, and no additional intervention was necessary.

The next interview was the following week. The session started with the therapist's asking what had been helpful about the previous session and what had not. The couple identified the progress made on working out issues as having been particularly helpful, and both hoped to continue in that line in this session. The therapist asked the couple once again to focus on what the pair needed to do to solve their problems. Again, the therapist did not have much direct participation in the discussion.

By the third and final session, the couple stated that things were tremendously improved. Once again, the therapist did not intervene other than to encourage Bob and Mary to continue their problem solving. The therapist and couple planned ways for the pair's problem-solving discussions to continue without the therapist.

In the case of Bob and Mary, the importance of "doing what works" led the therapist not to intervene in a structured or strong way but merely to encourage the very successful problem solving that the clients naturally fell into. The therapist considered issues of protection, unit, sequence, and hierarchy, but these considerations were not needed to guide the intervention. This encouragement of already displayed competence in handling natural life transitions is what Minuchin refers to as a "coaching" case (personal communication, November, 1993).

Coaching is commonly used when a previously successful marriage has been interrupted by the stress of work and children or by an issue such as normal grieving or normal family life-cycle transition. These problems tend not to heavily involve third parties (as might be the case with an affair). Significantly, such couples quickly move from the "Who is to blame?" conversation to the "What do we do about it?" discussion.

The indication that coaching is sufficient is that clients get what they want from the therapy, continue improving, and end therapy easily and happily. If the couple does not get the desired results, then a more active clinical intervention is called for.

Case 2: Carol and Larry

Carol and Larry, a couple in their early 50s, set up an appointment for marital therapy. The couple had two daughters, a 20-year-old in college and a 17-year-old who, though still at home, was very socially active and spent little time with the parents. Larry worked as a midlevel corporate bureaucrat, and Carol described herself as a dance teacher who had chosen to stop working in order to dedicate herself more fully to the children. In the first interview, Larry stated that his primary goal was to get his wife to nag less. Carol said that she knew that she nagged and had tried unsuccessfully to stop for extended periods. She also added that her primary goal in coming to therapy was to get her husband to communicate more and to follow through on tasks around the house. The husband admitted that he had a problem with communication and follow-through but that he was unsuccessful in changing for more than a week at a time. The husband noted a tremendous backlog of household items that he had agreed to fix as an example of his failure to follow through.

The couple described their communication as previously having been completed to a large degree through their older daughter, a role that the second daughter had not assumed. For the last 7 years that the older daughter had lived in the house, she had the job of relaying messages back and forth between her parents. Larry and Carol currently did not view this as healthy but were unsure of how to stop this established pattern when their older daughter returned home for vacations.

Larry and Carol could be viewed as coming to therapy to develop a new system of communication. The couple had tired of the former method that was, at any rate, no longer feasible with their older child away at college. In the context of the family life cycle, this may be viewed as a problem relating to the weaning of parents from children (Haley, 1973).

The couple was unable in the therapy session to talk constructively about how to solve their difficulties. The spouses kept turning to the therapist in hopes that the clinician would say who was correct. In other words, the problem-solving strategy exhibited in the therapist's office was to triangulate with a third party rather than to solve the issue by staying within the marital dyad. Significantly, the conversation never moved beyond the discussion, "Who is to blame?" to the discussion "What do we do about it?" without very direct intervention by the therapist.

Using an idea from the work of Don Jackson, the therapist reframed the problem as being a breakdown in the negotiating process (Jackson, 1965; Lederer & Jackson, 1968). Each spouse was frustrated by an inability to get cooperation from the other; Larry complained that his wife nagged him, and Carol complained that she could not get her husband to do work around the house.

The therapist defined nagging as an incomplete attempt at negotiation. A negotiation was defined as a conversation about an exchange that ends in a "this for that" (*quid pro quo*) trade. For a negotiation to progress, the therapist explained, one party needs to make a request, and the other party needs to name or agree to a price. But in the case of nagging, something is requested without the other partner's responding by naming a price. So the initiating party keeps repeating the request, waiting for the other side to name a price.

This reframing allowed the wife to make requests of her husband without thinking of herself as a nag. The reframing also allowed the husband to think of his participation in a negotiation as an equal rather than as a brow-beaten husband who was "giving in" to his wife.

The therapist asked the couple if the pair wanted to try a fun exercise that was designed to get a couple back on track with their negotiations. The couple asked to give the exercise a try. The therapist then offered a handout describing a very formalized negotiating technique with 14 points (see Figure 11.1).

The exercise consists of negotiations using a particular structure. The first step of the exercise is to have the spouses read the points to one another and discuss them. The second step is to have the couple experiment with tiny, fun negotiations in the therapist's office. The third step of the exercise is to have the couple experiment with tiny, fun negotiations at home. The fourth and fifth steps involve employing this exercise to negotiate more emotionally charged subjects in the therapist's office (Step 4) and then at the couple's home (Step 5). Some couples can move through two steps in a single week, while others need more time.

The therapist emphasizes that this exercise, in its formalized totality, is not meant to be a description of how couples should normally work out problems. This exercise is successful when it allays the spouses' fears that the negotiation will be "win–lose" and leads the couple to playful experimentation with "win–win" discussions instead.

With some amusement, Larry and Carol read the 14 steps, and the

FIGURE 11.1. Negotiation handout. (Have couple read out loud and discuss before trying.)

1. Negotiation draws on the reserve of good will that loved ones store for one another. This reserve must be replenished by the couple's having fun together and enjoying each other's company *outside the household* Negotiation only works when those involved have had enough fun together. This is why good business negotiators are often big spenders when it comes to entertaining those they plan to do business with.

   [Therapist's explanation: Intimate communication involves the directing of intense amounts of attention to one another. Couples' homes are so habitually distracting that often partners are unable to give each other the attention they need. This is especially true if there are children in the house. It is therefore recommended for most couples to get out of the house.]

2. Some negotiations take one discussion, others five, and others 200. Have a style that allows negotiations to start, break, and restart easily. If one ends a negotiating session nicely, one can come back to it nicely.

3. Never say "No" during a negotiation unless there is an ethical problem with what is requested. The closest one should come to saying "No" is "I will seriously consider that."

   [Therapist's explanation: In our culture, "No" simultaneously denies a request and blocks future discussion. Blocking future discussion is contrary to the spirit of cooperative negotiation. A phrase borrowed from Japanese business negotiating, "I will seriously consider," is understood to momentarily deny a request while leaving open the possibility of discussing the request again in the future.]

4. Negotiating is only about the present and future. Avoid bringing up the past except as an example of what is being requested.

   [Therapist's explanation: This is one of the most important rules in many communication courses. One of the leading causes of failure in negotiation is getting side-tracked. Talking about the past is the best way to avoid completion of a negotiation.]

5. Avoid explanations as to why one wants the package being negotiated. These will only side-track conversation.

   [Therapist's explanation: Requesting an explanation not only side-tracks the negotiation but also may be perceived as patronizing.]

6. In negotiation, assume that one knows only what is best for oneself, and not for others.

   [Therapist explanation: This type of discussion side-tracks negotiation. Additionally, no matter how well-intended, questioning the validity of another's request is usually received as being patronizing.]

7. Each party owes the other a "price" for the request in negotiation as long as what is being requested is moral.

8. Avoid only doing those activities that both enjoy. Use negotiation to get one's partner to try something new, and be prepared to do the same in return.

9. Each party in a healthy romantic relationship is benevolently trying to change 2% of one another while accepting the other 98%. If one is trying to change much more than 2%, the relationship is one characterized by nagging. If one is not trying to change the other at all, the partners grow apart over time and do not feel an adequate amount of intimacy.

[Therapist's note: Oddly enough, the perception that one's spouse is interested in changing one is part of the perception of intimacy.]

10. Define time parameters of what is being requested. Be very specific about terms.

[Therapist's note: Couples should start by only negotiating for time segments of 1 week at a time and *slowly* build up the amount of time involved in transactions. Also, requests should be described in very behavioral terms, especially early in the therapy. For example, "be more loving" is too general a request, where as "hugging and cuddling" are appropriately specific requests. Global requests for change must be broken down into simple behaviors.]

11. Hold hands continuously through difficult or emotional negotiations. The physical closeness is a reminder of the love that underlies all discussions.

[Therapist's note: This is an especially effective approach for a couple whose arguments quickly spiral out of control even in the therapist's office. Negotiation is not a time for couples to fight, and such unproductive disagreements must be quickly blocked. Therapists know that they should intervene quickly to stop an argument if the pair, in the midst of a disagreement, disengage in their hands.]

12. Seal all negotiations with a kiss. Write all negotiations down in a specific place such as a blank book of the type often sold as a diary.

[With emotional negotiations, individuals tend to later confuse the memory of their starting position with the final agreed-upon compromise. Spouses tend to confuse where they started in a negotiation with where they ended. Writing negotiations down addresses this almost inevitable problem.]

13. The negotiation should not end until each partner feels that a "win–win" situation exists whereby each is happy with the negotiated arrangement.

14. When a couple learns to negotiate explicitly, it is at first more troublesome than helpful. Have patience!

therapist gave an explanation as to why this type of explicit, "win–win" negotiating would work in the near future to help each change the other. The initial coaching by the therapist about negotiation included frequent shifting of sides as he joined with one spouse and then the other. The couple successfully completed several small negotiations involving fun and household chores during the first interview. Carol requested that Larry talk to her for 15 minutes each evening during the week; Larry agreed to do so in exchange for being able to have 15 minutes of uninterrupted rest upon return from work each evening. Larry then asked what his wife wanted in return for "happily" supporting his taking a 3-hour fishing trip that weekend. Carol agreed to encourage the fishing trip in return for his completing 3 hours of trim painting in the house. The couple negotiated issues related to sex, time spent with children, and other issues. The pair also negotiated "penance" after the husband, on one occasion, did not follow through with his side of the negotiation. After six sessions, Larry stated that the nagging was no longer a problem, and Carol stated that he was more communicative with his family and contributed more at home.

The couple expressed fear that their older daughter, Sylvia, might try to regain her role as communication hub for the parents. The therapy then progressed to helping the couple deal with other issues related to their change in life cycle. The therapy then was suspended until the older daughter returned for summer vacation and tried to resume the role of intermediary between her parents. Having discussed with the clinician that Sylvia might lovingly try to regain this inappropriate role, the couple returned to therapy as soon as the pair realized what was happening.

In order to deal with Sylvia's role confusion, the therapist asked the husband to buy a gift of lingerie for his wife and to give it to her within eye-sight of, though not directly in front of, Sylvia. The wife was instructed to give her husband a very sexy kiss. This task caused the couple to laugh as they explained that they were never physically affectionate in front of their children. The therapist explained that romantic affection between parents is one of the best ways to emphasize to a child that she is not an equal to the parents. The couple carried out the task, and the older daughter immediately responded to the sight of the lingerie and her parents kissing by asking her father why he hadn't bought her a piece of lingerie as well. As the wife proudly told the therapist, the husband responded by saying "because I'm not married to you." The couple reported in a 1-year follow-up that they were more comfortable handling problems with Sylvia after this incident.

From the perspective of a clinician of the Washington School, the intervention in Case 2 facilitated change in numerous ways, but the changes can most practically be described by using the PUSH construct.

Protection. The therapist viewed the effort of the older daughter as an attempt to be helpful to the parents. This view evoked more empathy from the clinician and led to the daughter's being seen as carrying on a job that was no longer necessary rather than as an individual who was inappropriate and nosy with her parents. This view of the daughter as trying to be helpful led the therapist to coach the parents to present themselves in a more relationship-competent fashion to the daughter.

Unit. The marital triangle involved in the presenting problem included the daughter, and, thus, the goal was to facilitate direct communication between husband and wife. The therapist temporarily replaced the daughter as the point of triangulation in the marital relationship (Haley, 1976).

Sequence. The sequence of the presenting problem was that of request followed by noncooperation between the spouses followed by triangulation with the older daughter. At the start of the therapy, the parents were already working on communicating without the help of the older daughter, but they were not able to change the sequence whereby each was not cooperating with the other's requests for collaboration. The negotiating exercise resulted in the couple's shifting into a cooperative mode. Thus, the couple went from noncollaboration with triangulation of a child to collaboration with triangulation of a therapist to collaboration without significant input of a third party.

Hierarchy. The hierarchy or balance of influence of the couple started with each spouse being rather closed to the influence of the other. If either made a request of the other, one felt like an ogre, and the one being asked felt oppressed. If a couple desires a marriage between equals, each spouse needs to be able to exert open influence from a position of equality (Schwartz, 1995). This was achieved with Larry and Carol through the negotiation intervention and through the detriangulation of the older daughter. Hierarchical equality is openness to influencing and being influenced in overt and ethical ways by one's spouse.

Case 3: The Treatment of Marital Violence

The Washington School approach to marital violence is addressed in the books *The Violence of Men* (Madanes, Keim, & Smelser, 1995) and *Sex, Love, and Violence* (Madanes, 1990). The therapy of abuse and violence is usually more therapist-inspired than that of other problems, and these books offer chapters detailing issues that will be touched on below.

For the purpose of describing the range of the Washington School, let us suppose that Larry and Carol had the additional problem of marital violence. *Given that the first priority is preventing harm, stopping additional spousal abuse would take priority over other presenting problems.*

In Case 3, let us hypothetically change the story of Larry and Carol to include monthly drinking bouts by Larry that, three or four times a year, involve violence against his wife. The violence includes slapping, punching, and pushing. Carol has had two black eyes in the last year. The goal of Carol, expressed in individual interview, was to stay in the marriage and to work on the violence.

Case 3 might involve the following interventions from *The Violence of Men* (Madanes et al., 1995):

1. After considering the history and type of violence, the therapist might recommend a physical separation of the couple until behavior and substance abuse is under control and until there is appropriate involvement of significant others in a safety plan.

2. An apology ritual would be used in which the husband would, in the therapist's office, take full responsibility for violence and would express sorrow and repentance to his wife in front of all available significant others. For example, the apology might take place in front of Larry's widowed mother, his father-in-law, and his two siblings. Preceding the apology, there would be a discussion involving the whole family as to what violence transpired (in exact and detailed language), why the violence was wrong, and ideally both a senior woman (Larry's mother) and man (father or father-in-law) would explain the pain of domestic violence to him.

3. Planning for a possible return to the household, Larry might return to the house after the following conditions have been met:

   a. Carol feels safe with the idea of Larry's returning home.

   b. Larry expresses sorrow and repentance to his wife in front of a group of significant others. His statements must include a full acceptance of responsibility for the violence, and Carol should not be put in a position of having to respond (for example, saying "I forgive you.").

   c. The substance abuse is being addressed (substance abuse therapy, Alcoholics Anonymous, etc.), and there are significant consequences for future drunkenness.

   d. A plan is made for how to address violence should it occur in the future. The consequence of future violence usually includes police intervention and legal charges (Jacobson & Gottman, 1998) and an additional consequence that is more personally significant to the victim and offender (Madanes et al., 1995). Financial consequences are often used, as this has been found to be an effective addition to police involvement. An example would be that Larry would be required to remove $10,000 from his retirement and place it in an account in his wife's name. Should he assault her again, she would, in addition to other consequences, remove the money and spend it in a way that would be particularly irritating to her husband. Research by Schmauk (1970) suggests that potential loss of money is a stronger inducer of avoidant learning in sociopaths than shock, and the use of financial fines in therapy can be quite powerful for a range of people (Madanes & Madanes, 1994).

   e. A relative, perhaps Larry's mother, might move in with the couple for an agreed-upon period to help monitor Larry.

4. All through the therapy, the couple would work on their communication skills. Avoidance of violence is not only achieved through consequences but also through increasing the couple's ability to gain each other's cooperation through benevolence rather than blackmail.

Toward this end, the negotiation exercise described in Case 2 would be employed.

Comparing Cases 1, 2, and 3

Compared to Case 1, Case 2 resulted in more therapist-inspired interventions. The following characteristics in Case 2 suggested a more therapist-inspired approach:

1. The inability of the couple to move from the discussion of who or what is to blame to the discussion of what to do to solve the problem
2. The habitual involvement of a third party in the pattern of interaction that the couple wanted to move away from
3. The couple's perceptions that the pair were unable to stop a behavior that is not helpful
4. The couple's initial low confidence that the pair could change the problem

Case 2 did not, however, involve the following factors that Case 3 contained, which led to an even more therapist-inspired therapy:

1. Substance abuse
2. Physical violence or other situation where gradual reduction in the frequency of the problem is not acceptable; the problem must *never* occur again
3. Lack of experience by clients in dealing with this type of problem successfully

Strategic marital therapy may thus be described as having a range of therapist-inspired directiveness. The therapy tends to be more therapist-inspired to the degree that the following characteristics are present:

1. The inability of the couple to move from the discussion of who or what is to blame to the discussion of what to do to solve the problem
2. The habitual and overt involvement of a third party in the pattern of interaction that the couple wanted to move away from
3. The perception on the part of a client that the pair are unable to stop a behavior that is not helpful, or initial low confidence by the clients that they can change the problem.
4. Lack of experience or confidence by clients in dealing with this type of problem

5. Physical violence or other harm-threatening situation where gradual reduction in the frequency of the problem is not acceptable;
the problem must *never* occur again
6. Substance abuse

The therapy tends to be more client inspired to the degree that the goals
of therapy can be met by encouragement and coaching of already occurring conversations.

DISCUSSION

Is Therapeutic Change Unique?

Change in therapy is not viewed as being qualitatively different from
change without the help of therapy. For any intervention used by strategic therapists, one can find parallels in everyday life. Therapy is inspired
by and mimics the way change occurs in other facets of human interaction. This is perhaps why therapists of all schools have sought inspira-
tion in technique, theory, and ethics from such diverse sources as reli-
gion, anthropology, and international diplomacy.

Is the Therapist an Expert?

The strategic therapist is viewed as an expert when the term implies an
individual who has substantial training and experience. Since the rise of
"postmodernist" language in therapy, the term "expert" has taken on an
unpleasant additional meaning; an expert for this latter group is someone who views him- or herself as being superior to the client and who is
denigrating to the client's experience and worldview. Strategic ascribes to
the first meaning of expert (having special training and experience) and
joins others in abhorrence of clinicians who practice in the second sense
of the term (superior and disrespectful).

The Code of Ethics[1]

A strategic therapist should adhere to the following ethical code:

1. The first rule of strategic therapy is an adoption of the age-old
medical maxim, "Do no harm." Simply stated, therapy should not hurt
the clients, society, or therapists. One guidelines recommended by Haley
is that a therapist should only use therapeutic procedures that the therapist is willing to experience or have his or her children experience. No

therapist may ask a client to undertake any harmful, immoral, or illegal action, even as a paradoxical intervention (Haley, 1989). Part of not doing harm is careful evaluation of the harm caused by giving an individual a diagnostic label.

2. The therapist must practice in a competent manner and must accept responsibility for creating change in therapy. Not accepting responsibility for change results in blaming clients for failure in therapy. Blaming the clients results in patronizing treatment of clients, decreased effort on the part of the therapist, and perpetuation of blame cycles that are part of the pathology of the client's social context.

3. Therapists should assume that they wield tremendous influence. Clients are safest when therapists assume they yield too much rather than too little influence. The therapists must take responsibility for the intended and unintended effects of their direct and indirect influence on clients and clients' social systems. A therapist is not the equivalent of a classroom lecturer whose audience is relatively free to accept or reject his or her teachings. A client in therapy should be considered to be in an extraordinarily vulnerable position, much like that of a hypnotic subject in a trance, and such unusual openness to influence should not be taken advantage of.

4. Therapy must be respectful of the clients. Because of their influence, therapists are in a uniquely powerful position to denigrate clients and, therefore, must be all the more sensitive. Live supervision is especially helpful in training therapists to notice their inadvertent insults.

5. Therapists should have a minimalist view of changing clients' worldviews; this ensures maximum respect of the worldview of the client. In successful therapy, the therapist instigates a change in the clients' worldviews. However, attempts to change a client's worldview should be limited to the presenting problem that the therapist has contracted to change. Consciousness raising, here defined as influencing a client for a purpose not directly related to solving the presenting problem, must not be confused with therapy. For example, the Nazi ideology of a Mr. Smith would have to be addressed when the presenting problem is the violence of his son. However, the Nazi ideology would not necessarily be addressed if Mr. Smith came to therapy for help in dealing with normal grieving issues relating to the natural death of his 80-year-old mother.

A minimalist view of changing clients is a consequence of recognizing that the therapist's construction of reality serves the very specific function of helping another party in the context of therapy. For example, it is helpful for a therapist to view problems in terms of hierarchy and sequence; however, it could be a terrible idea for clients to forsake their own constructions and adapt these terms. Different constructs of reality can potentially be simultaneously valid and helpful (Haley, 1963; 1973; Watzlawick, 1984).

6. Therapists must maintain an awareness of the advantages and disadvantages of the use of overt versus indirect directives. The following discussion compares skillfully given overt and indirect directives. With an overt directive, the therapist's influence is overt and clearly identifiable to the clients. Dependence on the therapist is more likely to occur with the use of overt directives if clients credit the therapist instead of themselves as responsible for change. However, the intent and influence of direct directives are open to review by the clients and are thus less likely to lead to abuse. With an indirect directive, the therapist's influence is not clearly identifiable and may even be invisible to the client. The client receiving the indirect directive is more vulnerable to bad interventions because the directive is not as easily reviewed. The advantage of indirect directives is that the clients' feelings of self-determination and self-confidence tend to be increased more by indirect than by overt directives. Clients internalize more quickly and take more credit for change resulting from indirect directives. Thus, both overt and indirect directives have their advantages and disadvantages that must be monitored in each case.

7. Common sense is as important as theory when determining what might harm clients. Therapists should trust their gut feelings about appropriateness of interventions and discuss uneasiness with a supervisor before proceeding.

8. The therapist is responsible for using the most dignified, least intrusive intervention that will work within a reasonable time frame.

9. Therapy must not be oriented toward blame, nor should it collude in irresponsible or dangerous behavior or in the forfeiture of individual responsibility.

CONCLUSION

Strategic marital therapy is practice in a pragmatic, interactional, and constructivist fashion. Problems are described in a language that makes their solution readily apparent, and protection, unit, sequence, and hierarchy are the major terms of diagnosis. Flexibility is valued, and the goal is to solve the presenting problem by doing what works.

The most important part of therapy for the Washington School is the therapeutic contract. This not only defines the presenting problem but also defines the roles of the clients and therapist. The therapist is viewed as "an expert servant" who helps as directed by the clients and who has special knowledge and experience in facilitating change.

Erickson emphasized that a therapist must work with a wide assortment of people, problems, and situations and, thus, must have a wide assortment of approaches. This sort of flexibility is inspired by ideology but is created by training. Although the Washington School has traditionally trained using videotaping and live supervision with one-way mirrors, the most important training tool is a group of committed therapists who are willing to meet regularly over time, talk, and support each other in the pursuit of practical therapy.

The Washington School has been one of the most influential models of brief and family therapy, but it views itself as having a great deal in common with other approaches. Strategic therapy has been highly influenced by other models and continues to integrate ideas and practice from other schools. Well-trained therapists should be able to attend a training for any other model of therapy, pick out a helpful idea, and integrate that idea using the language of their own model of therapy.

NOTE

1. *The Family Therapy Institute Handbook for Trainees* (Keim, 1992).

REFERENCES

de Shazer, S. (1991). *Putting difference to work*. New York: Norton.

Erikson, E. H. (1959). Identity and the life cycle. *Psychological Issues, 7*, 1–171.

Fisch, R., Weakland, J., & Segal, L. (1982). *The tactics of change*. San Francisco: Jossey-Bass.

Grove, D., & Haley, J. (1993). *Conversations on therapy*. New York: Norton.

Haley, J. (1963). *Strategies of psychotherapy*. New York: Harcourt Brace Jovanovich.

Haley, J. (1971). *Changing families*. New York: Grune & Stratton.

Haley, J. (1973). *Uncommon therapy*. New York: Norton.

Haley, J. (1976). *Problem-solving therapy*. San Francisco: Jossey Bass.

Haley, J. (1980). *Leaving home: The therapy of disturbed young people*. New York: McGraw-Hill.

Haley, J. (1984). *Ordeal therapy*. San Francisco: Jossey-Bass.

Jackson, D. D. (1965). Family rules: The marital quid pro quo. *Archives of General Psychiatry, 12*, 589–594.

Jackson, D. D. (1967). Aspects of conjoint family therapy. In G. H. Zuk & I. Boszormenyi-Nagy (Eds.), *Family therapy and disturbed families*. Palo Alto, CA: Science & Behavior Books.

Jacobson, N. S., & Gottman, J. M. (1998). *When men batter women: New insights into ending abusive relationships*. New York: Simon & Schuster.

Keim, I., Lentine, G., Keim, J., & Madanes, C. (1990). No more John Wayne: Strategies for changing the past. In C. Madanes (Ed.), *Sex, love, and violence: Strategies for transformation* (pp. 218–247). New York: Norton.

Keim, J. (1992). *The Family Therapy Institute training handbook.* Unpublished manuscript.

Keim, J. P. (1995). Strategic therapy. In M. Elkaim (Ed.), *Panorama des thérapies familiales.* Paris: Editions du Seuil.

Lederer, W. J., & Jackson, D. D. (1968). *The mirages of marriage.* New York: Norton.

Mabrey, L. (1995). *An ethnography of family change: The experience of strategic therapy.* Unpublished doctoral dissertation, College of Education and Human Ecology, Texas Women's University.

Madanes, C. (1981). *Strategic family therapy.* San Francisco: Jossey-Bass.

Madanes, C. (1984). *Behind the one-way mirror.* San Francisco: Jossey-Bass.

Madanes, C. (1990). *Sex, love, and violence: Strategies for transformation.* New York: Norton.

Madanes, C., Keim, J., & Smelser, D. (1995). *The violence of men.* San Francisco: Jossey-Bass.

Madanes, C., & Madanes, C. (1994). *The secret meaning of money.* San Francisco: Jossey-Bass.

Miller, S., Duncan, B., & Hubble, M. (1997). *Escape from Babel.* New York: Norton.

Minuchin, S. (1974). *Families and family therapy.* Cambridge, MA: Harvard University Press.

Minuchin, S. (1984). *Family kaleidoscope.* Cambridge, MA: Harvard University Press.

Price, J. (1996). *Power and compassion: Working with difficult adolescents and abused parents.* New York: Guilford Press.

Satir, V. (1964). *Conjoint family therapy.* Palo Alto, CA: Science & Behavior Books.

Schmauk, F. J., (1970). Punishment, arousal, and avoidance learning in sociopaths. *Journal of Abnormal Psychology, 76,* 325–355.

Schwartz, P. (1995). *Love between equals.* New York: Free Press.

Watzlawick, P. (Ed.). (1984). *The invented reality* New York: Norton.

Watzlawick, P., Beavin, J., & Jackson, D. (1967). *The pragmatics of human communication.* New York: Norton.

Watzlawick, P., Weakland, J., & Fisch, R. (1974). *Change: Principles of problem formation and problem resolution.* New York: Norton.

Wedge, M. (1996). *In the therapist's mirror: Reality in the making.* New York: Norton.

12

◄◦►

NARRATIVE SOLUTIONS IN BRIEF COUPLE THERAPY

Joseph B. Eron
Thomas W. Lund

LITERATURE REVIEW

The narrative solutions approach developed at the Catskill Family Institute (CFI) integrates concepts and techniques from strategic, solution-focused, and narrative therapy. The conceptual basis for the approach was first presented in an article that proposed a framework for how problems evolve and dissolve (Eron & Lund, 1993). Its principles and practices were further elaborated in a recent text entitled *Narrative Solutions in Brief Therapy* (Eron & Lund, 1996).

In the 1980s, we were drawn by the simplicity and practicality of the brief therapy approach developed at the Mental Research Institute (MRI) in Palo Alto, California (Watzlawick, Weakland, & Fisch, 1974; Weakland, Fisch, Watzlawick, & Bodin, 1974). The MRI approach differed from the structural family therapies of the 1970s and 1980s in its inherent optimism about the nature of problems. Symptoms were *not* seen as caused by defective family systems or as serving a function in preserving the stability of relationship structures. An MRI brief therapist wouldn't assume that a boy with behavior problems was trying to detour conflict in his parent's marriage; nor was a man who acted depressed and withdrew from decision making necessarily intending to protect his wife's authority in the relationship. Problems developed *inno-*

cently from the mishandling of ordinary life transitions. How people viewed their difficulties and what they did about them determined the course of problems (see Wile, Chapter 9, this volume). The therapist's job was to interrupt problem-maintaining solutions and get people back on course, on to, and over the next hurdle in life.

In the early development of our approach, we were intrigued by the technique of "reframing" and tried to improve upon its effectiveness (Eron & Lund, 1989). Introduced by the MRI group as a "gentle art" (Watzlawick et al., 1974) reframing was a way "to change the conceptual and/or emotional setting or viewpoint in relation to which a situation was experienced and to place it in another frame which fits the 'facts' of the same concrete situation equally well or even better" (p. 95).

Although reframing was originally defined as a technique to alter the meanings people ascribe to events and behavior, this important cognitive element got lost in an emphasis on behavioral prescription. Also, MRI brief therapists applied reframing to the *immediate interactional context that surrounded the problem.* They rarely talked with clients about the preproblem past or asked about their vision of the future without the problem. In practice, reframing was confined to spin-doctoring, designed to get people to go along with therapeutic directives aimed at changing here-and-now patterns of behavior.

Although it was designed primarily to gain leverage for task assignments, we discovered that reframing was helpful in and of itself. We noticed swift and dramatic shifts in interactional behavior when people found new ways of understanding their stuck situations and how these took shape over time. Once therapists helped clients revise their perspectives on their problems, they often figured out for themselves what to do differently (Eron & Lund, 1989). Our shift away from the prescriptive practices of strategic family therapy paralleled the growth of the solution-focused and narrative therapies in the late 1980s and 1990s.

The solution-focused approaches of Steve de Shazer and Insoo Kim Berg (de Shazer, 1985; de Shazer et al., 1986) and William O'Hanlon and Michele Weiner-Davis (1989) shifted the therapist's focus away from talk about problems and toward talk about solutions. Solution-focused therapists reoriented family members to exceptions to the present problems and to the future without the problem by emphasizing people's strengths and competencies.

Narrative therapists Michael White and David Epston (1990) spoke about problems in a profoundly different way than their predecessors. They observed that as problems came to dominate people's lives, the stories they told themselves became negative and problem saturated. "Externalizing conversations" were designed to separate persons from problems and help them marshal their own resources against the problem. The broad spectrum of life experiences—times when people fell under the influence of problems and when they did not—were incorporated into helpful conversations.

With "collaborative inquiry," "co-created meanings," and a "non-hierarchical" therapeutic stance, narrative therapists stepped down from the lectern and became a part of the conversation. Harlene Anderson and the late Harold Goolishian (Anderson & Goolishian, 1988) rejected the therapist as expert role and instead promoted the idea that therapy should be a "collaborative conversation" in which therapist and family "co-create" alternative narrative constructions.

Over the past 15 years at the CFI, we studied conversations between CFI's therapists and the families they tried to help. We attempted to discern the key ingredients of helpful conversations that brought out the best in people and inspired solutions across the life span. The result was an approach that interweaves elements common to strategic, solution-focused, and narrative therapy that empower people to access the resources needed to resolve problems efficiently (Eron & Lund, 1989, 1993, 1996, 1997).

CONCEPTUAL AND TECHNICAL APPROACH

The cornerstone of the narrative solutions approach is that people have strong preferences for how they like to see themselves, how they like to act, and how they like to be seen by others. We call this constellation of preferences a person's "preferred view." The power of preferred view lies in its simplicity yet its profound impact on understanding the nature of human problems and how to resolve them through planful conversation. People are at their best when they act, think of themselves, and imagine that others regard them in ways that confirm who they wish to be. People are at their worst when they act, see themselves, and see others seeing them in ways that contradict preferred views of self.

We subscribe to the premise of the MRI approach that problems develop innocently from the mishandling of life transitions. A careful assessment of the mishandling of ordinary life difficulties takes into account shifts in how people think, feel, act, and interact during times of flux. Problems evolve and intensify when people experience a gap between preferred views of self, their perception of their own actions, and their thoughts about how important others regard them. Problems resolve and solutions emerge as the gap narrows between how people prefer to view themselves, how they act, and how they think others regard them.

Narrative solutions therapists use the following guidelines in managing helpful conversations (Eron & Lund, 1996, 1997).

1. The therapist maintains a position of sincere interest in the client's preferences and hopes. He or she pays particular attention to stories and experiences, both past and present, that reflect how people prefer to see themselves, to act, and to be seen by important others.

2. The therapist explores the effects of the problem on each family member. The emphasis of inquiry is on how the problem interferes with people acting in line with their preferences and being seen by others in preferred ways.

3. The therapist locates stories from the past and present that are in line with people's preferences and contradict the narrow range of troublesome views and actions that maintain the problem.

4. As part of collaborative goal setting, client and therapist discuss what the future will look like when the problem is resolved.

5. The therapist asks "mystery questions." For example, how did a person with X preferred attributes (hard-working, productive) wind up in Y situation (acting listless and feeling depressed) and being seen by others in nonpreferred ways.

6. Therapist and client often piece together an alternative explanation for the evolution of the problem that fits with how people prefer to be seen and inspires new action.

7. The therapist encourages clients to speak up about their preferences, hopes, and intentions with significant others. Helpful conversations inside the treatment room generate helpful conversations outside the treatment room, consolidating solutions.

Preferred view is the navigational beacon that guides helpful conversations from the outset of therapy to its conclusion. Joining with clients involves connecting with how they wish to act and be regarded and is key to the process of change. There's a stand-taller, sit-straighter form of power that gets sparked when a truly caring person—one you've engaged as an authority—understands you, respects you, and sees you as capable.

When clients see their therapists seeing them in preferred ways, they're apt to speak more openly about their difficulties and feel invigorated to consider alternative solutions. They're increasingly likely to notice their own strengths and resources. They may begin to perceive the current problem more as a mystery that commands an explanation than as a truth that speaks to who they really are. People often rethink (or "restory") how the problem evolved with less blame and negativity toward self and others. They reconsider (or "reframe") their immediate situation from a more empowered perspective. A unique aspect of our approach is the interweaving of restorying (a technique linked to narrative therapy) and reframing (a technique linked to strategic therapy).

PHASES OF TREATMENT

The phases of treatment involve *starting, continuing, and concluding* the therapeutic conversation.

Starting the Conversation

The starting phase focuses on joining with people and building a therapeutic alliance. This process begins with the first phone call, when we arrange the initial appointment and decide whom to see. The first phone call is our original contact with the person defining the problem and presents an opportunity to connect with that person's preferences, hopes, and intentions.

By "connecting with preferences," therapists forge an empathic link with people and set in motion the process of change. As therapists align with how each person in the relationship prefers to be viewed, this also sets the stage for people to discuss how they would like to be seen by their partners, highlighting troublesome gaps. For example, a wife may talk more openly about her career achievements once she notices that the therapist regards her independent spirit as a strength. As she does so, she feels empowered and contrasts this experience with the feeling of deflation that's come from concealing her independent aspirations from her partner. In this way, connecting with preferences can have a motivating effect in helping the person target what needs to change in the relationship and to move toward these goals.

Continuing the Conversation

The continuing the conversation phase focuses on goal setting and initiating change. We establish goals by inviting each person in the relationship to clarify how he or she would like to act, be seen by his or her partner, and how he or she would like the relationship to be. When people describe problematic behaviors (e.g., he loses his temper), we then explore the *effects* these actions have on self, others, and the relationship. How does your partner feel when you lose your temper? What does he or she do? How about you? Do you think better of yourself or worse?

Identifying gaps between preferences and effects helps to establish goals *and* motivates people to change. For example, a husband may clarify that he'd like to be in control (a preference), yet indicate that losing his temper has negative effects ("My wife and kids keep their distance." "They see me as out of control."). As therapists highlight the gap between preferences and effects, clients often become more committed to goals ("I need to get my temper under control." "I'd like my wife to have more confidence in me."). Another nonimpositional approach to establishing goals is to invite each member of the couple to describe a future vision of the relationship without the problem. The husband in our example might project a future vision of having greater control over his temper and of his partner trusting him.

The therapist maps the evolving problem and pinpoints key views and actions linked to the current problem. He or she pursues *when* views of self and other *shifted* in a manner that challenged preferred views of self. We explore the preproblem past—when each person felt good about the marriage, liked how he or she was acting, and liked how he or she was being seen by the other partner. The therapist also inquires about exceptions in the present, times when people act in line with their preferred view.

Change is initiated by locating "key stories" that resonate with preferred views of self and other and contradict the narrow range of troublesome views and actions that maintain the problem. For example, a wife who now complains of feeling distant from her husband might be asked to recall times when she felt more connected. In response, she may relate a story that captures images of herself feeling supported by her husband and responding with warmth and affection. The therapist then probes the mystery of how this account of warmth and support evolved into the current experience of disconnection. Such "mystery questioning" inspires the couple to reconsider how their relationship went astray—and to figure out how to get it back on track.

Often the therapist and couple develop an alternative explanation for the evolution of the problem that permits current problem-maintaining behavior to be reframed. This empowering explanation fits with how people prefer to be viewed and inspires new action. Change occurs as people begin to adjust their behavior to accommodate the new narrative framework. In our case example, the husband, now reassured that his wife's withdrawal was based on her growing distaste for his temper and *not* her distaste for him, begins to bring his temper under control. He also expresses interest in her independent pursuits, which alters how she views him viewing her. As she gains confidence that her husband now sees her as competent and worthy of support, she speaks up about what she'd like, shares her successes, and becomes more affectionate. The more confidence he gains that his wife regards him as attractive and worthy of affection, the more supportive the husband becomes. A positive feedback loop is set into motion.

Concluding the Conversation

Therapy draws to a close as couples develop less reliance on the therapist as a resource in strengthening their relationship and more reliance on each other. Couples leave therapy knowing how to initiate helpful conversations that bring out the best in each other. Equipped with an understanding of how the problem evolved and resolved, the couple is better able to negotiate future difficulties.

Although these phases of treatment have been described as distinct, in practice they are interconnected. The common thread from the start of therapy to its conclusion is that the therapist attempts to conduct conversations that close the gap between how people prefer to be viewed, how they act, and how they imagine their partners regard them.

SELECTION OF PATIENTS

There are no exclusionary criteria for selecting patients based on diagnosis or severity of problem. The decision about whom we talk with and when is based on the clients' preferences as well as those of the therapist.

The case featured in this chapter involves a man (Jim) who has acted aggressively toward his wife (Rita) and their children. Should the therapist feel that Jim's behavior makes it such that he or she cannot inquire about his preferences, hopes, and intentions with respect and empathy, then it's best to refer the couple to a colleague. Successful outcomes in narrative solutions therapy hinge on the therapist's ability to follow the principles and practices of helpful conversations, regardless of the nature of the problem the couple brings.

The beginning of therapy may be seen as a minitrial to determine whether therapist and clients can connect on preferences. Therapists should consider whether they feel capable and maneuverable to be helpful to the client. Over the telephone they decide whether there's a sufficient fit between their own wishes and the client's preferences to arrange an initial meeting.

In selecting clients for treatment, therapists might ask themselves this question: "Can I remain a good detective ?" "Can I talk with clients from a position of curiosity and respect and engage them in piecing together the puzzle of how the problem became a problem?" "Can I probe the problem (whatever its nature) as a mystery that *may not* represent the truth of who people really are and commands an explanation?"

Therapists need not *feel* neutral about the presenting problem. A therapist who is passionately opposed to violence in relationships may be particularly inspired to be helpful to such a couple. The key issue in deciding whether to take the case is gauging whether the therapist's personal passion renders him or her unable to connect with preferred views, to identify gaps between who people would like to be and how they behave, and, in general, to manage a respectful conversation.

The First Phone Call

A therapeutic conversation begins with the first phone call. This is when we arrange the first appointment and decide whom to see. Whether to see the couple together or separately is an issue on the therapist's mind as he or she talks with the caller.

When Rita Jensen first called to arrange an appointment, she sounded hesitant.

RITA: I'm calling as a last resort. I went to my lawyer today to see about a separation. He convinced me that I should give marriage counseling a try.

ERON: What did you think about the advice?

RITA: (*hesitating*) I guess he's right . . . I suppose I shouldn't give up so easily.

ERON: Did your husband go with you to the lawyer?

RITA: No. He didn't even know I made the appointment. He doesn't know I'm calling you.

ERON: What would he think about the idea of seeing a lawyer?

RITA: I don't think he wants a separation.

ERON: How about counseling?

RITA: He'd probably be okay with counseling, but I don't want to talk with him until I figure out what I want to do.

ERON: Should you and I meet the first time and take it from there?

RITA: Yes.

The therapist chooses not to pursue the issue of why Rita would prefer to keep private the meeting with the lawyer. He simply respects the client's preference to meet with him separately. He does not impose alternative rules for conducting couples counseling (e.g., "I can't set up an appointment with you until one of us talks with your husband." "I can't proceed when there are secrets.") These rules might evoke more caution and result in an already hesitant client failing to keep her appointment.

In this telephone conversation, therapist and client preferences converge, and both feel comfortable arranging an initial meeting. Let's consider an alternative scenario in which preferences clash.

Say that Jim had called to make an appointment with Rita at his side. When Jim declares that he wants to meet together, the therapist asks what Rita would like. Jim hands her the telephone, angrily saying, "Talk to the doctor." The therapist asks Rita whose idea it was to seek therapy. She says it was Jim's idea. When the therapist explores Rita's view, she sounds fearful and doesn't assert a clear preference. "Whatever Jim wants is okay with me," she says. When the therapist suggests that he would like to meet with Jim and Rita separately to understand each person's point of view, Jim interrupts and repeats his demand for a joint session. Jim explains that he wants a third party present to mediate between the couple and wants to make sure that Rita hears what he has to say.

At this stage, the therapist may not feel in a maneuverable position to conduct a first session. He might again offer to meet with Jim individually, respecting Jim's wish to talk, Rita's reluctance, and his own discomfort with the role of referee. Should Jim accept this offer, the door remains open to talk with Rita at a later time when the terms suit her better. Should Jim reject the offer, the therapist might clarify his preference to be helpful and stick to the arrangement that suits him. He might end the conversation by encouraging Jim and Rita to think things over and get back to him, keeping the door open to helpful conversations in the future.

It's important for therapists to arrange conversational formats that allow each of the conversants (including the therapist) to feel empowered, not overpowered. It's unlikely for therapists to be helpful in managing issues of coercion or aggression in a relationship when they themselves feel coerced.

Should the therapist and client(s) agree on terms for a first meeting, then the therapist can take the time to explore further people's preferences, hopes, and intentions. Usually, the initial focus is on help seeking itself. What are the client's views about therapy? Is seeking professional help compatible with his or her preferred view? The client's ideas about therapy provide a window into understanding who he or she wish to be.

The First Session

It was a warm mid-September day when Rita arrived for her first appointment. She was dressed professionally in a business suit and greeted the therapist warmly. Rita was a petite woman, well-mannered, and soft-spoken. Despite the temperature outside, Rita wore a shawl around her shoulders and clutched it tightly when the conversation became uncomfortable.

ERON: Have you ever gone for marriage counseling before?

RITA: No, never. This is very hard for me. I like to solve my own problems (*smiles*).

ERON: I got the impression that you wanted to think things through independently from Jim. Did you decide to talk with Jim about our appointment?

RITA: No. I still want to keep this to myself until I figure out what I want.

ERON: Would you be likely to speak with Jim about what you've thought through independently?

RITA: I don't know . . . Sometimes he gets really angry. I don't want to deal with his temper.

Rita responds to the question about previous counseling by asserting that she likes to "solve her own problems." Coupling this statement with what she said over the telephone, the therapist seeks to understand Rita's preferred view. Rita confirms the therapist's impression that she'd like to "think things through independently."

When the therapist then inquires into the effects of talking openly with Jim about her appointment, Rita brings up the issue of Jim's temper. Thus, by connecting with preferred views and discussing the effects of open discussion, the conversation moves quickly into a serious concern. Nonimpositional inquiry into preferences and effects gives therapy a *focus*. We are now poised to learn more about Jim's temper and its influence on Rita, Jim, and the marriage.

FINDING THE FOCUS

The therapist maintains a focus throughout the therapeutic conversation on people's preferences. The therapist's questions are designed to zero in on problematic gaps—between who Rita would like to be and how she acts, between who she'd like Jim to be and how he acts, between what she'd like the relationship to be and what it was and is, between how she'd like to regard herself and how she thinks Jim regards her. These gaps become the focus of the therapy. They represent the basis of relationship difficulties, and we aim helpful conversations at closing them.

In the first session, the therapist's focus on preferences has led quickly (and nonimpositionally) to the identification of a serious problem—Jim's temper. For obvious reasons we now want to focus on this issue of how Jim's "temper" may have been a factor in Rita's decision to talk with an attorney about a separation. Rita may need reassurance from Jim about "controlling his temper" before she speaks openly with him or proceeds with couple therapy. By the close of the first session, the therapist will need to consult Rita's preferences, and his own, about how to continue. Does Rita think it would be a good idea to talk with Jim? Would she prefer that the therapist meet with Jim separately? Does the therapist feel he must talk with Jim in order to be helpful to Rita?

The conversation continues with a focus on the effects of Jim's temper on Rita.

ERON: When Jim's temper takes over, what happens?

RITA: I lose Jim. He becomes someone else . . . someone I don't like very much (*hesitates*). . . . He rants, raves and carries on. (*Rita's* face appears more intense *as if to mirror Jim's intensity or reflect her own fear.*) He gets an intense look on his face like he's about to explode.

ERON: Does he?

RITA: He doesn't explode as much as he used to.

ERON: What does he do that feels scary?

RITA: He used to drink, but he stopped a year ago. He's better now, but he still gets suspicious. He thinks I'm doing things behind his back. Last week I was on the phone with my friend. He barged into the room, grabbed the phone from me, and started firing all these questions at me (*holds tightly to the shawl, pulling it closer to her*). He was two inches from my face . . . (*hesitates*). I'm never sure what he's gonna do (*composing herself and rearranging shawl*). You know. This is terrible. All I'm doing is talking about Jim . . . as if all our problems are *his* fault. I'm making him out like he's a horrible person. He's not . . . and I'm not perfect.

ERON: Actually, I don't think you've said an unkind word about Jim. You're helping me get a picture of *what you'd like.* It sounds like you don't like the effect Jim's temper has on him or you. You chose interesting words. It's like you "lose Jim" when he acts that way.

RITA: I guess that's true. . . . But I think we should start talking about me. All I'm doing is talking about Jim.

In this segment, the therapist tries to get a clear picture of what Jim does and what effect his actions have on Rita and the marriage. Note that the therapist frames his questions in an externalizing manner. Instead of asking what happens when Jim "loses his temper," he asks what happens when Jim's "temper takes over." The therapist avoids suggesting that Jim *is* his temper or that violent behavior is synonymous with his character. This allows Rita and the therapist to discuss what Jim *does* without feeling as though she has to judge Jim. In fact, Rita *herself* describes Jim's behavior in an externalizing manner. She says "she loses Jim," and that he "becomes someone else."

After telling a story about a recent incident of Jim's aggressive behavior, Rita asks to switch the subject. The therapist chooses to respect this preference, even though he's concerned about the issue of violence in the marriage. Rita has offered clues about a possible transition point in the relationship. She mentions that Jim stopped drinking, yet he didn't stop acting aggressively. At some point, the therapist will try to return to the subject of "Jim's temper" and to focus the conversation around a mystery question: Why would a man who got control of his drinking still have difficulty controlling his temper? By focusing on times when Jim acted in control (investigating the story of recent sobriety), we may obtain a preferred picture of Jim through Rita's eyes. This should help lessen Rita's concern about blaming Jim or portraying him in a negative light.

The therapist closes this segment of conversation by connecting with Rita's preferences. He emphasizes her sensitivity to Jim (a preferred view) by reminding her that she never judged Jim in describing his behavior. The therapist also reassures Rita that she was *helpful* to him by clarifying what she'd like in the relationship. Rita's wish to be helpful to family members becomes a key theme in her account of the history of her 20-year marriage and her own family background. By framing Rita's frank discussion about Jim's behavior as caring, the therapist increases the likelihood that the first session will end with a clear focus.

PLANNING THE TREATMENT

The primary goal in planning treatment is to be helpful to people, not to be brief. Brevity follows when therapists engage people's strengths and resources in rethinking their life circumstances and empower them to initiate solutions. Neither clients not therapists are likely to feel empowered, however, if artificial time limits are imposed on the conversation.

By suggesting that positive outcomes can be achieved in 10 sessions or less, we set the stage for clients and therapists to experience failure. "Whoops, it's now Session 5, and our sex life hasn't improved. I guess that proves our marriage is dysfunctional." "Uh-oh. It's now Session 5, and I haven't fixed the couple's sexual problems. I guess that means I'm an incompetent therapist."

Decisions about planning treatment pivot around a careful assessment of the evolving problem and of the key views and behaviors that sustain current relationship patterns. Let's summarize what the therapist learned from Rita Jensen in the first session that helped to plan the next steps in treatment.

Rita's Story

As we left the conversation with Rita, she indicated that she wanted to talk about herself and not just about Jim's temper. The therapist took this opportunity to learn more about Rita as a person.

Rita perked up as she spoke about her children. Andrew and Julia were doing well at college, and a third son, Mark, a football star, was preparing to go off to college the following year. Rita expressed pride in her ability to "keep things normal" for the children, shielding them as best she could from the effects of their father's drinking.

Jim's recent sobriety and the looming prospect of an "empty nest" left Rita thinking about herself for the first time in years. She wanted to pursue opportunities in her career and socialize with her fellow elementary school teachers. She hoped to reclaim passion for horseback riding. While she wanted to spend more time with Jim, she also wanted "breathing space to be herself."

During their 20-year marriage, Rita wasn't accustomed to talking about herself or bringing attention to her own needs. If she had experienced disappointment at giving up horseback riding, Jim wouldn't know about it. When she felt exhilaration with an achievement at school, she'd keep it to herself. As Rita became interested in pursuing new activities, she did so privately. For example, she'd telephone an old friend who shared her passion for horses but wouldn't discuss these exciting conversations with Jim. He might then discover a phone bill listing a series of long distance calls. "How come you're spending all this money calling Pennsylvania?" he'd demand. Sheepishly, Rita would reply that she was making plans to go horseback riding with Ellen and let Jim know he too was invited. "You know I hate horseback riding," Jim would say, and "What's with you calling Ellen all the time? Since when are you two such close friends?" Feeling rebuffed, Jim would decline Rita's invitation, then accuse her of never wanting to do anything with him. Feeling restrained, Rita would cancel her plans with Ellen. Following these hurtful exchanges, the couple would typically retreat into silence for a few days, although Jim would continue to pursue Rita sexually. At first, Rita might reject Jim's overtures, then she'd accede, more to appease him than to please herself.

Rita mentioned that she had recently gotten close to a male friend through work. She enjoyed talking with him about her aspirations and, when lonely, wrote letters to him. Rita said she had no interest in a romantic relationship with this man but felt comforted by their conversations. She said that Jim was extremely jealous of this relationship and read more into it than there really was. The therapist learned that Rita was talking with her friend on the telephone the day Jim barged into the room, seized the phone, screamed and cursed at her, then left in a huff, after kicking a hole in the door.

When asked whether this incident reminded her of times past, Rita admitted that there had been three instances over the course of the marriage in which she worried about her safety. In all three situations, Jim was drunk, jealous, verbally abusive, and physically menacing. Although Rita claimed that Jim never struck her in the course of their marriage, he had in fact grabbed her, shaken her and warned her that she'd "get hers" if she ever "snuck around on him." Suspicion about unfaithful behavior was a common theme surrounding Jim's past temper outbursts. His recent return to aggressive behavior, and the painful memories it evoked, was enough to motivate Rita to make an appointment with her attorney to discuss a separation. Fearing Jim's wrath, she had done so secretly.

Based on Rita's story, we can draw a diagram of the problem cycle for Rita (see Figure 12.1).

Although we refer to Rita's indecision as an "evolving problem," it is, in fact, the start of a solution. Alcoholism and violence have been long-standing problems in the relationship. Rita became motivated to speak up about her preferences, once protecting the children from Jim's irresponsible behavior ceased to be her major focus. In the next segment, note how the therapist frames the presenting problem in the context of this time of transition and joins with Rita's hopes and aspirations for the future.

ERON: It seems like you saw the last year as a time of opportunity for you and Jim to bring out the best in each other, and you wanted to take advantage of it.

RITA: Yes, I'm really proud of Jim, that he stopped drinking, but I'm disappointed in what's happened between us. I think he can do so much more for himself. I guess I can too.

ERON: Sounds like you'd like to see Jim take control of his temper like he did with his drinking.

Doing

- Withdraws from partner (Jim).
- Maintains secretive plans, including talking with attorney.
- Conceals preferences from Jim. Discusses hopes and aspirations with friends.

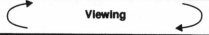

P.V. Independent, responsible, energetic, successful, a caring and loving mother

D.V. "I'm acting irresponsibly (secretive) and insensitive to Jim."

D.V. "My husband thinks I'm irresponsible, insensitive, uncaring."

D.V. "He is threatened by my independence."

FIGURE 12.1. The problem cycle for Rita. *Note:* This diagram links current behavior ("Doing") with key views of self and other ("Viewing"). In the "Viewing" box, we highlight preferred views of self and the views of others that contradict the client's preferences. The designation "P.V." is used to refer to preferred views, while "D.V." refers to disjunctive views. The arrows connecting "Viewing" and "Doing" show that the experience of contradiction between how people prefer to be seen and how they see others seeing them is what propels problematic behavior.

RITA: I feel I can't talk with Jim about what I want. I can't trust him not to explode. I hope I haven't made it sound like Jim's got all the problems. I know I contribute ... I've been keeping things from him, and I know I've really hurt him.

ERON: When you say you'd like Jim to control his temper, I think you're talking about Jim being the best person he can. Jim had the strength to take control of his drinking, why then wouldn't he take control of his temper and support you in pursuing what you'd like?

RITA: I can't imagine Jim supporting my independence. I'd settle for a little breathing space (*smiles*).

ERON: I feel like the next step for me might be to talk with Jim and get his sense of things. Would that be okay with you?

RITA: Yes. But I'd rather he come in and talk with you alone. I don't think I'm ready for us to come together.

ERON: I'd be happy to do that. Would you mind if I mention some of the things I've learned about you to Jim? I wonder if Jim knows what effect his temper has on you when it gets the best of him.

RITA: That's fine. I think you can do a better job talking about me than me talking about me at this point (*smiles*).

ERON: How should we proceed? Would you like me to call Jim? Would you like to talk to him?

RITA: I think it's time for me to talk with Jim. I want to tell him about our meeting and my meeting with Mr. Englehardt [the lawyer]. I know Jim doesn't want a separation, and I'm sure he'll want to see you. I think despite all these things I've said about Jim, you'll like him. He's really a good man.

ERON: I look forward to hearing from him.

BUILDING THE ALLIANCE

The therapist attempts to build a *separate alliance* with each person in the relationship. By the end of the first session, Rita sees the therapist seeing her as a competent, loving mother who successfully raised three children, helping them focus on their own independent aspirations rather than be burdened by their father's out-of-control behavior.[1] Rita might also regard the therapist as sharing in her enthusiasm for a new stage of family life in which she focuses on her own independent aspirations. She sees the therapist as interested in her stories about horseback riding, her commitment to bringing out the best in her elementary school students, and in her desire to make new friends.

Rita also sees the therapist as on her side in wanting an end to in-your-face confrontations, yelling, cursing, pushing, threatening, and kicking holes in doors. Rita notices that the therapist regards her preferences for nonviolence as consistent with wanting what's best for Jim—as fitting with his commitment to sobriety and self-control.

Building an alliance with Rita helps in building an alliance with Jim. The therapist enters the conversation with Jim understanding Rita's preferences for a loving marriage, understanding what she sees as strong in Jim, and knowing what Jim might do to rebuild his alliance with Rita.

Jim Jensen called to arrange an appointment 2 days after the therapist's meeting with Rita. When Jim arrived for the first meeting, he seemed a contrast to Rita. Wearing a tee shirt and jeans, he seemed unconcerned about his appearance. Although only slightly taller than Rita, he was imposing, muscular, and his intensity filled the room. When upset he'd show it, his face crinkling as he strained to find the right words to express his emotions.

Consider these excerpts from the first session with Jim that further illustrate our approach to alliance building.

Jim's Story

ERON: I guess Rita spoke with you about our meeting last week. I felt she and I had a good talk.

JIM: I didn't know about her appointment with you. I was upset. It's typical of Rita to do things that way, but I'm glad she told me about her meeting with the lawyer and with you. I don't want a separation. I'm not ready to give up on 20 years of marriage.

ERON: Rita mentioned that you're not the kind of person who gives up. [preferred view]

JIM: (*smiles*) That's true. I can be stubborn.

ERON: She talked about how you stopped drinking in the last year. She's admired your self-control.

JIM: Once I put my mind to something I usually stick to it.

ERON: What do you think led Rita to change her mind about a separation and give counseling a try?

JIM: I don't know. I think she's confused. She doesn't know what she wants. I think she felt good about her talk with you. Maybe she rethought things and wants to give the marriage a chance. I hope so.

ERON: Is that what you'd like?

JIM: Yes. I don't think giving up is the thing to do. We've raised three kids who are ready to be on their own. I thought this would be the time for us finally, but Rita seems to try to keep away from me as much as she can.

ERON: How does that affect you?

JIM: What do you mean?

ERON: When you sense Rita is keeping her distance from you and you don't know why, what effect does that have on you?

JIM: I suppose she told you about my temper.

ERON: I tried to get a picture of what happens when your temper takes control. What you do, how Rita feels, what she does, but it took me a while to get the details. I think Rita was concerned that she might be describing you in a negative light.

JIM: I hate it when she beats around the bush like that. I wish she'd just come out with it. Tell me what bothers her.

ERON: You'd prefer straightforward talk.

JIM: Yes. Whatever it is. Even if Rita didn't love me anymore or if she wanted to be with someone else. I'd be upset, but I could deal with it. It's not knowing what's going on that drives me crazy.

ERON: Is that when your temper gets the best of you?

JIM: Definitely.

ERON: Maybe you can help give me a straightforward picture of what happens? What do you do?

The therapist uses the information gleaned from the first session with Rita to align with Jim's preferred view. He starts by portraying Jim at his best through Rita's eyes. He mentions that Rita described Jim as a person who doesn't give up easily and then alludes to her pride in his self-control and determination to stop drinking. By emphasizing Jim's strengths and resources, the conversation moves swiftly and nondefensively into a discussion of the presenting problems—Rita's indecision about the marriage and Jim's temper.

The conversation is guided by the therapist's curiosity about preferences and effects. The therapist inquires about the *effect* on Jim when Rita appears distant or keeps information from him. Jim immediately brings up the subject of his temper. The therapist then mentions his own *preference* to get a clear picture of "what happens when Jim's temper takes control." He also mentions Rita's reluctance to describe Jim in a negative light. Jim recasts Rita's behavior as a form of misguided protection, asserting his own *preference* for "straightforward talk." In keeping with Jim's stated preference, the therapist invites him to give a "straightforward" picture of what happens when his temper takes control. After getting Jim's description of what he *does* and under what circumstances, the therapist will then inquire whether Jim's aggressive behavior fits with his own preferences, and what effects he feels his actions have on Rita and the relationship. At this point we can diagram the problem cycle for both Rita and Jim (see Figure 12.2).

In asking preference and effects questions, the goal of therapists is to discern whether a gap exists between who people would like to be, how they act, and the effects their actions have on others. If a gap is identified, therapists have motivation to work with. When clients describe feeling unsettled about their own behavior, concerned about its effects, and distressed about how important others regard them, they often want to do something about their situation. In this case, the conversations with Rita and Jim reveal that both persons experience gaps, which can be portrayed diagrammatically (see Figures 12.3 and 12.4).

What do therapists do when they inquire respectfully about people's preferences and effects and find that there is no gap? Say that Jim had replied that he enjoyed the fear-injecting, distance-creating effects he has

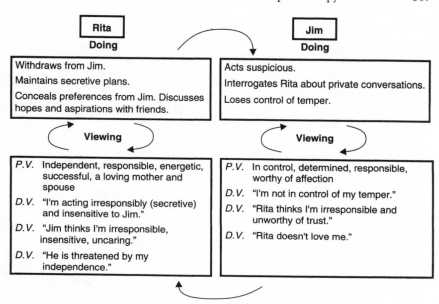

FIGURE 12.2. The problem cycle for Rita and Jim.

on Rita and liked the feeling of power he derives by expressing his emotions through rage. In such an instance, the continuation of couple therapy may be harmful to Rita, and the therapist should feel free to change the agenda.

The therapist might shift the focus to helping Rita access resources that promote her preference for nonviolence and self-affirmation. As a consequence, Rita might recontact her attorney to advise her about a separation. In turn, the therapist might continue the conversation with Jim to ease the transition through separation, suggesting that Rita's initiatives are understandable given the gap between the couple's preferences.

Jim may be more likely to accept the idea of a separation if he were to view this event as an extension of his own intentions rather than as an indicator or Rita's defiance or rejection. Thus, the therapist might maintain a conversation with Jim that holds him accountable to his preference (for rageful communication) and might suggest that by articulating this preference, he has helped Rita reach a difficult decision.

Using preferred views as a navigational guide, therapists can be planful yet flexible in steering the conversation. They can do what fits. They needn't feel committed to a contract for couple therapy or feel "lost at sea" when fixing the relationship seems untenable.

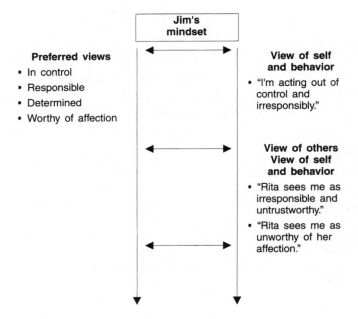

FIGURE 12.3. Jim's gap between preferred views and disjunctive views. The greater the gap, the greater the client's distress.

In this case, the first two sessions end with an alliance built between the therapist and both partners in the relationship. After speaking with the therapist about what they'd like for themselves and their marriage, Rita and Jim are now more likely to speak with each other about what they'd like for themselves and for their marriage.

CORE TECHNICAL MANEUVERS

The steps described thus far set the stage for *restorying, mystery questioning*, and *reframing*. These core techniques are extensions of the principles of helpful conversations outlined earlier. The central feature of a helpful conversation is *narrowing the gap* between how people prefer to be viewed, how they act, and how they think important others regard them. From the first phone call with the client through the first meeting and the various stages of the therapeutic conversation, the therapist focuses on closing these troublesome gaps, thereby inspiring solutions (see Figures 12.3 and 12.4).

Helpful conversations are generative. The therapist's interest in each person's preferences (inside the therapy room) sparks the couple to talk with each other about their preferences (outside the therapy room). In the third session, Jim arrived looking more cheerful. The basis of his optimism was a *different conversation* that occurred over lunch at the couple's outdoor picnic table. Jim said that he spoke with Rita about what he'd like for their marriage and that she did the same. The gist of Jim's appeal was for more physical affection. He said that he pictured the two drawing closer after he got sober and the children left home and was disappointed that they hadn't. According to Jim, Rita responded that she was having trouble feeling close to Jim because she was afraid of his temper. She also said she wanted to "have her own thoughts" and to feel free to pursue her own interests in the marriage.

In the third and fourth sessions the therapist followed up with Jim and Rita on the effects of this new conversation. The therapist's aim was to focus Jim and Rita's attention on what was helpful about their conversation and build upon their initial success.

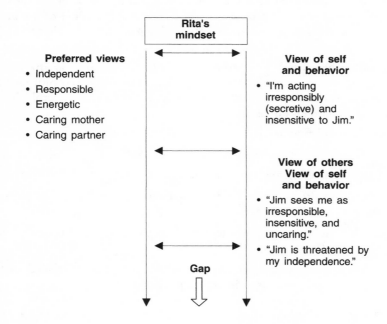

FIGURE 12.4. Rita's gap between preferred views and disjunctive views.

Session 3 (with Jim)

ERON: How did you feel about your talk with Rita?

JIM: Pretty good. But I'm still not sure what Rita means when she says she wants to have her own thoughts.

ERON: Were you pleased with how you came across?

JIM: Yes. At least I didn't blow up or lose my cool. I guess that's good.

ERON: Sounds like you helped Rita understand what you want in the marriage.

JIM: I think *I* was clear, but I'm still not sure what Rita wants. She confuses me.

ERON: You'd like to understand better what Rita wants? Would that be helpful?

JIM: Yes.

Session 4 (with Rita)

ERON: Jim told me about a conversation you and he had over the picnic table. He seemed encouraged. (*Rita describes her version of the picnic table discussion, which is compatible with Jim's version.*) How did you feel the conversation went?

RITA: Better than usual. Jim told me he wanted more physical affection. I felt more comfortable talking than I usually do. I told him that I need to think for myself and do things for myself. I also told him that I don't like his temper.

ERON: How did that feel?

RITA: Good. It felt better to tell him than to keep everything inside.

ERON: And Jim listened?

RITA: He seemed to. At least he didn't lose his temper. He stayed pretty calm.

ERON: Jim told me that it would help him to understand better what you want.

RITA: (*shrugs, looks skeptical*) That's a surprise. At least we talked with each other. That's a step in the right direction.

The picnic table discussion was "helpful" because it narrowed the gaps diagrammed earlier (see Figures 12.3 and 12.4). Jim was "pleased with himself" because he acted in line with his own preference to be in control, responsible, and worthy of trust. Rita felt relieved because Jim talked with her in a way that fit within her preferred image of Jim and the marriage. Rita felt that she had acted in line with her wish to think and act independently. She also experienced herself as "responsible" (a preferred view) because she had spoken with Jim *directly* rather than talking *about him* with others or talking to herself.

This helpful conversation outside the therapy room set the stage for further exploration into the mystery of the problem evolution, which is the basis of restorying and reframing. Whereas reframing applies to the immediate interactional predicament, restorying applies to a broader context of meaning that embraces past, present, and future dimensions of experience. In introducing this technique, White and Epson (1990) describe a story or self-narrative as follows: "In striving to make sense of life, persons face the task of arranging their experiences of events in sequences across time in such a way as to arrive at a coherent account of themselves and the world around them. Specific experiences of the past and present, and those that are predicted to occur in the future, must be connected in a lineal sequence to develop this account. This account can be referred to as a story or self-narrative" (p. 10).

At first glance, helping Jim and Rita to "arrive at a coherent account of themselves and the world around them" that integrates past, present, and future, seems a daunting task. After all, isn't brief therapy about changing what people are doing *now* so that they can move on to the next hurdle in life? Restorying becomes more purposeful and precise, however, if we know what stories to look for and emphasize to promote change in here-and-now patterns of interaction.

Selecting Key Stories

In this case, the therapist chooses the story of Jim's decision to seek sobriety as a centerpiece of collaborative inquiry. There are several reasons to select this key story.

1. This story represents an exception to the present problem, portraying Jim at his best—as a person who *can* set behavioral limits, act responsibly, and seize control of his life and relationships.
2. This story provides a vehicle for future *mystery questioning* with Jim and Rita. How is it that a man who was able to set limits on his drinking is not exerting control of his temper and jeopardizing a marriage he wants to keep?
3. The juxtaposition of this story of sobriety with accounts of past and present aggression helps to transfer accountability for the future relationship over to Jim. The therapist's purpose is to *lift*

the burden from Rita to prove that she is a loving and affection- ate partner and *shift the burden* over to Jim for reclaiming Rita's trust.

As the conversation continues in the fifth session, the therapist explores with Jim the story of his sobriety and uses this story to *connect with preferred views.*

ERON: I'm interested in what inspired your decision to stop drinking. Rita told me how impressed she was with your determination.

JIM: It was kind of a sudden decision. I just looked at my life and where it was heading and felt I had to do something different.

ERON: Not everyone can take a hard look at his life and redirect its course. I'm not an expert on alcoholism, but don't some people wind up drinking themselves to death?

JIM: I think I was one of those (*smiles*). I'm not sure I'd be talking with you know if I hadn't stopped.

At this point, Jim told the therapist his version of a story already told by Rita in the first session. Jim's decision to stop drinking followed a dangerous car ride with his two younger brothers. Jim's youngest brother, Bill, was driving the car. Jim was in the front passenger seat and his older brother, Art, was in the back. Art and Bill had been drinking at the family party, and the three were on their way to Jim's house. Jim, who had experienced petit-mal seizures as a result of a head injury from a drinking and driving accident five years before, was sober only because he had an appointment with his neurologist the following morn- ing. Art and Bill were screaming and cursing at each other, while Bill, the driver, picked up speed. Somehow, Jim was able to convince Bill to pull over to the side of the road. Then he took the wheel and drove everyone home safely.

Jim described this event as a kind of epiphany. He hated the fighting that was going on between his brothers and wanted it to stop. He thought about his appointment with his neurologist and felt lucky to be alive. He didn't like what drinking had done to his brothers or to him. He experi- enced an aura similar to the kind induced by the petit-mal seizures, but this time there was no loss of control. His life flickering dream-like before him, Jim felt strangely composed. His approach with his brothers was calm and matter of fact; a stark contrast to their reckless behavior. He decided it was time to stop drinking. He attended AA meetings for 6 months following the episode, then maintained sobriety on his own.

In this next segment, the therapist uses Jim's dramatic story of sobriety as a vehicle for *mystery questioning.*

Session 5 (with Jim)

ERON: I was interested in your reaction to your brothers' fighting in the car, both under the influence! You took charge, somehow got them under control and drove everyone safely home. You took a stand *against* violence and *for* safety.

JIM: Yes (*looking proud and confident*).

ERON: (*looking puzzled*) Maybe you can help me out with something. How is it that a man who is against violence—who had the where-withal to grab control of the steering wheel, then grab control of his life by stopping drinking—finds himself in a situation where he loses control of his temper and is seen as out-of-control by the person he most loves? [mystery question]

JIM: (*looking thoughtful and subdued*) That's a good question. I need to think about it.

Jim responded to the therapist's puzzling question by becoming thoughtful. His reflections took him back in time. He then told a story about his violent background, about living with an alcoholic father and frightened mother who fought intensely. It was as if Jim retrieved this past story to explain the contradictions posed by the mystery question. The therapist followed up asking Jim to describe the *effects* his parents fighting had on him. Jim said he hated it when his parents bickered. Feeling frightened and alone, he and his brothers would go off to their separate rooms. Jim said he felt compassion for his mother who didn't drink, yet "put up" with his father's abuse. The therapist noted that "Jim's *preference* for compassion and nonviolence had firm roots in his growing-up years." Although Jim seemed moved by this comment, he was also challenged by the contradictions it implied to his current situation. The comment may have inspired Jim to ask himself a mystery question: "Why if I hated my parents fighting, am I acting aggressively in my own marriage?" The therapist then remarked that "becoming sober *and* taking a stand against violence seemed to *fit* for Jim," again emphasizing a current preference.

Jim, growing more thoughtful, had what seemed another epiphany.

JIM: I think I've got to change my approach to Rita.

ERON: What do you mean?

JIM: I get in her face and scare her when I think she's doing things behind my back. Maybe that's why she keeps things from me. [a softening, see Johnson, Chapter 2, this volume]

ERON: I think you're on to something. Sounds like you'd like to find a way to help Rita feel more confident about speaking up about her preferences. You've said she has difficulty doing that.

JIM: It sure doesn't help when I blow up. I'm gonna have to count to 10, stop and think, do something to get myself under control.

In the context of restorying, Jim decides to change his current approach to Rita. He *reframes* Rita's secretive behavior as based in fear rather than a rejection of him. Perhaps she has isolated herself just as he isolated himself as a child—for purposes of self-protection. Jim also begins to weave an *alternative explanation* for current relationship difficulties that holds him accountable for change. (Perhaps Rita finds me worthy of love and affection, but my own actions interfere with her ability to freely express herself. I must earn her trust by acting in line with my own preference for self-control, that is, "I've got to change my approach to Rita.")

Psychodynamically oriented therapists might be curious about the emphasis on the past in this approach. Narrative solutions therapists use the past, present, and future to gain insight into who people aspire to be, not to impart insight about who they are. The past stories Jim tells about driving in the car with his brothers and growing up in a violent household reveal a *preference for nonviolence*. The therapist brings this preference out of hiding and places it into bold relief, inviting Jim to examine it against his present behavior and Rita's cautious approach to him. As a result, Jim becomes motivated to rethink his current actions within a richer narrative—who he *was*, *is*, and *hopes* to be. The therapist does not probe the past to delve into the origins of Jim's mistrust or rage. Such an inquiry orients the conversation around what's wrong in Jim; and bypasses what is strong in Jim. Instead of rethinking his present approach as a *contradiction* to his preferred view, Jim might merely justify his current actions as *consistent* with unresolved rage or mistrust. The therapeutic conversation might remain frozen in the past rather than using the past to introduce fluidity or movement into the present and future.

Session 6 (with Rita)

Rita arrived for Session 6 excited to describe a recent incident. She said that she left her diary open by accident, and Jim began reading it. In the diary was a passage she had addressed to her male friend about her hopes for the future and her fears that her marriage might not survive. More recent notes reflected Rita's dream to pursue horseback riding and eventually purchase a horse. She also wrote about her wish that Jim reconnect with their son and daughter in college. She wanted her grown children to know Jim as the sober person he was becoming, rather than the reckless person he was when they lived at home.

Rita was astonished at Jim's reaction to reading the diary. At first she was upset with his intrusiveness and girded herself for the explosive reaction that seemed certain to come. Somehow, however, Jim read the passage written to her male friend and contained his rage. Looking shaken but determined to control himself, Jim asked Rita's permission to read more, saying that he wanted to understand what was in the diary so that he could better understand Rita. Rita told Jim that if he felt compelled to read the diary, he should go ahead. Jim then went off into another room and read it. He returned saying that it was difficult for him to read the diary but helpful. He had learned more about what Rita wanted for her life and apologized for not paying attention to her. He said he wanted to talk with her more about horseback riding. Rita, still appearing bewildered, said that she couldn't believe this transformation in Jim, but it was clear she liked this "new Jim" far better than the "old Jim." And it was also clear that she felt that Jim "had it in him" to be a responsible person. "Perhaps I wasn't a fool," she said, "when I married Jim, knowing his background and thinking he could change."

Session 7 (with Jim)

In Session 7, the therapist followed up on the diary incident with Jim.

ERON: I remember last time we met you told me you were committed to changing your approach to Rita. Sounds like you meant business. [preferred view]

JIM: What do you mean?

ERON: Rita told me how impressed she was with your reaction to reading her diary. (*Jim tells his version of the story of the diary incident.*) How did you manage to contain your anger when you read Rita's entries in the diary? Particularly that note to her friend.

JIM: I was determined to do what I said. Blowing up wouldn't have helped. I decided to count to 10 and go in the other room and read the diary on my own. I kept telling myself that whatever the hell was in there it would help me to know what was going on.

ERON: Did reading the diary help?

JIM: After I thought about it, yes. Don't get me wrong. I don't trust the guy she's been talking with, but I'm pretty sure there's not much going on there.

ERON: Why are you more confident?

JIM: Rita and I got close this week. The next day I talked with her about horseback riding. I told her I'd like to see her be more involved with it.

ERON: How did Rita react?

JIM: She seemed really happy and seeing her happy made me happy. I encouraged her to call her friend in Pennsylvania and make plans. I told her I'd go see Andrew [son] that weekend. We could go to the football game at his college.

ERON: What do you think about all that?

JIM: I think it's a good idea. My kids know me as a drinker. They need to know me for who I am now.

ERON: You said you and Rita got closer this week. What did you mean?

JIM: I think we got closer than we have in years. A really amazing thing happened . . . (*hesitates*). . . .

ERON: What was it?

JIM: Rita kissed me (*smiles*). It sounds weird, but it's been a while since she's kissed me when we have sex. I've been really upset about it.

ERON: What do you think changed things?

JIM: I think she's beginning to trust me more.

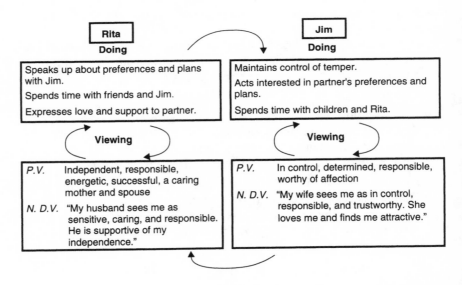

FIGURE 12.5. A narrative solution. *Note:* The designation "N.D.V." refers to nondisjunctive views. Solutions emerge when there is no contradiction between how people prefer to be viewed, how they act, and how they see their partner viewing them.

Seven sessions had now been conducted with Rita and Jim—three with Rita individually (Sessions 1, 4, and 6) and four with Jim individually (Sessions 2, 3, 5, and 7). The changes reported by the couple may be portrayed diagrammatically (see Figure 12.5).

This diagram illustrates the basis of narrative solutions in short-term couples therapy. Each person in the relationship is behaving differently and in ways that confirm preferred views of self. Jim is exerting control of his temper and demonstrating to Rita that he is interested in her thoughts, hopes, and aspirations. These new behaviors are in line with Jim's preferred view to be in control, responsible, and worthy of trust. As Jim acts more trustworthy, Rita begins to speak up about her own preferences. She suspends talking with friends privately and begins sharing with Jim her conversations with others. These new behaviors are in line with Rita's preferred view to be a caring, responsible partner.

Jim supports Rita's pursuit of horseback riding and even encourages her friendships around this activity. As Rita sees Jim seeing her in ways that confirm preferred views of self, she begins to feel more loving toward him and expresses her affection openly. Jim sees Rita seeing him as trustworthy, in control, and worthy of affection, which promotes more of the same responsible behavior. Each person sees the current relationship as fitting within his or her preferred vision of a fulfilling marriage. Because helpful conversations are occurring between the couple outside the therapy room, they are able to rely more on each other as a resource in sustaining change, and less on the therapist. Given these demonstrable changes, it becomes possible to discuss the idea of ending therapy.

PLANNING TERMINATION AND FOLLOW-UP

Session 8 was held with the couple together to summarize what had been accomplished and to plan future steps.

ERON: Sound like things are a bit different for the two of you than when I first spoke with you.

RITA: I'm amazed actually. Jim seems like a different person. The way he responded to the diary really impressed me. I was really afraid of his reaction. But he kept calm. It's strange. It actually seemed to help Jim to read the diary. I thought this would be a disaster, and it's like it became a turning point for us.

ERON: Do you see it that way, Jim?

JIM: Well, I probably shouldn't have looked at the diary in the first place. I didn't like what I read, but I wanted Rita to see that I can control my temper. I need to do that. It helped me to understand what she's thinking.

RITA: I'm beginning to see that now. Jim gets all worked up when he doesn't know what's going on. I don't like when he gets that way. When he's suspicious, he asks me all these questions, and I don't have the answers. All I want to do is get away.

JIM: (*to Rita*) I don't want to do that anymore (*smiling*). Yeah, I told Dr. Eron you were so relaxed you kissed me.

RITA: You're right. I felt more relaxed; I could be myself.

The conversation soon shifted to horseback riding. Rita described a recent day in which she had a great time riding in the backwoods. Jim had encouraged her to take the day off. He made dinner that evening and they talked about the pleasurable day. It was that evening that Rita kissed Jim while making love. Jim left the session with a deeper understanding of Rita's kiss and what he had done to inspire it.

In this conjoint session, Jim and Rita talk with each other in a way that underscores the changes outlined earlier (see Figure 12.5). The therapist simply helped the couple to notice what they were already doing to bring out the best in each other and to explain how they now saw each other. Rita shows that she viewed Jim's suspicious behavior from a different perspective when she said "Jim gets all worked up when he doesn't know what's going on." She then explains to Jim that when he gets suspicious and fires questions at her, all she wants to do is "get away." Jim's response suggested that he now views Rita's secretive behavior differently. He says "I don't want to do that anymore," in reference to acting suspicious and menacing. Hearing Jim take responsibility for his actions should bolster Rita's confidence in his commitment to change.

The therapist steered the conversation to other positive developments. He inquired about whether the couple had followed through on their weekend plans discussed in the previous sessions and learned that they had. Rita reported having a fine time horseback riding with her friend, and Jim enjoyed his visit with his son. Rita spoke about the collaborative planning that went into this weekend as a milestone in their marriage. She couldn't get over how Jim supported her in doing something she loved and could now picture doing things separately from Jim without feeling pressured. She was also pleased that Jim chose to do something with their son. It was as if this weekend represented a structural shift in their relationship. During Jim's drinking years, Rita had been the one focused on the children, while Jim caroused. Now, Jim was helping Rita to focus on having fun while he spent time with the children.

Four criteria for concluding therapy had been met:

1. The problems originally presented by the couple were no longer being presented as problems. Rita felt more confident about staying in the marriage, more trusting of Jim, and more emotionally connected. Jim was controlling his temper and sharing in Rita's preference for a loving (and nonviolent) relationship. Both partners were satisfied with their sexual relationship.
2. The couple was engaging in helpful conversations outside the therapy room.
3. The couple had an explanation for how the problem evolved and dissolved that might help them negotiate future difficulties.
4. The couple were crediting themselves, and not the therapist, with the changes that had occurred.

CONSOLIDATING SOLUTIONS

In light of the changes reported by the couple, the therapist raised the question of stopping therapy.

ERON: You both seem clear about what is working between you and how to make that continue. Have I outlived my usefulness?

RITA: I'm feeling great about things. It would be okay with me to stop for a while. We can always call you if we get stuck.

JIM: I'm a little nervous about stopping. It's only been a short time that we've been doing things differently. I want to make sure I stay on track and our marriage stays strong. I'd like to continue.

RITA: I'm glad that Jim wants to continue. Maybe I can come in once in a while or with Jim as needed.

ERON: How would that be, Jim?

JIM: That's fine with me. I'd like to have regular meetings and maybe leave some time in between so I can work at things. I think Rita could still use your help in speaking up about herself. I know that's a problem for her, and I think it goes back to her family. But I'd like to leave that to her.

RITA: I agree with you, Jim, but as I told you, Dr. Eron, I'd like to work things through for myself. I feel now I can talk with Jim about my issues. [preferred view of independence]

ERON: How about if we meet in a month, Jim, and then we'll take it from there?

The therapist continued meeting with Jim at 4- to 8-week intervals over the course of the following year (a total of eight sessions). Rita came in for two individual meetings and one conjoint session during that time. (The total therapy therefore comprised 20 sessions.)

There were times that Jim had difficulty with Rita's independent pursuits. She wanted to attend evening seminars but wouldn't let Jim know of her plans until after they'd already been made. Jim would become angry. The therapist would often remind Jim of his preference for nonviolence and open conversation. Typically, Jim would collect himself, then let Rita know that he'd like to support her professional pursuits. He'd then convey his wish that she discuss her plans with him ahead of time so that they might work things out together.

Gradually, Rita spoke more openly with Jim about her professional development. In turn, Jim began talking more with Rita about his frustrations with the monotony of his 20-year job as senior mechanic of a local plant. He revealed that he was envious of Rita's excitement in her work and her advanced education. Rita explained that her sensitivity about these differences had restrained her from talking openly with Jim about her work. The couple identified this "misguided protection" of the other as an old pattern that needed to change. With Rita's encouragement, Jim started to consider alternative career possibilities and eventually interviewed for a new job as a groundskeeper at a resort (he loved the out-of-doors). The summer following the couple's entry into therapy was marked by triumphs and potential disaster. Early in the summer, Rita bought a horse. She credited Jim with this decision, because she felt reluctant about the responsibility and the time away from home. Jim advised Rita during the negotiations and helped her get a good price. He was on Rita's side throughout, encouraging her to follow her passion. After tending to or riding her horse, Rita would come home feeling happy and warm toward Jim. Jim noticed that these were the times when he and Rita were closest.

In the late summer, Jim decided to try drinking again. Rita scheduled an appointment to express her concern and to consider how she wanted to approach the issue. In the past she had withdrawn from Jim when he drank, suppressing her worries and fears. This time she chose to talk with him. She told him how uncomfortable she was when they went to dinner and she ordered a gin and tonic, and he did the same. When Jim had a second drink, she said it really concerned her. She encouraged Jim to talk with the therapist, as she had done.

When Jim met with the therapist, he did not hesitate to discuss the recent drinking. He also mentioned two other incidents that Rita didn't know about. He said he had been purposeful in ordering a drink in

Rita's presence and curious about her reaction. He was pleased that Rita spoke up about her discomfort, even if not at the moment.

The therapist inquired about Jim's reaction to his own behavior, asking the usual preference and effects questions. What effect did his experiments with drinking have on Jim and the relationship? Did he feel comfortable and in control? How did he feel about himself after drinking with Rita, and how did he feel when concealing his drinking from Rita? Jim responded by saying he felt worse when concealing the drinking from Rita and better when discussing the issue with her. He also mentioned that, in all three episodes of drinking, he felt little control. He preferred to consider the episodes as an "experiment" that were proving to him that he was not able to drink under control. By the conclusion of this therapy session, Jim decided to return to AA meetings. He recalled the messages he had received about "alcoholic pride," the inclination of alcoholics to think they can control something they can't control. He also recalled helpful advice about making amends to loved ones and felt it was time to complete these steps.

In a recent follow-up 6 months after Jim's drinking experiment, he was still attending AA meetings. As part of his recovery, Jim apologized to Rita and the three children for his past out-of-control behavior and repeated his commitment to sobriety. He and his oldest son had a heart-to-heart talk about drinking during another father and son college weekend. Jim had been concerned about Andrew's excessive beer drinking during the summer and wanted him to know about his own experiences as a recovering alcoholic. Jim said that the conversation had gone well.

CONCLUSIONS

Although significant progress had been made (and the conditions for concluding therapy had been met), the therapist didn't impose termination in Session 8. Instead he consulted the clients' preferences. The focus was on how the couple wished to utilize their own resources and those of the therapist. Jim elected to continue meeting on a regular, though less frequent, basis to "stay in touch." Rita chose to come in, if she "felt stuck," reiterating her preference to figure things out for herself. Fittingly, it was Jim who took responsibility for maintaining positive momentum in the relationship.

Had the therapist chosen to terminate therapy after eight sessions, one wonders how the couple would have weathered Jim's return to drinking. In the context of Jim's continued commitment to open communication and self-control, however, this event became an opportunity for consolidating solutions. Jim reevaluated whether he could drink under control and reengaged AA as a resource. Rita and the therapist also became resources to Jim in this reevaluation process.

The narrative solutions approach is based on principles of helpful conversations that empower people to take ownership of their lives and seek solutions that fit within preferred modes of being and behaving. Couples in distress often experience a gap between who they'd like to be as persons, how they behave with their partners, and how they imagine their partners perceive them. It is by helping couples to close these gaps that creative solutions become possible.

NOTE

1. The therapist does not refer to Rita's approach to Jim's drinking in dysfunctional terms, for example, as a form of "codependency" or "enabling." Instead, he focuses on her strengths as a protective parent.

REFERENCES

Anderson, H., & Goolishian, H. A. (1988). Human systems as linguistic systems: Preliminary and evolving ideas about the implications for clinical theory. *Family Process, 27,* 371–393.

de Shazer, S. (1985). *Keys to solution in brief therapy.* New York: Norton.

de Shazer, S., Berg, I. K., Lipchik, E., Nunnally, E., Molnar, A., Gingerich, W., & Weiner-Davis, M. (1986). Brief therapy: Focused solution development. *Family Process, 25,* 207–221.

Eron, J., & Lund, T. (1989). From magic to method: Principles of effective reframing. *Family Therapy Networker, 13,* 64–68, 81–83.

Eron, J., & Lund, T. W. (1993). How problems evolve and dissolve: Integrating narrative and strategic concepts. *Family Process, 32,* 291–309.

Eron, J. B., & Lund, T. W. (1996). *Narratives solutions in brief therapy.* New York: Guilford Press.

Eron, J. B., & Lund, T. W. (1997). Narrative solutions couple therapy. In F. M. Dattilio (Ed.), *Cases studies in couple and family therapy: Systemic and cognitive perspectives* (pp. 371–400). New York: Guilford Press.

O'Hanlon, W. H., & Weiner-Davis, M. (1989). *In search of solutions: A new direction in psychotherapy.* New York: Norton.

Watzlawick, P., Weakland, J., & Fisch, R. (1974). *Change: Principles of problem formation and problem resolution.* New York: Norton.

Weakland, J. H., Fisch, R., Watzlawick, P., & Bodin, A. M. (1974). Brief therapy: Focused problem resolution. *Family Process, 13,* 141–168.

White, M., & Epston, D. (1990). *Narrative means to therapeutic ends.* New York: Norton.

13

—◄o►—

A TIME-EFFECTIVE, SOLUTION-FOCUSED APPROACH TO COUPLE THERAPY

STEVEN FRIEDMAN
EVE LIPCHIK

Working effectively with couples is a complex and challenging endeavor. Differing perceptions between partners requires great sensitivity in acknowledging often strongly held yet divergent points of view while maintaining a working alliance with each member of the couple. In addition, faced with sometimes volatile and emotionally charged communications and affects, the couple therapist must manage high levels of reactivity in ways that offer the couple a path out of its members' problem-saturated reality. To meet these challenges, the time-effective, solution-focused therapist acts as a facilitator of the therapeutic conversation in ways that open space for the couple to move toward a preferred future. Working from a perspective of competencies and strengths, we take a nonpathologizing approach that respects the clients' goals and utilizes the clients' own resources and "expert knowledges" in reaching these goals (Friedman, 1997; Lipchik, 1993).

The work we do can be considered "minimalist" in that we aren't looking to reconstruct relationships by delving into partners' past individual histories to find relevant themes. While gathering information is part of any clinical contact, we envision our role less as "information gatherers" and more as facilitators of the therapeutic conversation, using questions to help the couple construct new meanings and understandings about their relationship. Our attention is focused primarily on the here and now, and even more importantly, on the future, since the future provides a blank canvas on which the couple can paint a picture of the pair's wishes and hopes.

BACKGROUND/HISTORICAL CONTEXT

Our clinical practices are situated in a postmodern or social construc-tionist frame—in that we view the conversational process in therapy as a forum for meaning-making (e.g., de Shazer, 1994; Rosen & Kuehlwein, 1996). Rather than uncovering objective truths, the therapeutic conver-sation allows the therapist and client to co-construct realities in ways that open space for new perspectives (Anderson & Goolishian, 1988; Friedman, 1993b; Gergen, 1985). Within any conversation there are multiple opportunities (i.e., ambiguities) for meaning making about events in people's lives. It is this conversational process and its ambigu-ities that offer client and therapist the maneuverability to create new sto-ries.

Our approach grows out of the solution-focused tradition that dates back to the early 1980s and the pioneering work of the Brief Fam-ily Therapy Center (e.g., Berg, 1994; Berg & Miller, 1994; de Shazer, 1982, 1985, 1988, 1991, 1994; Kiser, Piercy, & Lipchik, 1993; Lipchik & de Shazer, 1986; O'Hanlon & Weiner-Davis, 1989; O'Hanlon & Wilk, 1987).[1] Solution-focused therapy builds on and complements the innovative work of the Mental Research Institute (MRI) (e.g., Fisch, Weakland, & Segal, 1982) and the "uncommon" psychotherapy of Mil-ton H. Erickson (e.g., see Haley, 1973). While drawing primarily on solution-focused methods, Friedman's work with couples (e.g., Fried-man, 1996, 1997) also incorporates ideas from the domain of narrative therapy (White & Epston, 1990).

The solution-focused therapist joins with the couple in a collabora-tive relationship that builds on previous successes and problem "excep-tions." While validating and respecting each partner's needs and wishes, our work aims to open space for "both/and" solutions (Lipchik, 1993; Lipchik & Kubicki, 1996). Since action outside the therapy room is nec-essary for change to occur, homework suggestions are used as a way for the couple to carry the work of the session into their day-to-day lives at home. Throughout the therapy process, we emphasize client strengths and resources. Rather than becoming immersed in the couple's problem-saturated story or in a litany of negative complaints, we redirect attention to those aspects of the relationship that are working and tailor homework assignments to the specifics of each couple's situation. This doesn't mean that the problem, or those affects that accompany the problem, are ignored, only that the problem story does not get central focus in the therapy. It's clear to us that staying in the "problem" frame can quickly lead to a sense of hopelessness and demoralization for both client and therapist (Friedman & Fanger, 1991). Because our goal is to engender hope and encourage movement, our attention stays focused primarily on ways the couple has found to take steps toward a more preferred future.

In many instances, fortuitous events in the life of the couple have a major impact on the change process (see Miller, Duncan, & Hubble, 1997). By spacing contacts between sessions, the therapist allows the "normal restorative processes of life" to operate (Hobbs, 1966). In addition, allowing time between sessions provides an opportunity for the couple to implement homework suggestions. In general, because movement and change in therapy are unpredictable, the solution-focused therapist does not contract for a fixed number of sessions. Instead, plans for each future session are negotiated at the conclusion of the current one.

Research on the solution-focused therapies (summarized by De Jong & Hopwood, 1995; McKeel, 1995) supports their usefulness and effectiveness in a wide variety of clinical situations. These competency-based approaches place the client in the driver's seat in establishing goals and in deciding when these goals have been reached. This collaborative and cooperative stance is a primary factor in achieving successful outcomes in therapy (Whiston & Sexton, 1993).

As we will see, two primary ingredients influence the generation of positive outcomes in solution-focused therapy: (1) the language the therapist uses (to both develop a cooperative and collaborative relationship and engender hope) and 2) the use of tasks that engage the client in activities or actions that lead to new perspectives and behaviors.

CORE CONCEPTS

The basic assumptions of solution-focused, time-effective couple therapy are as follows:

- Every human being is unique.
- All relationships are unique.
- People have inherent and potential resources to help themselves.
- Change is constant and inevitable.

- You can't change the past, so concentrate on the present and future.
- Problems are experienced individually but can change interpersonally.
- There is no true cause and effect of problems.
- No situation is totally negative.
- A small change can lead to bigger changes.
- If something works don't fix it; if it doesn't, do something different.
- Therapists don't have the power or knowledge to change clients.
- You catch more flies with honey than with vinegar.

These assumptions can be translated into five major processes that define a time-effective, competency-based therapy (Figure 13.1).

1. *Connection*: Listening, affirming, and acknowledging each partner's story while joining with both around a set of mutually agreed-upon goals.

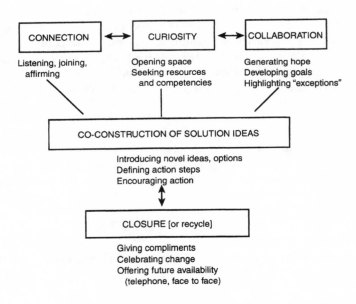

FIGURE 13.1. A competency-based model of time-effective therapy. From Friedman (1997, p. 234). Copyright 1997 by Allyn & Bacon. Reprinted by permission.

2. *Curiosity*: Opening space for a discussion of multiple perspectives while attending to the couple's resources.
3. *Collaboration*: Working together with both members the couple in the direction of *their* preferred futures. Highlighting successes ("exceptions") and generating hope.
4. *Co-Construction of solution ideas*: (a) Introducing novel ideas that emerge from the clinical conversation; (b) defining action steps ("homework").
5. *Closure*: Giving compliments; celebrating and applauding change; offering each partner an opportunity to acknowledge and comment on changes in the other; offering future availability.

THE PROCESS OF THERAPY

Establishing the Emotional Climate

The therapy process requires that the clinician establish a working alliance with the couple. To establish this alliance, and to maximize positive outcomes, we find the following actions on the part of the therapist necessary: respect for the client's point of view, empathy for the client's predicament, the engendering of hope and positive expectations, and genuineness and authenticity in the clinical interaction (Duncan & Moynihan, 1994; Frank, 1974; Miller et al., 1997). As Friedman (1997, p. 3) points out:

> All therapies . . . require sensitivity, patience, compassion, and an ability to listen for subtleties (Lipchik, 1994). Applying a set of principles blindly without attending to these aspects of the relationship will inevitably lead to clinical dead-ends. . . . Therapist flexibility is vital. The steps in the therapy cannot be neatly and algorithmically mapped out. As Milton Erickson emphasized, each therapy encounter must be *invented* based on the client's presentation. Therapy, being a recursive process, requires meeting clients at their points of readiness and shifting gears in light the subtleties of the clinical conversation.

Basically, the therapist uses the clients' reality about their situation as the basis for collaboration. The speed and success of solution construction depend on the therapist's ability to stay connected with the clients' reality throughout the course of therapy. This is the underpinning for the whole collaborative process, the grease that keeps the axles turning. Figure 13.2 provides an overview of the factors that contribute to establishing and maintaining a positive emotional climate (adapted from Lipchik, 1992).

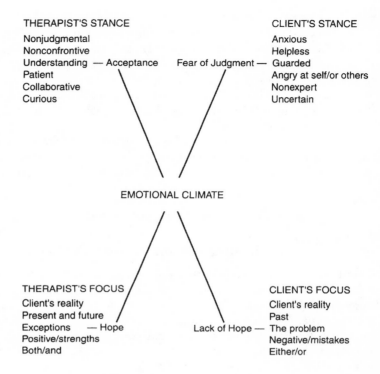

FIGURE 13.2. The climate and context of therapy.

Asking Pivotal Questions

The manner in which solution-focused therapists speak with clients (the questions used) both influences clients' expectations and optimism and directs the clients' attention to aspects of their lives that are indicative of change (Lipchik & de Shazer, 1986). When clients experience a sense of hopefulness and a positive expectancy about change, positive outcomes are more likely (see Friedman & Fanger, 1991; Miller et al., 1997; Whiston & Sexton, 1993). When, for example, a therapist asks about changes that happened prior to coming for the first session, he or she is already setting the stage for the client to tune into positive developments (Weiner-Davis, de Shazer, & Gingerich, 1987).

As we see in the transcript of Phil and Sherry below, a number of pivotal questions are used in the initial session, and thereafter, that support a positive, collaborative, and resource-oriented perspective (see Lipchik & de Shazer, 1986). The therapist keys in on "exceptions," that is, times when the problem isn't happening and uses these "sparkling moments" as building blocks for encouraging further change. The therapist also maintains a future focus by asking questions that allow each member of the couple to consider what his or her desired changes will look like (Kiser et al., 1993). For example, the therapist might ask,

> "How do you usually solve problems like this? What percentage of the time is this situation problematic compared to when things are working fairly well? What would a small change toward the goal look like? When this change begins to happen, what will you notice first? What might I notice about you (both of you) that would indicate that a change has happened? Who else might notice this change? When you're feeling loved (appreciated, respected, etc.) by your partner, what is he or she doing differently? How do you feel differently since you and your partner began to fight less?"

If the members of the couple aren't able to generate any "exceptions" to the problem, it's useful to ask the "miracle question" (de Shazer, 1988): "If a miracle happened tonight and you woke up the next morning and your problem were solved, how would things be different?" This question opens space for the couple to project a new future, one that doesn't include the problem. The partners' responses to this question provide a road map to the couple's preferred future.

When members of a couple are stuck in a blaming mode or pattern, it can be useful to externalize this "problem" or "pattern" (see Zimmerman & Dickerson, 1993) as a force that is creating distance and conflict. Here the therapist aligns with the couple "against" the dominance of the "pattern." In effect, the person or couple is separated from the "problem." For example, the therapist might ask questions such as "How did this pattern of conflict take hold of your lives?" "In what ways have you acted contrary to this pattern?" "If this pattern continues to dominate your relationship, what do you anticipate will be the outcome?" "What would your relationship look like when this pattern is no longer dominant?," and so forth. If a couple continues in a negative mode, it can be useful to ask: "How come things aren't worse?" "What have you done to keep things from getting worse?"

In the course of therapy, it is also helpful to employ "scaling questions" (e.g., Berg & de Shazer, 1993). Scaling questions allow the members of a couple to place themselves along a scale from 0 to 10 on some dimension of their relationship. For example, partners can be asked to place themselves on a scale regarding their commitment to the relationship or to indicate their hopefulness in turning the situation around or to tell you about where things were when they called for the appointment and where things are now.

Concluding the Session: The Summary Statement

Solution-focused therapy is often practiced as a team approach with one therapist in front of a one-way mirror interviewing the couple and one or more therapists behind it, observing. Sessions usually last about 1 hour. Whether working alone or with a team, the interviewing therapist usually takes a 5- to 10-minute consultation break about 40 to 45 minutes into the hour. The therapist reviews the session and composes (with the team or alone) a summary message to communicate to the client when the therapist returns to the room. The consultation break was first described by Selvini Palazzoli, Boscolo, Cecchin, and Prata (1978) using a different theoretical model.

The summation message consists of (1) feedback to the client (couple) on what the therapist heard during the session about why the two are coming for therapy and what their goals are; (2) compliments on positive steps already taken; (3) a framework or context in which to place the couple's predicament, (preferably one that emphasizes normal developmental processes); and (4) the suggestion of a task or homework assignment for the couple to experiment with between this session and the next. This suggestion is made tentatively, and clients are encouraged to modify the task as they wish.

The overall goal of the message is to provide the couple with a new or different perspective on their predicament while creating a comfortable emotional climate that engenders hope and positive expectations. So, for example, the therapist might begin by saying, "What I heard you say today is. . . . " This statement includes what the therapist heard the clients say (using the clients' language as much as possible), their goals, progress, and comments about their feelings or emotions. Next, the therapist offers compliments, reinforces positive changes, normalizes, reframes, or presents information from a developmental perspective. Finally, a suggestion is made. This can be as simple as "Continue doing what you're already doing" or one more specifically designed to guide the clients toward doing something different. In the transcript to follow, we present several examples of summation messages and therapeutic tasks.

PHIL AND SHERRY: A COUPLE IN DISTRESS

The following are excerpts from a series of interviews with a couple who were struggling, in an early stage of their marriage, to find a balance between their individual needs for autonomy and their wishes for closeness. The therapist is Eve Lipchik, who provides personal commentary on the therapy process. Steven Friedman also adds his thoughts at various points in the transcript.

The Initial Interview

Sherry, 27 and Phil, 39, were married only 9 months when Phil called to initiate couple counseling. Phil had been married previously, while Sherry had not. Six years ago, Phil, who had formerly been a flight instructor, changed careers and began his own commercial art business. He was recently experiencing a lot of stressful competition in this new line of work. Sherry supervised and trained in-flight personnel for an airline and was attending night classes to becomes certified as a school teacher.

Sherry signaled Phil to start talking about why he wanted counseling:

PHIL: For me its all about the nurturing I get, the kind of support that I get, and when I'm not supported, then I kind of have this little conversation like, "Why should I support her, if I'm not going to be supported?"

[Phil has offered some valuable information about himself at this point; he is aware of his pattern, and it is "tit for tat."]

LIPCHIK: Of course . . . and by support, you mean . . . ?

PHIL: Just encouragement or acceptance. If she doesn't attack or doesn't criticize.

LIPCHIK: So nurturing means being warmly accepted or supported?

PHIL: Uh huh.

LIPCHIK: And how about you, Sherry?

SHERRY: For me it's just not doing the things that could make it good. It's, you know, being highly critical, or feeling like I'm under attack or feeling like my opinion doesn't matter. And again, it's all feelings, but it's very real to me.

LIPCHIK: Sure.

SHERRY: Part of it is communication . . . we both approach communication differently. Where if I ask a question, and I ask, uh, "What are you hungry for?" or "Where do you want to go for supper?" Phil might say, "Oh, I'm hungry for pizza, let's go to the pizza place," and I say, "Oh, gee, I'm not really hungry for pizza, I'm hungry for something else"—Phil will say "I don't want to argue about it." Well, I'm not arguing, I'm discussing. Is he, like, really hungry for pizza and just couldn't do for anything else, or is he just kind of neutral? Or am I kinda neutral and just kind of leaning toward something versus really wanting something.

[The focus should now be on defining a goal both partners can agree on. This was difficult for Sherry and Phil. At first they only agreed on the fact that they argue 80% of the time. Also, both acknowledged that the other was hurting equally as a result of this arguing. This admission was chosen as the "resource" upon which to build the goal.]

LIPCHIK: So you both agree, the other one feels as bad as you do?.... Any ideas what the solution might be?

[Since I believe that clients, generally, have good ideas about creating change, I asked them directly about potential solutions.]

PHIL: I have a real clear idea what the solution is.

LIPCHIK: Yeah?

PHIL: Uhm. (*Looks at Sherry, who is laughing.*) Is it okay if I say?

SHERRY: Yes. Just laughing to myself.

PHIL: Why?

SHERRY: 'Cause . . . you know everything, so go ahead.

PHIL: So it's not out of my knowing everything that I speak it's . . . it's answering the question. Uhm, I guess I forgot what you said.

LIPCHIK: What the solution might be?

PHIL: Yeah, the solution to me would be . . . uhm . . . simply acceptance.

LIPCHIK: On Sherry's part? On your part?

PHIL: Well, for both of us.

LIPCHIK: Oh, for both of you.

PHIL: If we both . . . got rid of the shields and armor and weapons for protection . . . and got rid of the fears . . . any quick reaction or fright or, "You didn't do this 'cause," or "I didn't get that," or any of those things, just leave them aside.

LIPCHIK: (*to Sherry*) What do you think?

SHERRY: Uhm, I guess it's a similar idea but uhm . . . the only solution I see, because, there is a lack of . . . I have lost a lot of trust in our rela- . . . in Phil, in our relationship.

LIPCHIK: Trust . . . in terms of . . . ?

SHERRY: . . . His judgment, trusting that he's really my partner, trusting that he's in this relationship to be my partner and not to criticize me or be cynical . . .

LIPCHIK: And if by some miracle that trust would [be] there tomorrow . . . how would you know . . . What would the signs be?

[Here I asked a modified form of the "miracle question" in the hope that Sherry would be more specific about signs of change.]

SHERRY: There would be that respect. . . . I wouldn't be criticized. . . . he would recognize my accomplishments. . . . Yes . . . I would feel really respected, and he would also get that from me.

LIPCHIK: Can you give me an example of a time when that happened?

SHERRY: It's his attitude. . . . it would just be different.

LIPCHIK: What do you think, Phil?

PHIL: I will feel pretty much loved and trusted . . . when there is a sense of love or caring.

LIPCHIK: What will Sherry be doing when you feel that?

PHIL: It's not any one thing . . . I will feel support.

[These clients seemed not to want to talk about positives but only to complain about each other. To persist asking about positives could lead to them feeling misunderstood. I chose to ask them when they thought the problem started. This line of questioning requires careful monitoring to avoid becoming immersed in problem-talk.

Both partners dated the beginning of the tension back to the end of summer. Sherry admitted that at that time she began not to like being married because "I was feeling the extra responsibility and that I had to live up to . . . all these expectations and standards." She also recognized that some of those expectations were hers, not Phil's.]

SHERRY: I started school in September, and Phil began to take seminars, and all of a sudden we started to have more problems. It got very demanding. . . . I started requesting more, requesting that certain house things stay this way, because I don't have time to pick up any- more; I don't have time to clean the house. Time became a real issue for me, and so Phil would make these promises and then not keep them and then act like it was no big deal that he didn't keep them. . . . I was angry that he made promises he didn't keep. So it started with the little things like that, and it just grew to the point where at the end of November I decided to stop smoking—after 10 years of smoking—thinking I would have this hugely supportive husband who's always wanted me to—I mean we've seen each other for 7 years, and he's wanted me to stop smoking—so I'd finally made this big decision "Okay, I'll stop smoking," and the day I stopped, he started ragging at me over some other thing. I asked him to be understanding and try to be nice to me anyway. . . . so when he didn't do that, when he got nasty anyway and belligerent, that really broke down the trust. Maybe it's school and the holidays. Maybe it's those things combined just causing so much stress and anxiety. I always thought that we would just work this out, you know, that it would calm down. I think when I was out of school we got along better, you know, because there's less stress. Less things to do. He wasn't taking any seminars. We were home together more.

[As Sherry spoke, Phil had been nodding in agreement. It turned out that their schedules were so full that they had little time together during the week and many chores to do on the weekends. At this point, I was experiencing both partners as increasingly discouraged but less eager to complain. This suggested to me that they might be ready to work on defining a goal based on positives and avoid further problem-talk.]

LIPCHIK: What's enjoyable about being together?

SHERRY: We laugh, and we share stories and ideas.

PHIL: There is so much spontaneity, fun, craziness. [He describes an elaborate birthday dinner she had prepared for him recently.]

[As the couple relaxed and talked about the positives in their relationship, I tried again to get them to delineate some small behavioral shifts that would indicate positive change.]

LIPCHIK: Can you give me a little bit of an idea what will be the first thing you notice when things get better?

SHERRY: I would notice, uhm, it's hard to explain. . . . but I would notice Phil was accepting what I was saying without arguing or fighting or being corrected or rephrasing what I'm saying. General acceptance, I guess I would notice something like. Is that . . . ?

LIPCHIK: Yeah.

PHIL: For me it would be ... willing to be free.... I don't know, this isn't coming out right. Just give me a moment.

LIPCHIK: You would notice ... ?

PHIL: No, just wait, wait a minute.... That Sherry would be supportive ...

LIPCHIK: Could you tell me what that would look like by giving me a specific example?

PHIL: (*long silence*) I'm having a hard time with this.

LIPCHIK: Well, you don't have to answer.

PHIL: (*to Sherry*) To me it looks like you're just friendlier.

LIPCHIK: Uh huh, you'd see a smile on her face?

PHIL: Well I enjoy sharing my day or sharing my frustrations, and sharing my joys, and I like those to be nurtured and for an exchange to take place.

LIPCHIK: Paid attention to?

PHIL: Sort of, more or less. I mean, I don't like talking to the air, you know.

Phil obviously had a hard time translating his feelings into behavioral terms. In order to be helpful to him I will have to work on understanding his way of cooperating. At this point in the interview, I took a break and left the room to develop a summation message. By removing myself from the intensity of the session, I was able more easily to get perspective to formulate a feedback statement that captured the spirit of the interview while providing a context for the therapy. The couple was also left in a state of anticipation that may increase their openness and receptivity to the message.

LIPCHIK: What I heard you say today is that you've been married for about 9 months, and you've come because your relationship is increasingly conflictual. You, Sherry, said you feel criticized and attacked that your opinions don't count. Phil, you described your dissatisfaction as not getting the kind of nurturing and support you want. You both seem to feel your communication needs improvement and that you need to be less reactive to each other.
    My response is that I found both of you to be very clear and open about how you described your situation. It struck me that, in spite of your differences, you both want the same thing in the rela-

tionship—understanding, respect, and support. . . . and both of you seem to be hurting a great deal. I was impressed that you acknowledged each other's pain. Often people are so focused on their own pain, they don't even notice that the other person is hurting too.

One thing I was thinking is that you're in a transitional stage in your relationship. You may be moving from the romantic stage—where love is blind—and people just try to be what they think their partner wants—toward more emotional intimacy. A lot of people get stuck at that point, and it feels really scary because suddenly differences seem to come out. But for love and trust to grow, people have to be themselves and accept each other with differences . . . and negotiate them in a way that works for both of them.

These transitions in relationships are normal. . . . You may just have experienced it more intensely because you got so busy in the fall and suddenly couldn't spend much time together anymore. It's a good thing you're coming for help early, rather than letting it go too long.

What I usually do when I see a couple is to see them each alone one time before I see them together. It just gives us a chance to connect individually. Is that all right with you? (*They both nod in agreement.*) I would also like to suggest something for you to think about. Think about and notice what is happening in your relationship that you want to continue to have happen. You told me a lot about what you want to change, now it would help me to learn from you about what you don't want to change. I would suggest you do this separately . . . don't share it.

The couple decided that Phil would be interviewed first, and this appointment is scheduled for 2 weeks later. I always see couples separately one time after the initial conjoint session for several reasons: (1) It allows for closer joining with each partner; (2) the individual session can help clarify the amount of responsibility each partner is willing to assume for the problem and solutions; (3) if a confession of an affair or interest in another person is made, it serves as an opportunity to educate the partner about the impossibility of working on the marriage while one is engaged in a competing relationship. When such information is disclosed and the person insists he or she wants to improve the marriage, I tell the client that one cannot work on one relationship while having another. I suggest the client consider ending the other relationship, or at least agree to a period of no contact, while the marital therapy is occurring. If this suggestion is refused, I inform both partners in a conjoint session that I recommend that they seek separate help until they're both clear about their commitment to improving the marriage.[2]

Individual Session with Phil

Phil came in carrying a pad, prepared to take notes during our session.

LIPCHIK: How are you doing?

PHIL: Good.

LIPCHIK: I just want to explain to you why I have these separate sessions. Sometimes people like to tell me things without their partners present. This is an opportunity to do so. It may be helpful to you, and it is often helpful to me. What we discuss is confidential. If there is something I would like to discuss with your partner present I would ask your permission to do so first. Okay?

PHIL: That's fine.

LIPCHIK: So is there anything like that on your mind?

PHIL: Well, not really right now. But since the last time we saw you, it's been. . . . 50–50 in terms of good and bad.

[Since this move from 20–80 to 50–50 is a positive development, I took this as an opportunity to explore what made the difference.]

LIPCHIK: What accounts for this improvement?

PHIL: We're making a more conscious effort to get along better. That exercise you gave us cut through the negative stuff that was accumulating for us. It got both of us beyond all that junk that was going on—that was nice ground to begin on and helped both of us.

[Phil then went on to discuss Sherry's frequent complaint that he's not a real "partner." It was apparent that they had very different ideas of what that meant. For her it seemed to mean that he was thinking of her as well as of himself, while for him it seemed to mean he should give up doing what he wanted to do in order to please her.

He reported that they had, however, had a good talk after going to church. He had asked her to start telling him when he is being the partner she wanted instead of when he wasn't. On Monday she did something different: She called him from the office and shared her week's schedule with him. He reported that he told her how much he appreciated that and that it made him feel cared for. I tried to build on this, but he did not want to pursue further positives.]

PHIL: I feel I get verbally beaten up. I see things differently than she does. She doesn't let me in on what she *likes*, but she flares up about every little thing she doesn't. I have to choose my words carefully to avoid flare-ups. . . . At the end of the session last time you said we are both hurting. We really are similar in many ways, and we both take a stand to show the other how wrong they are. Maybe a good way for me to approach things would be to think of her side of things?

LIPCHIK: Well, that's something to consider. . . . It's always good to speculate about her side as well as yours, but it might lead to your making assumptions that aren't really so. What works well for many people is to actually ask your partner where they're coming from . . . what they are feeling or thinking.

[Phil confessed that in his first marriage he had been a "controlling jerk." He was determined not to make the same mistakes in this marriage. He wanted to be "truthful and honest and express emotions clearly and talk about them . . . everything I didn't do then. . . . " In this marriage he has been trying to accommodate in order to avoid conflict rather than to control and manipulate. He has found that this isn't working with Sherry, who considered his direct statements authoritarian and negative when they weren't meant to be.]

PHIL: If I stop believing that behaving *this* way is wrong, too, I have nothing . . . where am I going to go with it then?

LIPCHIK: It may be a question of different perceptions, not right or wrong. It doesn't have to be either/or . . . win/lose. . . . it's supposed to be win/win. You have different but complementary styles of expressing yourself. You are more direct; she's more tentative. What will you have to know about her style so you can express yourself in a way that doesn't cramp your style?

PHIL: That's good . . . that's good. If you put it in terms of different style . . . that clicks for me.

At the conclusion of the session, I excused myself and prepared a summary message to present to Phil.

LIPCHIK: What I heard you say today is that you found the exercise to be useful and that you noticed it had some positive effect because it helped both of you to try harder to improve things. You also said that you had put a lot of work into figuring out what went wrong in your first marriage, and you're determined to not make the same mistakes in this one. However, you said that the approach you're trying with Sherry, not to be controlling and to be honest with yourself and with her, isn't working either, and you are very discouraged about it.

My response is that you both seem to want respect and love from each other, not criticism and disdain ... but because you are different people ... have different styles ... you may have *to express it* in a different way than you want to have it *expressed to you*. You're certainly on the right track in trying to learn what Sherry wants in a partner by asking her to let you know when she thinks you're meeting her expectations. My suggestion would be that you keep on asking for more positive feedback from her and let her know, as well, when she's acting in a way that makes you feel good.

Individual Session with Sherry

Two weeks later I met with Sherry, who also came with a notebook ready to take notes. I introduced the reason for the individual session to Sherry. She said she really didn't know what to say because counseling was really new to her.

LIPCHIK: So what's been different?

[The purpose of asking this simple yet pivotal question is to cue Sherry to select and recall happenings in her life that reflect some change from the status quo. Since change is ever present, this question provides an opportunity for Sherry to recall or remember what has been different over the past 2 weeks.]

SHERRY: I think—maybe we're paying more attention to things so we're getting along a bit better—more good moments. At the same time, some of the bad things are more explosive. I think, for me, when I get frustrated, there are moments when I wonder if this [marriage] is right.

LIPCHIK: What's your gut feeling?

SHERRY: My gut feeling is that we can work it out.

[She described some improvement in their ease of talking with each other and a general lessening of tension. But she wanted to get back to the theme of Phil not acting like "a real partner."]

SHERRY: We're both home ... going to have breakfast. He fixes what he wants to eat and doesn't ask me what I want. I might as well live alone. When we came home from visiting my parents at Easter, he unpacked his things and left mine in the trunk . . .

I found out a while ago that he just says "Yes" to everything in order to avoid arguments. I didn't notice it at first until he started getting shorter with me and more sarcastic. I was furious. He made the decision to be that way with me without telling me. This is not partnership. I didn't like it. I asked him to stop doing that, but he still does it once in a while . . . He gives me short answers. I don't think it's funny. He uses those short answers or "okays" as pacifiers. That's not a partnership! It's a put down. It just ignores who I am.

[I attempt to broaden her view to "both/and."]

LIPCHIK: I see your point. On the other hand, people usually have to make choices about how to respond to others, especially when it's someone they care for a lot. Sometimes putting your needs aside can be loving . . . giving of yourself. I can see that in this situation it makes you feel he wasn't respecting your needs. . . . including you. How will he have to behave in the future for you to feel validated and for him to be able to express his side of things?

[Individual sessions can facilitate change for both partners because they offer an opportunity to address individual and/or couple issues in a less threatening manner.]

Sherry continued by sharing her confusion about the boundary between herself as a woman and her role as Phil's wife. I asked her several questions about this. For example: What would be going on if she were able to describe herself as a wife and feel positive about it? What would have to be different for her to feel okay both as an individual and a wife? In what respect is this happening already? At the end of this discussion, I excused myself and prepared a summary message as follows:

LIPCHIK: What I heard you tell me today is that sometimes you have doubts about your relationship, but that in spite of that, you're invested in making it work. You seem not to have been able to figure out yet how you can assume the role of a wife without giving up aspects of yourself that define you as a woman separate from being a wife. On the other hand, Phil's attitude toward you—how he affirms your opinions and how considerate he is of you—seems to be an important part of figuring that out for yourself. You also told me that, when you focus on the positive things in the relationship, things go better for you and Phil and are more relaxed.

My response is that you seem to be on the right track and, in order to stay on the right track, have made the decision to come for some help sooner rather than later. I am impressed with how well you know yourself and Phil and how much thought you give to finding a solution. You have some good ideas about what you might do differently to help the situation . . . like letting Phil know how you feel sooner before you get so angry. You are right that some of the things you value about each other—the competitiveness, the strong opinions—are the very things that also cause problems. I have a suggestion you might want to try until we meet again . . . Notice what you do to overcome the urge to react to Phil in an emotional, competitive way and what you are doing differently when you respond in a way that works for both of you. Don't expect instant success, this will take time. It's all about changing habits.

[Again, I used Sherry's motivation and her own ideas to suggest a task that would lead toward greater acceptance of each partner's differences.]

Second Conjoint Session

The second meeting with both members of the couple took place about 2 weeks later. Sherry and Phil looked very upset and tense as they entered the room and sat down. They both reported that things had been "terrible." Phil said they had been doing very well for about 1 week after their individual sessions: Communication was better; they were having good conversations. He had felt a sense of "freedom and support" until the past weekend when they had had a fight that wiped out any progress. Phil described that he had wanted to talk to Sherry on Saturday morning about some of the difficulties with one of his clients. They were in the kitchen making breakfast. She was just in the process of making pancakes and sausages and arranging them on the plates when he was describing the situation. He felt she had responded critically and told him what he should have done before she even heard the end of the story. He felt invalidated. Sherry's side of the story was that the minute she asked a question he became defensive. She felt invalidated first by his not wanting to answer her questions and then by his "rudeness." As their interaction escalated, he had taken his plate of food and went into the living room to eat by himself. They didn't talk for the rest of the weekend.

Sherry, too, expressed her feelings of discouragement. She had begun to hope they had left the past behind and were on a new path because things had been going so well for over a week. It's quite common for clients to report some positive changes after the first session and then come back with more complaints instead of reports of progress. That's why it's always useful to suggest going very slowly and not expect too much change too soon. The therapist's task is both to communicate acceptance for what clients are reporting and to search for difference to promote hope and motivation.

LIPCHIK: It sounds like you're both very angry and disappointed that things didn't continue to go so well. I wonder, though, if you could tell me what was different about this fight than past ones?

PHIL: Nothing. . . . nothing. . . .

SHERRY: It was even more discouraging because things had been so good.

LIPCHIK: I know it may have felt the same—even worse—but was there anything about this fight that was different than past ones?

SHERRY: Well. . . . uhm . . . it felt . . . uhm . . . well actually, in the past when we fought I'd ask him to leave . . .

PHIL: (*interrupting*) The first thing is always "Why don't you just leave!"

SHERRY: . . . but this time we just stewed . . .

PHIL: She didn't throw me out as usual . . . I stayed in the other room most of the day . . . We didn't talk.

SHERRY: Maybe it was different . . . we gave each other enough space to get it together by Sunday night.

The couple described the small, but significant, difference in this situation and began to appear more hopeful again. I asked them both to scale their level of confidence that their relationship will work out. Sherry said 75%, while Phil said 50%. One thing that became increasingly clear to me in talking with this couple and watching them take notes during sessions was that they both had a background in teaching and that they saw themselves as "students" in this situation. Their way of cooperating for change was to want to "learn" how to get along. They had responded well to the first task and expected more homework assignments. Their competitive manner was something that had originally attracted them to each other and had to be utilized in a positive manner instead of being seen as a liability. The following is the summation message I gave after this session.

LIPCHIK: What I hear today is that you're both disappointed that some of the gains made after our first sessions didn't continue at the same level. You both reported how happy you felt when there was less tension and you could talk with each other in a relaxed manner, but then you found yourself again in an argument that made you feel as though you hadn't made any gains. Both of you reported on how hurt you feel when your partner is not valuing what you have to offer. However, you did report that, while very similar to other fights, this one was a bit different because you found a way to stay in the apartment *together* until you could work things out.

My response is that you are both strong, emotional people who value your individualism but that you need each other to affirm that individualism. When you're able to do that for each other, it's really good. But when you have even the slightest doubt about the other's belief and admiration for your individual self, you react very strongly, and things break down. While it's normal and healthy for partners in a relationship to want to be very close while maintaining a sense of separateness—Both an "I" and a "we"—some people find that when things go well too long in terms of their closeness, their individuality begins to feel threatened, and they need some distance for personal comfort. Many people aren't quite aware when they need that distance, and they may create it in a negative way by fighting without wanting to do that. I was wondering if you may want to see if that's the case for you?

An exercise I would suggest is to predict separately, and without sharing with each other, whether you think the next day will be a good day or a bad one in terms of your relationship. The next evening you get together and share whether your prediction was right or wrong. You must accept the other person's decision without asking how they reached it or why. If you find that for three nights in a row you predicted things would be good, you must toss a coin and the person who wins the coin toss must do something the next day to create distance. Then you begin the process all over again.

[For a homework assignment to be effective, it needs to emerge from the clinical conversation and be specifically tailored to the ongoing themes presented. The task presented here was designed to counteract the couple's reactiveness toward each other and to provide, in a playful yet planned way, an opportunity for this couple engage in an activity that would allow them to regulate their closeness/distance. The task also served to normalize "bad days" as something that can be expected from time to time in any relationship.]

Third Conjoint Session

At this session, held 2 weeks later, the couple came in relaxed and smiling. They reported that they had done the exercise and had had some good days and some bad days. This is the solution-focused therapist's cue to attend to the changes as carefully as possible in order to reinforce them. Phil said he never actually predicted any bad days, whereas Sherry had predicted 2 days and that was right after they had left the last session. Sherry reported that they had had to create distance twice. One day she had the opportunity and one day Phil did.

SHERRY: But that was interesting because now I think we saw how much we react to one another.

LIPCHIK: Did you?

SHERRY: Well, yeah, because someone's creating distance, and all of a sudden you find yourself reacting to whatever they're doing even when you know that it could be on purpose ... But, I don't know ... I'm so wired I'm babbling.

PHIL: Go ahead.

SHERRY: It was funny because when I left I didn't know how that conclusion was drawn, that our space or our person was invaded at some point in our relationship, and I still don't know where that came from. Uhm, or what we said that would make you think that or whatever. But I thought well, I'll still do the exercise and I did, and at the very least it got us talking about how our days are going. And we agreed then not to talk about whether it was bad or it was good, and there was no huge discussion because at times it probably could have gotten into another ...

LIPCHIK: You didn't argue about whether it was good or bad?

SHERRY: No. We just decided and then if, if someone said it was bad, it was bad, and that was it. And we didn't discuss why it was bad.

LIPCHIK: But that's sort of different from your normal ways of saying that "It's my way." How come you just agreed and not argued about whether it was either/or?

SHERRY: Well that was part of the instruction, first of all. Or how we both understood the instructions. And, it's funny, the first day that I got to create distance was the first day we really wanted to talk about it. 'Cause Phil said the next day, "Now were you really trying to create distance, or were you just doing that, or ... ?"

PHIL: Or reacting?

SHERRY: "Which was it, was it just you or were you trying to do that?" And I said, you just have to take it as me creating distance and that's it, and of course I wanted to go on and talk about something else, but he said, "But Sherry we can't talk it about too much." But that was good because then we didn't have to get to that point of beating a dead dog. Because we'll each go on and on about what we thought.

LIPCHIK: So was that better for the relationship?

SHERRY: You can answer this time.

PHIL: I think so. I guess it's better for both of us which I guess means it's better for the relationship. I want to talk about the exercise for a minute. I found it very difficult to create the distance when I was supposed to. I had to first stop and look at what it feels like to be close, what was I doing that was caring. So I had kind of an opposite reaction, and when I had to create distance, I had to really think about what I had to do to create distance. And then I tried some things and I found it so humorous that I couldn't really. . . . So I kind of removed the cloud over the relationship in terms of the volatility of it. I see that this is a great exercise for us. 'Cause we told you that things go really good and all of a sudden *cabam*! Everything explodes. And the line between the beauty and the beast is so fine that we never notice it.

SHERRY: Wow.

PHIL: I mean that's how I see it. We told you also that we can get along about a week, and your reaction to us was good. Three days. If we can get through 3 days . . .

LIPCHIK: A week is too long?

PHIL: Yeah. And so, we go "Okay, we'll do 3 days," and I wanted to talk about stuff. We have a good day; we have a bad day.

SHERRY: You wanted to talk about what made those bad days?

PHIL: (*speaking to Sherry*) Yeah, I wanted to know what your reaction was or what your thoughts were on just purely how you evaluated that as good or bad. I wanted to ask well, what percent you were actually creating distance and what percent you were . . .

SHERRY: Right.

PHIL: 'Cause I had a really hard time creating distance. I mean I just found it very amusing.

SHERRY: I did have a hard time too. I thought, "How am I going to do this?" because everything was going really nicely. But it wasn't just 3 good days. Each day preceding the 3 in a row got better and better.

But like I said, if one of us thought it was a bad day for one reason or another, then that was that, even though 90% of the day could have been good. Anyway, I had to think about "What am I going to do to create distance?" "How can I make it noticeable?" It was humorous only in the way that I knew exactly what I could do to do that. It was, uhm, like well "I know this topic," or "If I bring this up, I know that kind of pushes one button." "Or if I have this topic . . . " But then again, I didn't just want an argument. If I wanted to create distance, I had to do it a little more carefully.

PHIL: It was interesting to be on the other end of it too because I know what her goal is! I'm monitoring myself 'cause I don't want to be manipulated because I know that she's supposed to create distance.

SHERRY: (*laughing*)

PHIL: So I checked myself out on how I'm acting and reacting. It's pretty amusing.

SHERRY: But you'd be reacting so quickly. That's what I found most amusing . . .

PHIL: Uh huh.

SHERRY: It's like, boy, it doesn't take much. Even when we know what each other's doing, we still can be set off like that.

PHIL: Also I found another good thing about it, was that I felt a success. You know you go 3 days, we had a target, we had 3 days where we had to achieve something . . .

SHERRY: Right.

PHIL: So just setting it up in that framework, I found myself being more cognizant of how I had to react . . . 'cause I wanted to achieve the 3 days. When we achieved the 3 days I acknowledged myself, and I acknowledged Sherry, and we acknowledged each other and said "Well, this is good," and then we flipped the coin either way and that was it.

LIPCHIK: So there was a push to accomplish the 3 days?

PHIL: Well, for me, that was something I felt.

LIPCHIK: (*to Sherry*) Okay, okay. Did you feel that way?

SHERRY: No, uh uh. Especially at the beginning, and we went through quite a few days before we even got to 3 days. I guess on those three days I thought, "Oh well, if this is good, we're pretty distant," and then it became more of a playful thing. Like, "Careful, this is the 3rd day." You know, something like that.

LIPCHIK: Yeah.

SHERRY: No I guess I didn't have that goal. It was more that I wanted to see . . .

LIPCHIK: At 3 days did you think you could do 4 or 5 without distance?

PHIL: Uh huh. I thought it would be a logical progression that we would do 4 [days] next and then do 5 next and then do 6 and 7 and just start thinking about that . . .

SHERRY: Ha ha! Don't think!

PHIL: So much for what I think is logical! (*laughing*) It might be asking for disaster too, you know, how long can you go.

SHERRY: The last time we had the 3 days though—I don't remember when it was . . . The last time you got to create the distance, I was really ready for some distance. It wasn't because of our relationship necessarily, but at work I was starting to feel real bogged down, so with distance, I felt like I could be more just by myself, to myself.

LIPCHIK: What does that say about what you need from each other at times even when things are going well in the relationship?

SHERRY: It's a time issue. When we're creating distance or even arguing, I can just, not can, but do, go off into my own thing.

LIPCHIK: Uh huh.

SHERRY: I may not leave the house, but I do my school work, or I just completely block everything out. Where if there isn't distance, and everything's going fine, I guess I feel an obligation to talk more or to communicate more . . .

LIPCHIK: Well do you think you can have both? . . .

SHERRY: Yeah.

LIPCHIK: How can you do that without Phil taking it personally?

During the rest of the session, the couple also discussed how the two could communicate differently so that they do not take the need to have some space as personal rejection. Phil also said that he learned to accept Sherry more for who she was because he could not ask for reasons for her predictions, and Sherry agreed that she felt more accepted and had become more accepting of herself. They also spent time in the session discussing their different styles of closeness. They concluded that Phil had a greater need and tolerance for closeness than Sherry who withdrew when she had her fill. The more stress she felt on a daily basis, the more space she needed, whereas the more stress Phil experienced the more closeness he wanted.

At the conclusion of this session I prepared a summary message as follows:

LIPCHIK: What I heard today is how hard you worked on this exercise, how much you both got out of it. You both seem to have learned so much about how different you are in some ways, like about your need for closeness under stress, and your similarities in others. You really should pat yourself and each other on the back for working so hard on this. It isn't easy to learn to control your urges and curiosity.

I was also impressed with how open and honest you were about all your reactions. Since the exercise was so useful, you may just want to continue to do it . . . but you may figure out a variation on the pattern . . . like 3 days, or 4 days . . . or whatever you can agree on. I do want to say though, it might be useful to think of this as a good beginning . . . like the beginning of a new pattern, as opposed to a solution that is in place. Sometimes it takes time to develop new patterns and new habits. If there are reoccurrences of problems, this should not be seen as a setback, but as an opportunity to learn more about how to prevent them in the future. So it makes sense to be patient and keep working at it.

Another session was scheduled for three weeks later.

Fourth Conjoint Session

Sherry and Phil were beaming when they entered the room. They reported that on a scale of 1 to 10, with 10 being excellent, they were at a 9 or 10, 95% of the time since the last meeting. "It's magic!" is how they described the changes.

LIPCHIK: What was different?

SHERRY: We had a couple of bad days . . .

PHIL: Yeah, uh huh.

SHERRY: . . . where we said, "Oh, it's just a bad day, we might as well start over again."

LIPCHIK: Now what about that?

SHERRY: In fact, it was our first 3 days after we saw you. We were on to our 4th day, and we decided the 4th day was a bad day, so then we had to start over again, and we had to only work with 3 days at a time. So we decided if we had a bad day before 4 days then we can handle that.

LIPCHIK: Uh huh.

SHERRY: But after that we got 5 days in.

LIPCHIK: Well what about the bad days? How is it different now having a bad day than it was before?

SHERRY: It didn't last for 3 days. (*laughing*) But that's the same as last time.

LIPCHIK: How is it different?

PHIL: You're the one who always gets the coin toss, coin toss, coin toss.

SHERRY: I don't think it's very different, but when I get the coin toss, you always end up starting to do it (*laughing*).

PHIL: That's interesting. I always get myself ready . . .

SHERRY: Yeah, but he'll actually do it . . .

PHIL: . . . for rejection or something (*laughing*).

SHERRY: Uhhm, what was the question? I'm really . . .

LIPCHIK: How are the bad days different?

SHERRY: Oh, I think that it's, they're not as bad.

LIPCHIK: How do you explain that?

SHERRY: It's not anger, well it's still anger. We each might raise our voice and we . . . Well I, in order to break away from an argument I have to get away from it for a while, and that's how one of them went, I know. And on another one, Phil came up to me before, before I would have said anything about it and just started talking about it . . . We seemed more receptive to each other in fixing it, don't you think? In talking about it and saying "Okay I'm sorry, I hurt your feelings, I'm sorry," rather than about why it hurt your feelings and how, you know . . .

LIPCHIK: Uh huh.

SHERRY: So, (*to Phil*) what do you think of that?

LIPCHIK: If your life were to go on in this pattern, would that be okay? Would you consider that a good relationship?

PHIL: Yeah, I would . . .

SHERRY: Uh huh, pretty good.

PHIL: What's interesting about where these little breakdowns have occurred is that prior to seeing you and this exercise, this could [have gone] on for days. You know this, yadda yadda, bickering . . .

SHERRY: Yeah, 4 or 5 days, pretty awful.

PHIL: So what's going on now is it's getting off [that pattern] real fast.

SHERRY: We do. I guess that's it.

PHIL: And seeing what, where it is, what's going on and what you're committed to, and is it really important or what's the issue . . .

SHERRY: Yeah. I find myself asking myself . . .

PHIL: And after that it's like some silence, hmm, you know, what's the cost, and this is ridiculous. So I find that we get off, we get away from the junk and start talking and start hearing yourself and hearing the other person, and then you say, what're we doing here, this is really pretty stupid, where are we trying to go with this conversation?

SHERRY: And this far, we're both receptive to that. If one of us says something to bring it in another direction like, "We don't really want to do this," the other person always seems to be receptive to that, where before we weren't. "Did you mean to talk about that?" "Yes I did, and I meant to say this too!!" Uhm, I don't know why we're not doing that though.

LIPCHIK: It sounds like you're not angry at each other.

SHERRY: Pardon?

LIPCHIK: Is it because you're not as angry at each other?

SHERRY: That could be . . . Good answer.

(*at the end of the session*)

LIPCHIK: Well, should we stop at this point, should we have more sessions or is this good enough?

[I raise the issue of termination here, since the relationship is now on a more positive trajectory, and both partners seem satisfied with their progress. As the reader may have noticed, the amount of laughter and general, good-natured bantering has significantly increased in the third and fourth sessions—a very positive sign.]

PHIL: Well, I wouldn't mind just having a 6-week . . . what do you think of that . . . ?

LIPCHIK: Quality check . . .

PHIL: Just sort of . . .

SHERRY: (*laughing*) Four- to 6-week checkup.

PHIL: Just to do it. I mean this is sort of new, it really is sort of new considering that we've had extreme up and downs, and this is probably the most balance that we've had in our interactions . . .

SHERRY: Uh huh.

PHIL: Controlled balance. And I wouldn't mind coming back, in say 4 to 6 weeks. (*to therapist*) I don't know what you think of that.

LIPCHIK: It might be a good idea to come in one more time . . . and certainly you could cancel the session if you felt you didn't need it.

In the summation message, I acknowledged and applauded the progress they had made. I made one suggestion:

> "Every time you have a negative thought about the other, and there's no way that doesn't happen in the best of marriages, that you follow it with a positive thought. Like, 'Ugh, he's irritable today, or she's cranky, but he was so considerate. . . . she was so supportive yesterday . . . etc.' You need to maintain your balance between the good and the occasional bad. There can be times when there are 2 or even 3 bad days in a row, and it doesn't mean the relationship isn't good. I'm hoping you can keep up your confidence and not get scared. So getting into the habit of thinking a positive thought along with a negative one can build up your strength to handle the more difficult times."

Follow-Up Contacts

Sherry and Phil canceled the follow-up session and said they were doing so well they didn't need to come in. Ten months later I saw them for one session. They appeared to be very angry with each other and recited similar complaints to those presented at the first session. It turned out that they were experiencing a time of extreme stress. Both of Phil's parents were ill, and the couple had been spending the past 4 weekends traveling 5 hours to Phil's hometown to cook and clean for them. Phil was very appreciative of Sherry's efforts but felt she had little energy left for him. Phil was also in the process of deciding to give up his failing business and to look for another job. Meanwhile, Sherry was feeling a lot of responsibility to support both of them.

I asked them what they believed had been most helpful to them as a result of our past sessions, and they immediately realized that they had fallen back into an old unsatisfying pattern: Phil needing extra support when he was under stress and Sherry needing more space. I used scaling questions to get them to evaluate the big picture of their relationship as opposed to the present crisis. They both said they had been an "8 to 9" until recently. They recognized that they had tuned in only to their feelings and had forgotten to be considerate of their differences. They left looking much revived and called 2 weeks later to say they were doing fine.

Fifteen months later Sherry and Phil came for a "consultation" session. They reported that things were going well for them individually and together. Phil had given up his business and was feeling successful at a good job. Sherry had finished her courses and was exploring starting a business of her own. They were ready to start a family and wanted to be sure their relationship was solid enough. They estimated that they had three to four fights a year at this point but that these were much less emotionally draining and resolved much sooner. On a scale of 1 to 10, they agreed they were generally at an 8 to 9. I wondered what their expectations were for a good relationship, and they both admitted they would like a guarantee of perfect harmony, if possible. I told them how impressed I was that they had reduced their conflict to so few times a year, and we reviewed what they needed to know and do to keep things as mutually satisfying as possible.

Four years later Sherry and Phil returned for one session. They now had a 2½-year-old son and had come because they felt "rejected and not respected" by each other. Once again, when I asked scaling questions, they quickly recognized that their lives had become unusually stressful but that, overall, their relationship was going well. Sherry had started a business of her own, which was doing well but required a lot of her time and energy. Phil was working full-time and was keeping books for Sherry's business on the side. They both wanted to spend as much time as possible with their son, and they had had no time alone as a couple for several months. This time I hardly had to ask a question. They realized what the solution was and said they would have to keep a sign on their refrigerator for the future to remind themselves that they have to make time for each other regularly, but especially when things got rough.

CONCLUSIONS

The following outlines 10 useful steps for achieving time-effective outcomes in solution-focused couple therapy (after Friedman, 1997).

1. Tune-in to the couple's affect and emotional experience; acknowledge and support the couple's struggle and desire for a more satisfying relationship.
2. Maintain a position of naive curiosity, optimism, and respect by actively listening to each partner's story; pay special attention to openings that create space for constructing a new story.

3. Be on the look-out for evidence of change or success. Listen for stories that offer hope.

4. Stay simple and focused, listening for exceptions (i.e., contradictions to the problem-saturated story). When a problem or pattern seems to have taken on a life of its own, engage in externalizing conversations, defining the pattern as an outside force that is oppressing, subjugating, or constraining forward movement.

5. Stay tuned to the couple's goal: What does each partner see as reflecting a positive outcome? What does each partner hope to accomplish?

6. Negotiate with the couple to frame the outcome or goals in clear observable terms.

7. Build on strengths, competencies, successes, and resources.[3] Invite the couple to tune in to exceptions to the problem.

8. Introduce ideas (tasks, homework) that create space for the couple to "do something different." Encourage small steps and support the couple's creativity.

9. Encourage action/practice outside the therapy room. Define the change process as hard work and applaud small steps taken in a positive direction.

10. Ask pivotal questions that embed changes in the couple's experience. Compliment the couple on positive steps taken. If the goal is not attained, begin the cycle again. Leave the door open for future contact.

Figure 13.3 presents some helpful "do's" and "don'ts" in solution-focused therapy with couples.

A WORD ABOUT MANAGED CARE AND THERAPIST ACCOUNTABILITY

As we're all aware, the managed care movement in the United States has had a major impact on the way mental health services are delivered. The move from therapy as a cottage industry to the industrialization of mental health care has been rapid indeed (Cummings, 1991). Issues of accountability, efficiency, and effectiveness have grown more prominent in the interest of containing costs.

One of our responsibilities as therapists is to be accountable for the work we do. To assure this accountability, we need to systematically monitor outcomes in therapy. One simple way to assess progress is by using the scaling questions discussed earlier. Here, the client provides a

DO

STAY joined with both partners at all times, and agree with both their points of view in the summation message.

FREQUENTLY ask each partner for his or her point of view about what the other said to keep them both involved and to keep yourself from becoming partial to one side.

TRY to find common agreement, no matter how small.

INQUIRE about their sexual relationship; they expect you to!*

HAVE them define goals in small steps and in behavioral terms.

BE sure to get agreement from both partners about the treatment plan.

DON'T

EVER believe a relationship is hopeless by the way a couple presents their situation.

SEE them together, if they have mutually exclusive goals.

SEE them together, if they fight continually.

LET one partner tell you secrets about the other over the phone.

HAVE a separate session with one partner without inviting the other in for a separate session as well.

WORK with a couple if one partner has confided in you about an ongoing affair that he/she does not want to end.

FIGURE 13.3. Do's and don'ts. Copyright Eve Lipchik, ICF Consultants, Inc., Milwaukee, WI. Reprinted by permission. *SF: This is a "don't" for me unless one partner brings it up for discussion. I have found that this subject will naturally emerge if it is relevant to our work and/or part of the couple's agenda in coming for therapy.

self-assessment of progress along a defined scale. Using scaling questions makes a great deal of sense, since it is the client's reported satisfaction with progress that should determine whether the therapy has been successful. We refer the reader to Ogles, Lambert, and Masters (1996) for information on a variety of useful instruments to track change in therapy and assess client satisfaction.

The solution-focused therapies, as exemplified in the clinical situation presented here, offer a set of principles and methods that allow us to practice with integrity while providing quality time-effective service. We understand that keeping people in therapy beyond what is needed is costly both financially and psychologically. As competency-based therapists who do not use the language of pathology and psychiatric diagnosis, we have learned to be bilingual (Hoyt & Friedman, 1998) by translating our terms and ideas into a language that the managed care company can understand.

By focusing, as we do, on alliance building, co-constructing goals for therapy, using specific and tailored homework assignments, and assessing outcome, we offer a "user-friendly" therapy that both supports clients' goals and meets the objectives of managed care companies.

NOTES

1. For examples of the application of solution-focused thinking to work with couples, see de Shazer and Berg (1985); Friedman (1993a, 1996); Hoyt and Berg (1997); Hudson and O'Hanlon (1991); and Weiner-Davis (1992).
2. SF: I don't, as a usual practice, see each partner separately. There are, however, two situations in which I would: (1) if one partner appears to be intimidated in the presence of the other; and (2) if there is a reasonable possibility that an affair is occurring.
3. We can learn a great deal about the importance of attending to strengths by listening to the voices of our clients. Chasin, Grunebaum, and Herzig (1990) present the interviews of four prominent therapists with the same couple. When that couple was contacted 6 months after these interviews, the following remarks were made. The wife reported: " . . . I think the major objection I had with the four interviews was that *nobody really emphasized any of the positive things in our relationship.* . . . It made me feel a little bit empty and insecure afterwards because they were always emphasizing 'Well, what are the problems in the relationship. . . . [which] led to a reiteration of all the problems' " (p. 367). The husband, agreeing with his wife, went on to say, that "One of the things that struck me was, Why didn't anybody ask us if we love each other or why we'd been together for 10 years? . . . I think that [the positives in our relationship] could have been stressed more that [they were]" (p. 367).

REFERENCES

Anderson, H., & Goolishian, H. A. (1988). Human systems as linguistic systems: Preliminary and evolving ideas about the implications for clinical therapy. *Family Process, 27,* 371–393.

Berg, I. K. (1994). *Family based services: A solution-focused approach.* New York: Norton.

Berg, I. K., & de Shazer, S. (1993). Making numbers talk: Language in therapy. In S. Friedman (Ed.), *The new language of change: Constructive collaboration in psychotherapy* (pp. 5–24). New York: Guilford Press.

Berg, I. K., & Miller, S. D. (1994). *Working with the problem drinker: A solution-focused approach.* New York: Norton.

Chasin, R., Grunebaum, H., & Herzig, M. (Eds.). (1990). *One couple, four realities: Multiple perspectives on couple therapy.* New York: Guilford Press.

Cummings, N. (1991, Spring). Out of the cottage. *Advance Plan,* pp. 1–2, 14.

De Jong, P., & Hopwood, L. (1995). Outcome research on treatment conducted at the Brief Family Therapy Center, 1992–1993. In S. D. Miller, M. A. Hubble, & B. L. Duncan (Eds.), *Handbook of solution focused brief therapy* (pp. 272–298). San Francisco: Jossey-Bass.

de Shazer, S. (1982). *Patterns of brief family therapy: An ecosystemic approach.* New York: Guilford Press.

de Shazer, S. (1985). *Keys to solution in brief therapy.* New York: Norton.

de Shazer, S. (1988). *Clues: Investigating solutions in brief therapy.* New York: Norton.

de Shazer, S. (1991). *Putting difference to work.* New York: Norton.

de Shazer, S. (1994). *Words were originally magic.* New York: Norton.

de Shazer, S., & Berg, I. K. (1985). A part is not a part: Working with only one of the partners present. In A. S. Gurman (Ed.), *Casebook of marital therapy* (pp. 97–110). New York: Guilford Press.

Duncan, B. L., & Moynihan, D. W. (1994). Applying outcome research: Intentional utilization of the client's frame of reference. *Psychotherapy, 31*(2), 294–301.

Fisch, R., Weakland, J. H., & Segal, L. (1982). *Tactics of change: Doing therapy briefly.* San Francisco: Jossey-Bass.

Frank, J. D. (1974). *Healing and persuasion: A comparative study of psychotherapy.* New York: Schocken Books.

Friedman, S. (1993a). Possibility therapy with couples: Constructing time-effective solutions. *Journal of Family Psychotherapy, 4*(4), 35–52.

Friedman, S. (Ed.). (1993b). *The new language of change: Constructive collaboration in psychotherapy.* New York: Guilford Press.

Friedman, S. (1996). Couples therapy: Changing conversations. In H. Rosen & K. T. Kuehlwein (Eds.), *Constructing realities: Meaning making perspectives for psychotherapists* (pp. 413–453). San Francisco: Jossey-Bass.

Friedman, S. (1997). *Time-effective psychotherapy: Maximizing outcomes in an era of minimized resources.* Boston: Allyn & Bacon.

Friedman, S., & Fanger, M. T. (1991). *Expanding therapeutic possibilities: Getting results in brief psychotherapy.* San Francisco: Lexington Books/Jossey-Bass.

Gergen, K. J. (1985). The social constructionist movement in modern psychology. *American Psychologist, 40*(3), 266–275.

Haley, J. (1973). *Uncommon therapy: The psychiatric techniques of Milton H. Erickson, M.D.* New York: Norton.

Hobbs, N. (1966). Helping disturbed children: Psychological and ecological strategies. *American Psychologist, 21,* 1105–1115.

Hoyt, M. F., & Berg, I. K. (1997). Solution-focused couple therapy: Helping clients construct self-fulfilling realities. In F. Dattilio (Ed.), *Case studies in couple and family therapy* (pp. 203–232). New York: Guilford Press.

Hoyt, M. F., & Friedman, S. (1998). Dilemmas of postmodern practice under managed care and some pragmatics for increasing the likelihood of treatment authorization. *Journal of Systemic Therapies, 17*(3), 23–33.

Hudson, P., & O'Hanlon, W. H. (1991). *Rewriting love stories: Brief marital therapy.* New York: Norton.

Kiser, D. J., Piercy, F. P., & Lipchik, E. (1993). The integration of emotion in solution-focused therapy. *Journal of Marital and Family Therapy, 19*(3), 233–242.

Lipchik, E. (1992). A reflecting interview. *Journal of Strategic and Systemic Therapies, 11*(4), 59–74.

Lipchik, E. (1993). "Both/and" solutions. In S. Friedman (Ed.), *The new language of change: Constructive collaboration in psychotherapy* (pp. 25–49). New York: Guilford Press.

Lipchik, E. (1994, March/April). The rush to be brief. *Family Therapy Networker,* pp. 34–39.

Lipchik, E., & de Shazer, S. (1986). The purposeful interview. *Journal of Strategic and Systemic Therapies, 5*(1), 88–99.

Lipchik, E., & Kubicki, A. D. (1996). Solution-focused domestic violence views: Bridges toward a new reality in couples therapy. In S. D. Miller, M. A. Hubble, & B. L. Duncan (Eds.), *Handbook of solution-focused brief therapy* (pp. 65–98). San Francisco: Jossey-Bass.

McKeel, A. J. (1995). A clinician's guide to research on solution-focused brief therapy. In S. D. Miller, M. A. Hubble, & B. L. Duncan (Eds.), *Handbook of solution focused brief therapy* (pp. 251–271). San Francisco: Jossey-Bass.

Miller, S. D., Duncan, B. A., & Hubble, M. A. (1997). *Escape from Babel: Toward a unifying language for psychotherapy practice.* New York: Norton.

Ogles, B. M., Lambert, M. J., & Masters, K. S. (1996). *Assessing outcome in clinical practice.* Boston: Allyn & Bacon.

O'Hanlon, W. H., & Weiner-Davis, M. (1989). *In search of solutions: A new direction in psychotherapy.* New York: Norton.

O'Hanlon, W. H., & Wilk, J. (1987). *Shifting contexts: The generation of effective psychotherapy.* New York: Norton.

Rosen, H., & Kuehlwein, K. T. (Eds.). (1996). *Constructing realities: Meaning making perspectives for psychotherapists.* San Francisco: Jossey-Bass.

Selvini Palazzoli, M., Boscolo, L., Cecchin, G., & Prata, G. (1978). *Paradox and counterparadox.* New Jersey: Jason Aronson.

Weiner-Davis, M. (1992). *Divorce busting.* New York: Fireside/Simon & Schuster.

Weiner-Davis, M., de Shazer, S., & Gingerich, W. J. (1987). Building on pre-treatment change to construct the therapeutic solution: An exploratory study. *Journal of Marital and Family Therapy, 13,* 359–363.

Whiston, S. C., & Sexton, T. L. (1993). An overview of psychotherapy outcome research: Implications for practice. *Professional Psychology: Research and Practice, 24*(1), 43–51.

White, M., & Epston, D. (1990). *Narrative means to therapeutic ends.* New York: Norton.

Zimmerman, J. L., & Dickerson, V. C.(1993). Bringing forth the restraining influence of pattern in couples therapy. In S. Gilligan & R. Price (Eds.), *Therapeutic conversations* (pp. 197–214). New York: Norton.

14

◄O►

COUPLES, CULTURE, AND DISCOURSE

A Narrative Approach

JOHN H. NEAL
JEFFREY L. ZIMMERMAN
VICTORIA C. DICKERSON

You are about to enter into some different kinds of ideas about people, relationships, and therapy. In this chapter, we talk about gender and power and couples from our particular bent on narrative theory and practice. Like other authors in this book, we describe some of the more important conceptual aspects of the work and illustrate these with a transcript. Throughout, we use an interview format in which John is interviewed by Vicki and Jeff about his work with a couple. This allows us to provide multiple perspectives on the thinking that organizes the work through a conversation among therapists of both genders. Our intent in using this format is to enhance the visibility of both the "thinking" and the "doing" of the work.

A second purpose of this chapter is to exemplify the ways narrative therapists think about and work with the effects of cultural discourse and—in the context of couple therapy—its operation through gender. These effects can be thought of in terms of certain attitudes and habits toward which men and women have been culturally shaped. However, the dominant culture is not neutral; to consider the effects of these attitudes and habits is to acknowledge a situation where there are real effects of power. Within this view, it is useful to understand and address relationship conflicts as effects of power. Narrative therapists treat so-called individual problems, like anxiety and depression, similarly. They often "understand" these problems as effects of being in positions of less power, sometimes thought of as marginalization (i.e., not living up to what is understood as "correct," not having access to resources, etc.). As narrative therapists, we also try to "walk the talk" of these ideas by conducting our therapies in a way that is consistent with an understanding of our position of greater power in the role of the therapist.

As we write this, we are also aware that many readers may have little or no familiarity with the thinking and practice of narrative therapy. Generally speaking, we believe that narrative therapists' view of persons and problems is radically different from the view of more traditional psychologies. As mentioned above, we "see" problems as existing in cultural discourse, so that when persons attribute meaning to their experience, they "story" their experience in certain well-prescribed ways specified by the culture. These stories are constitutive of persons; they create versions of persons, some of which fit the contradictory specifications of dominant culture and some that do not. When some of these versions do not fit the person's preferences and/or are outside what is considered "normal" by cultural standards, they may be experienced as problems. In narrative practice, the therapist works with the client to help him or her separate from the problem story; this is the well-known process of "externalization" and allows the client to notice that the problem is not about his or her "deficiency" but, rather, is an effect of cultural discourse. Once clients experience this separation, they can begin to notice other aspects of their experience that had gone unstoried. The next phase of the work thus becomes "reauthoring." These ideas will be made more available in the clinical example and transcript with the couple in the following pages.

So what do we mean when we talk about power? From our particular understanding of the world, how persons think, feel, behave, and experience themselves can be understood to be (1) organized in narrative form and (2) saturated with cultural beliefs and practices. What therapists usually think of as "intrapsychic" or "systemic" and "interactional" problems, we understand as *effects* of the contradictory cultural prescriptions people use to make sense of themselves and to guide them in their relationships. As people, our experience is of doing what makes sense. Yet, the results are not always what we want. This occurs often when what we want is different from what the dominant culture supports.

In and of themselves, these might not seem like revolutionary ideas. Everyone understands that we exist within culture and cannot be unaffected by it. The elements that makes this approach so different from other individual and family approaches to therapy are its view that these cultural prescriptions are what primarily support problems and its emphasis on how these cultural ideas and practices inadvertently operate as forms of power on individuals and relationships. A common example of this is reflected in the way that men often disqualify women's thinking. When a woman's experience (e.g., of his effects on her) is at odds with a man's experience of his own behavior, it is likely that he discounts what she is speaking of and may attribute a lack of "rationality" to her thinking. From our point of view, this is an effect of male entitlement, which encourages men to assume that their understanding is the one that "makes sense." Cultural practices that inform maleness and femaleness often operate in these circumstances to encourage women to distrust or doubt their own experience in order to get along—to "dissociate" from their experience as Gilligan (1990) would say.

> *Vicki:* I'd like to begin our commentary, but I'm wondering how odd the readers will find this conversational style? As a woman I pay a lot of attention to the effect I (we) might have on others.
>
> *Jeff:* As a man, my first thought was on doing this the way we think is "right," so it's good, I think, that you raise this issue. This way of writing does mirror, in some ways, our work with couples, as it puts the reader in the kind of reflexive position one member of the couple is in while we talk to the other. Somehow, listening to a conversation seems to trigger more new possibilities than taking part in one or certainly more than being talked at or lectured to. I'm wondering if we are really conveying what we mean about our emphasis on the effects of dominant cultural "stories."
>
> *John:* If we take seriously the ideas about power discussed in this chapter, we must explain how we think about what we do, not just assume its value will be taken for granted. My answer to your question, Jeff, about our emphasis on the cultural is that by making our thinking visible—enabling readers to notice how we arrive at certain ideas and clinical practices—we can illustrate the practice of transparency we use to address our relative positions of power. We will also be illustrating the point of view we are influenced by in our work.

The discussion that follows focuses on three aspects of narrative therapy with couples: (1) how to approach problems as effects of power and gender on individuals and relationships, including useful and not-so-useful ways for therapists to make visible the operation of culture and power and how these relate to the personal experience of each member of the couple; (2) how to think about and use the narrative metaphor;

and (3) how to think about and use "reauthoring" practices. By "reauthoring" we mean those clinical practices that help persons to remember preferred personal experiences of themselves and their relationships and to reclaim these in such a way that they are experienced as their "identity" and the "identity" of the couple's relationship.

We are aware that our focus on culture and power,[1] and therefore gender, may take some readers by surprise and make others uncomfortable. Some therapists avoid raising questions about power with couples out of the intent to avoid imposing their values on their clients. Other therapists, who make it a part of their work, struggle with how to explore and talk about it in the therapy without alienating one member of the couple (most often, but not always, the man). It is our experience that narrative therapy offers concepts and tools for addressing this operation of power within relationships and within persons in ways that honor and respect the experience of both members of the couple.

Jeff: Perhaps our passion for considering issues of power, including the effect of therapeutic conversation on clients, is misread as not appreciating the intentions of other therapists. We certainly take a strong stand against a pathologizing of relationships or constructing individual deficits.

John: I agree. And because we believe power is tacitly involved in most if not all problems, it feels right for us to proceed in these ways and wrong (for us) to avoid issues of power. I am also aware that, for many others, this is not the case.

Vicki: I believe it is important for others to appreciate that we see these ideas and this work as a metaphor for understanding persons and problems and therapy. There are, of course, many possible metaphors of understanding, some of which have better effects than others on those with whom we work. We happen to prefer the narrative metaphor, how it fits for us and our lives, and the effects it has on our clients.

We are also aware that some therapists interpret narrative therapy as an "individual" therapy. This interpretation may have developed because of the ways we tend to structure conversations in the room, talking to each member individually rather than encouraging conversations between members of the couple. Narrative therapy comes out of a tradition of therapies that focus on interactional and systemic pattern (cf. Zimmerman & Dickerson, 1994). While we structure conversations in certain ways, the ideas that organize what we do include an understanding of complementarity and pattern (Neal, 1996). Like systemically oriented therapists, narrative therapists orient to interactional pattern when we explore clients' experience (Zimmerman & Dickerson, 1993a, 1993b, 1994; Neal, 1998). However, we do not understand the complementarities and patterns we construct to reflect pathologies or other characteristics of individuals and their relationships. From our narrative perspective, complementarity and pattern are more usefully considered as reciprocal invitations to think and behave in certain ways. As such, understanding and behavior reflect personal and unique interpretations of culturally defined ways of knowing and behaving rather than characteristics of clients or their relationship. A couple's feelings, thoughts, and relationship patterns are organized and constrained by culturally dominant ideas and practices. As a consequence, the relationship "knots" familiar to systems therapists reflect the culturally available ways of making sense and behaving. A "narrative" therapy that ignores how cultural beliefs and practices influence women, men, and their relationships would not be recognizable to those who work from this perspective.

CONCEPTUAL AND TECHNICAL ASPECTS

It is important to distinguish our use of the narrative metaphor from applications of the ideas and practices that do not include consideration of how cultural beliefs and practices influence persons' relationships and experience of themselves. The "technique" of externalizing problems and the concepts of "narrative" and "story" may be very helpful for clients within the framework of other theoretical approaches (e.g., brief therapy, solution-focused therapy, collaborative language-based therapy, or other "systems" and individual approaches). However, the distinction between narrative therapy, as we understand it, and these approaches is that the latter typically include a perspective on persons and problems that does not address the operation of culture and power within and between persons (cf. Paré, 1996). Since we view the politicization of therapy and health care in general as a good thing, our concern is that these other applications of narrative ideas and practices render the links among culture, power, and couples' relationships invisible and less accessible for revision. Nor do these uses of narrative ideas and practices challenge the negative effects these (cultural) influences have on persons' identities. The narrative therapy we know and practice addresses these links among culture, power, and relationships.

From our point of view, the "default" (or dominant) cultural perspective on problems leaves people with little room to make sense of problems other than as reflecting some defect in them and their relationships. Thus, we believe that therapists who do not challenge this default view—by making visible the links between cultural "truths" and individual experience—tacitly reinforce these negative experiences of identity.

The view White and Epston (1990) introduced with the practice of externalizing conversations challenges this default view of problems. It makes visible the ways problems become constitutive of the narratives that organize the thinking, feeling, behavior, identities, and relationships of persons. This raises the questions: If problems don't reflect the characteristics of individuals and their relationships, what do problems reflect and where do they come from? This is where all our talk about culture and power becomes important for how one understands what is being said and what to do in the room.

In couple therapy, the operation of power has traditionally been approached by therapists in terms of differences in power between men and women. This view of power is valid and important but also unnecessarily narrow. It explains little about the particularities of how power operates on persons and within relationships. Nor does this view of power explain men's and women's shared experiences of helplessness in the face of conflict. It has been said that narrative therapy "unmasks" the operation of power. This is how we understand the practice of externalizing conversations.

Externalizing conversations begin with the exploration of each person's experience of the problem. This experience is explored as an effect of the problem that invites other experiences of the person, his or her partner, and the relationship. Rather than asking why a person feels a certain way, the narrative therapist pursues what the problem does to the individual and how it is able to accomplish this. Once the effects of the problem on a person's experience begin to become visible, we pursue how this experience invites other experiences of oneself, one's partner, and the relationship. Eventually, these conversations explore how particular cultural views and practices might help invite the behavior that supports the problem(s) that produce these negative experiences. That is, the direction of causality is *reversed* from conventional ways we understand the relationship between persons and problems: Negative experiences of self and relationship are understood to be effects of the problem, and the problem is understood to be an effect of the couple's (knowing and unknowing) participation in particular cultural practices.

This narrative postmodern approach to persons and problems also enables us to make visible the negative effects of the problem on the couple's relationship. The negative effects of problems usually invite each person to behave in ways that strengthen the problem and to view him- or herself and each other negatively. A conflict hurts a person's feelings and invites that person to respond in ways (e.g., out of the experience of hurt or anger) that hurt the other person and are at odds with who each experiences him- or herself to be (e.g., a caring person). Or, by exploring how one experience of the problem promotes others, a narrative therapist might make visible how dominant ideas about men's anger and frustration provide the justification for the ways men express anger destructively (e.g., they scare their partners). Cultural "truths" (e.g., anger is "automatic") support the belief that men are unable to control the problematic expression of these feelings. This makes situations in which these same men do express their anger in constructive ways invisible and meaningless. Consequently, men may typically believe they are unable to control how they express themselves and are unable to recall times in which they behaved in ways at odds with the problematic expression of anger. In short, narrative therapy helps clients to embrace preferred ways of experiencing themselves and to distance themselves from negative experiences by making visible the dominant cultural notions that support them.

> *Vicki:* John, what's our hope for how the readers will make sense of this dense information?
>
> *John:* My first hope is that our use of the narrative metaphor and externalizing conversations is distinguished from what therapists generally think of as "technique." Second, I want to emphasize that therapists who do not pay attention to the ways power operates risk keeping its negative effects invisible. And third, I want to make clear that these ideas and practices enable therapists to address the effects of power in ways that are respectful and collaborative.
>
> *Jeff:* I'm curious, too, if you have any ideas about how the readers will be able to use their own experience as they read further.
>
> *John:* I think these ideas become more experience-based in the transcript that follows. It is evident, for instance, how I understand the source of the couple's difficulties as existing within certain gendered cultural assumptions that affect all of us; and that by separating these culturally dominant "truths" from their respective identities, they are able to reclaim their relationship from the effects of the problem.

KEY PHASES OF THE WORK

Phase 1: Transparency and Situating of the Therapist—The Therapist as a Person

We usually begin with a couple by finding out a bit about each of them as persons. Next, the therapist offers the couple an opportunity to interview him- or her in order to "situate" him or herself as a person with certain kinds of experiences and background. The rationale for making the therapist known in this way comes from a postmodern understanding of power. It holds that persons in relative positions of greater power—as are therapists in relation to clients—should make the origins of their thinking and experience visible to those persons in positions of lesser power (White, 1993a). By privileging clients' perspectives on the therapist's thinking, the risk is lessened that therapists will misuse their power by imposing ideas and interpretations at odds with the life circumstances, values, and preferences of clients. With both heterosexual and same-sex couples, this conversation usually includes some acknowledgment of the therapist's gender and how the therapist believes this informs his or her work (Neal, 1998).

For reasons also having to do with the operation of power in therapy, we also use the related practice of "transparency" to make the thinking behind our questions visible to our clients. That is, when we ask a question, we generally accompany the question with the reasons for asking it. This enables clients (who are in a relative position of less power) to have a better sense about the experience and intentions of the therapist and the thinking that is guiding the work. Like Freedman and Combs (1996), we experience the practices of situating and transparency as "ethics in practice" (p. 275).

The following interview occurs with Elizabeth and Larry in the context of the Mental Research Institute (MRI) Narrative Therapy Training program. It included a reflecting team made up of mental health professionals participating in the program. For those of you who have been to MRI, we meet in the upstairs southwest corner rooms. Our walls adjoin the Brief Therapy Center where, until his death a few years ago, John Weakland worked along with Dick Fisch and Paul Watzlawick. Dick and Paul continue to see clients there on Wednesdays. Today is a Tuesday, so we do not have to worry about the noise we make. Like many of the rooms that many of you probably work in, this one is intolerably hot in the summer and surprisingly cold in the winter (at least by our thin-skinned Northern California standards). On this day, it is cold. And given that the wiring has not been upgraded since Don Jackson interviewed families here, we do not turn on the heater for fear of blowing a fuse. I am sure that Jay Haley must have been cold in this room more than once.

Married for 15 years, Elizabeth and Larry had consulted "lots of therapists" about continuing conflicts. They were referred to our training program at MRI by another therapist who had seen them a few times as part of an employee assistance program. They were experiencing financial difficulties, and the MRI Narrative Training Program offers services for a nominal fee. The couple had two children, a 16-year-old daughter and a 14-year-old son. At the time of therapy, Elizabeth was working as an administrator in a small office, and Larry was working as a technician in the electronics industry. I start the interview by getting some background from each of them to establish a sense of who they are as persons separate from a discussion of problems. Then I say:

JOHN: Okay. Is there anything you would like to know about me, either professionally or as a person?

LARRY: Yes, how long have you been doing this kind of thing?

This conversation continues for about 15 minutes. We are all nervous, and the pair pepper me with many questions. Larry, who appears the most nervous of the three of us, wants to know how long I've been practicing, how long I've been married, whether I've been divorced, the number and ages of my children, and other information that enables him to locate me socially and culturally. His questions are curt, and he appears uneasy. Elizabeth asks about my orientation to therapy and about MRI: What is it, and what are my roles here? She is interested in reading about narrative therapy and asks for names of books she can read. I am happy (then and now) to promote Jeff and Vicki's book (Zimmerman & Dickerson, 1996) as well as one by Jill Freedman and Gene Combs (Freedman & Combs, 1996).

Once their questions are answered, I review what I had explained on the phone in preparation for the meeting. This includes the setup with the one-way mirror and the structure of the interview that includes a "narrative reflecting team" (cf. Janowski, Dickerson, & Zimmerman, 1995; White, 1995; Zimmerman & Dickerson, 1996). I review this process by explaining that they will be interviewed by me for about 35 minutes. Next, the three of us will listen to the group discuss our interview from behind a one-way mirror. The group will then return behind the mirror, and the three of us will return to the therapy room to have a conversation about what we have heard. Finally, everyone who has been watching will come into the room with us to answer questions Larry and Elizabeth may have for me (or them) and to ask me questions about what I was doing in the interview. I also explain that during this last stage of the process, Jeff,[2] who is also present at this interview, may ask members of the group (and me) questions about our questions to make our thinking more visible.

JOHN: If there's anything else you'd like to know, please feel free to ask. One last thing that I like to say before going on is that if there is anything that I ask about or say that you find yourselves wondering about, for instance why I asked a particular question or what I'm thinking that would make me ask a question, please feel free to ask me to explain. We've found that sometimes the reasons that a therapist asks about this or that are more helpful than the questions themselves.

Here, I am introducing the practice of transparency mentioned above. People who have had previous experiences with other therapists often spontaneously comment how helpful it is to hear the thinking behind our questions. In her research on reflecting team process, clients reported to Anu Singh (1996) that it was extremely helpful for them to listen to therapists explain why they are asking what they ask and what it was in the therapist's own personal experience that made him or her interested in the particular aspects of the interview they asked about. Clients often find the reasons for asking a particular question more helpful than the question itself. If you think of power as the process through which the agreed-upon definition of truth is achieved—which is how I understand it—then how I am thinking and what I am thinking must be made continuously visible and open to question and consideration by clients. Without this kind of transparency, we therapists create even greater risks for ignoring important aspects of our clients' experience, and we keep the ways we are misunderstanding or not understanding invisible to ourselves and our clients. I think of it as honoring and respecting the experience of clients to acknowledge the inevitable limitations of the therapist's perspective and experience. I also think it has the effect of making people feel more respected and safe.

Jeff: When I do this, it also makes me feel I am engaging in the relationship more as a person.

Vicki: John, I noticed that you didn't situate yourself in terms of gender, that is, you didn't comment on your being a man, and how this affects your understanding of the man, and the woman, and your work. I know that at other times you do this (Neal, 1998). Why not here?

John: I suppose I could have. I know it is something all three of us always try to pay attention to with couples. But I guess I have come to think that to bring it up out of context, when it is not overtly related to something happening at that moment in the room, increases the risk of both members of the couple feeling that it is something I am imposing upon them. Certainly, bringing up the influence of gender risks alienating many men who experience such discussions as blaming. And, although acknowledging my gender is sometimes welcomed by women, at other times it makes them uncomfortable. How both men and women will react to this announcement depends a great deal on how they locate and explain the sources of their own personal experience. For those who do not understand themselves in terms of gender differences and the operation of power, I would rather find out a bit about their experience of the relationship, themselves, and each other in order to find ways that the operation of gender and power can be explored within their respective and shared experience. Since (in my mind) the operation of power always shapes what happens in the room, it is better addressed in a way that relates to the experience of the moment. Also, because the operation of power within and between people is so much a part of a narrative therapist's thinking, I do not believe I ever get through a first meeting without finding moments in which its influence is not brought into the room by me in one way or another.

Phase 2: Engaging Oneself in the Couple's Experiences of Problem(s) through the Exploration of the Effects of Problems on Experience

The work proceeds with the therapist engaging him- or herself in the couple's experiences of problem(s) in terms of their effects. In saying this we are suggesting that we are viewing each person's experience as effects of problem(s) rather than as the source of problems. As mentioned above, this is important to understand because it is counterintuitive to the ways most of us think and talk about persons and problems. It is also a key for engaging in "externalizing conversations."

We view, understand, and explore problems as the sources of the effects they have on persons. When a man, for instance, says his wife's behavior is the problem and that its effects on him are to make him angry, we are interested in how this anger affects him and the relationship. We do not wonder what it is about him, his wife, or their respective backgrounds that gets him angry or gets her to behave in whatever ways she does. We do not wonder whether or not his anger is "justified." Nor do we pursue whether he gets angry because of some "deeper" hurt. Instead, we explore how this anger affects his experience of himself, of his partner, and of the relationship. Then we explore the effects of these effects of anger on his experience of himself, his partner, and the relationship. We follow the effects of these experiences. While exploring these effects, we continuously ask about what he thinks and feels about them, looking for aspects of his identity and values that might be at odds with how the problem is influencing him, his partner, and their relationship. It is these alternative experiences, attitudes, and values that exist alongside and at odds with the experience of problems that later become entry points for beginning a reauthoring process.

Back to the interview.

JOHN: (*looking at both of them*) So should we get to it?

ELIZABETH: (*Nods.*)

LARRY: I guess so . . .

JOHN: Okay, (*looking at Larry*) so what's the thing that's gotten you to come here? What's the problem that you would like some help with?

> *Vicki:* How did you decide to start with the husband rather than the wife?
>
> *John:* Well, there are lots of ways to decide this. I may start with the man when I get some sense that the woman holds responsibility for the emotional welfare of the relationship, and I tend to start with the woman when I think the man seems to have greater say—and thus, silencing effects—on the woman's experience of the problem. So, I guess I am looking for ways to create experiences that enable the couple to step outside of the particular ways power is embedded within the relationship. I'll say more about this later.
>
> *Vicki:* John, I am thinking some readers might wonder how would you know the answers to these questions right at the start. Do you have any thoughts about this?
>
> *John:* I think it is usually fairly obvious. One person, usually the man, seems to possess greater (verbal or nonverbal) control over what might be described as the "truth" and what is deemed to be most "important" at any given moment. I suspect this is fairly transparent to women therapists who pay attention to gender politics. I don't think it's hard for male therapists once they start paying attention to the practices of power that we—men—use. In this instance I viewed Larry as taking control through the way he asked me questions and then looked to Elizabeth to indicate that it was her turn. It seemed that he gave her responsibility, though, for relationship issues. At that point, she asked me her questions. With other couples, it might be the way he responds verbally or nonverbally to what she says. Sometimes it's what he says (to assert his authority) or what he doesn't say (as in the practice of "stonewalling"). Or, it might be her response to what he says. But what are your thoughts, Vicki? As a woman who pays attention to men's uses of power, aren't the power relations quickly obvious to you?
>
> *Vicki:* Painfully so . . . That's why I usually start with the male member of the couple. In fact, John, I think that when we start by talking

with the woman, we may be inadvertently replicating the cultural message to women (i.e., they are responsible for the relationship). Although I must say, I learned this the hard way—but that's another story!

Jeff: John, some people might think of what you are doing as "rebalancing" the distribution of power. Is this how you are thinking about it?

John: I'm not thinking of it in this way, but in terms of how the use of power confuses and prevents members of couples from noticing and understanding each other's experience. I find that once men understand the negative effects of exerting power in their relationship and over their partners, they really do not want to continue doing so. The challenge is how to help make this visible—for men and not infrequently for women as well—in ways that are respectful and honoring of both partners' experience. But let's return to the couple:

JOHN: So what's the problem you would like some help with?

LARRY: (*With a combination of what seemed like irritation and vulnerability—almost as if his voice were about to crack—he replies in a curt tone.*) Well, ah, we have more than one problem. Let's see, ah, certainly money is a problem, a big problem. We're not bringing in enough to meet our needs. And that aggravates other problems. Um, communication is a problem. Sex is a problem. That's about it.

JOHN: So money is a problem, and it aggravates communication and sex?

LARRY: Yes.

JOHN: Larry, I'll want to come back and ask you about these in detail, but if it's okay, I am going to ask Elizabeth the same question before I do. Okay?

LARRY: Okay.

JOHN: Anything else that would be important for me to know—before I ask Elizabeth the same question?

LARRY: No, I don't think so.

Jeff: Why not spend more time exploring Larry's experience? You didn't really get much from him before you started to ask Elizabeth?

John: No, and even what I got was labored. I believe Larry was very uncomfortable. This was a potentially threatening situation in which there was a group of people watching the interview, and, while he appeared nervous, he also appeared to be trying to hide his nervousness. Although I would have preferred to continue to explore his experience, I did not want to make him even more uncomfortable by asking about or commenting on his nervousness. Even asking about his experience of the problem might be felt as an attack. So when I noticed his discomfort, I decided to speak with Elizabeth, acknowledging that I would return to him in a little while. I was hoping that he would feel a bit more comfortable after we got further into things. I suppose had I thought of a way to make him more comfortable in order to stay with him at that moment, I would have preferred to have done so in order to minimize the risk of reproducing the gendered arrangement of making her responsible for the relationship, as you commented on, Vicki. However, I find that it is more useful to try to make people feel comfortable rather than take an ethical stand before I understand their experience.

Jeff: So, don't you think some readers will see you as controlling? After all, you chose who you wanted to speak with first, rather than letting them choose, and when you noticed it made him uncomfortable, you switched. Perhaps the readers might want you to comment on this.

John: I am "controlling" of the process. From our point of view, it's impossible for therapists not to exert control. The notion that narrative therapists do not control the process of therapy reflects a naive view of power—that it is possible to make everything equal. From a postmodern narrative perspective on power, this is not possible. What is important is that we remain open to our positions of relative power, open to the fact that those who are less powerful are in a better position to see the effects of our power than those of us in positions of greater power. This understanding of power also requires us to maintain ways to make these effects visible and to address them. I could have commented on Larry's discomfort with the intention of making it a bit easier on him. However, as we were sitting down to begin the meeting, the three of us had discussed how the mirror and the group made them anxious. This was the first few minutes of the formal interview, and, because of the obviousness of his discomfort, I thought to ask or comment on it would have risked disrespect. By the way, we would want to ask Larry about his discomfort as part of the "deconstruction" of the therapy we routinely do at the end of meetings both with a reflecting team (White, 1995; Zimmerman & Dickerson, 1996) and when working alone (cf. Freedman & Combs, 1996). Narrative practices are designed to make this kind of information visible and in a way that enables clients to feel comfortable telling us about it.

Back to the interview.

JOHN: Elizabeth what's your experience?

ELIZABETH: All that's true. We went through about 5 weeks of counseling before, and we made some progress in communicating and barely started to make some accommodations to each other. The anger got less, and we started talking. And then we just slid back into our old ways of being, and started focusing on ourselves individually, and things just went back to square one. We just grow apart. It's just what we get into: coping and distance and not communicating.

JOHN: So there was a period when you were experiencing the anger as decreasing and felt some progress communicating with each other. Then it went back to the way it had been before?

[This experience is potentially a unique outcome. We note these to come back to later.]

ELIZABETH: We had been given some things, some real solid things to focus our energy on. Given the opportunity to not focus on each other, we don't. We just get distant.

JOHN: So together these things create *distance* between the two of you?

[Here, and in what follows, I continuously restate what she is telling me in an externalized form in order to facilitate an experience of the problem as separate.]

ELIZABETH: Yes.

JOHN: And when you notice that *distance*, how do you find it affects you?

ELIZABETH: I think it's sad, and I'm not quite sure what to do. And if I know that we have to go to counseling, then I put it on the back burner and wait to bring it up here. We can't really talk to each other at all unless we are sitting here talking with someone like you.

JOHN: So the *distance* makes you sad and not sure what to do about it, and gets you to put things on the back burner? Do you mean you put communication on the back burner?

ELIZABETH: I put the relationship on the back burner. We can do the day-to-day stuff in a habitual way, but I don't want our relationship to be like that. It's bad, but it's better than not getting along (*starts to cry*).

JOHN: Is it okay to keep going here?

ELIZABETH: Yes.

JOHN: You're not wanting it on the back burner, but the worse thing is not getting along?

[I am asking her about not wanting it to be this way as a possible entry (later) into preferred ways of being and relating to Larry.]

ELIZABETH: Well, I guess they're both kind of not getting along, but the arguing is worse.

JOHN: When the *distance* or the *arguing* take over, do they encourage you to view or see Larry in certain ways?

[I am assuming that the problem *creates* views she does not like and am wondering how it convinces her—what it makes her pay attention to in order to get her to believe—this is the "truth."]

ELIZABETH: Yes, I get real judgmental or negative. He calls it insulting, but that's not what I'm trying to do. I feel real judgmental and critical. I'm wanting more from him, and I'm not getting it.

JOHN: So you find yourself wanting more, and these feelings encourage you to see Larry in judgmental and critical ways. Do these feelings also get you to view the relationship in certain ways?

[I am again pursuing "effects questions," making a distinction between what the feelings get her to do and what she, herself, prefers. Then I ask about the effects of the problem on her experience of the relationship.]

> *Jeff:* This seems like a good example of the areas in which we want to help therapists learn how to ask "effects" questions; exploring effects and then effects of these effects. We ask them to explore how the problem affects the person, the relationship, the view of the other, and the view of themselves, as well as certain habits it creates. Are you purposefully asking these questions? Is it a map that you follow?
>
> *John:* Yes, I first focus on the "effects of effects" as critical for separating each person's experience of him- or herself and each other from the views and behaviors that problems "encourage." In so doing, people often can identify preferred ways of behaving and experiencing themselves. Aspects of experience in each of these domains exist on the "periphery," so to speak, outside the influence of problems. By pursuing such questions with each member of the couple through these questions, we can often construct the ways problems create difficulties in relationships.
>
> *Vicki:* At this point do you see the problem as distance, and are you mapping out the effects of distance?
>
> *John:* I wasn't thinking of distance as "the problem," but since Elizabeth used it, I was pursuing it to map out the effects of this experience. I wanted to explore the effects of distance as a vehicle to get

closer to each of their respective experiences of the relationship, each other, and themselves. This seemed to be an experience that would help me understand other experiences—the "effects of effects."

More interview.

ELIZABETH: Yes, they get me to wonder whether we're going to make it together. I have had those thoughts. And then it feels hopeless.

JOHN: And so these feelings make you doubt the relationship and feel hopeless? And do they try to make you feel certain ways about yourself?

[The attribution of intentions to problematic experiences often helps clients identify the rhetorical tactics that problems use to get clients to participate in them.]

ELIZABETH: I find myself putting most of it on Larry. I misdirect most of it on him. I start getting really depressed about my life. I try to take responsibility, but mostly I blame him (*begins to quietly cry again*).

[I am imagining that Elizabeth blames herself for getting upset at Larry, feels badly for feeling the ways she feels, and believes that doing these things reflects something negative about her as a person. I could comment on this, but comments of this kind often do not help people revise their understanding of how these experiences affect them. Instead I pursue the effects of these experiences in order to make their influence visible, believing that this will help to gradually separate her experience of herself from what the problem gets her to feel and do.]

JOHN: Is this okay to be talking about this? I know it's very hard.

ELIZABETH: It's okay.

JOHN: When you say you are being "blaming," is that like noticing the things that Larry does that you think are a problem?

ELIZABETH: Yes.

JOHN: And when you find yourself doing that, how does that affect you?

ELIZABETH: It makes me feel badly, I don't like it.

JOHN: So there's another part of you that doesn't want to be blaming, that doesn't like the way you find yourself seeing Larry?

[Separating clients from their problems often begins by identifying how their intentions are good and at odds with what the problem get them to do.]

ELIZABETH: Yes, definitely.

JOHN: So this has a lot of very painful effects on things between you— how these feelings get you to react to Larry, how they get you to blame him. And part of you doesn't want to be feeling about Larry in these ways, and seeing him in these ways? Am I understanding?

[I am summarizing how the problem affects her reactions (what it gets her to do,) how it colors her view of Larry, and how this does not reflect what *she* wants. Reviewing a problem's effects also facilitates the separation of the problem from the person.]

ELIZABETH: Yes.

JOHN: Is it okay if I turn to back to Larry and find out a little more about his experience?

ELIZABETH: Okay.

JOHN: So, Larry, you mentioned money, the communication between the two of you, and the sexual thing. Which of these should we be talking about?

LARRY: Finances are definitely a big issue. We never talk about it at home. We have a lot of trouble talking about it. We always have had trouble talking about it.

JOHN: Can you tell me a bit about this trouble?

LARRY: It's when Elizabeth is critical and judgmental. I just don't know what to say.

JOHN: So, what do you find yourself doing when this happens?

LARRY: I'm alone with the problem. You know, not that Elizabeth doesn't contribute financially, but I feel like the problem is mine to solve.

JOHN: So you feel like you're alone, and it's yours to solve, your responsibility to solve?

LARRY: Yes.

JOHN: And when you find yourself feeling that way, does that get you to do certain things, do you find yourself behaving or thinking in certain ways?

LARRY: No, I don't notice anything. I don't think it helps. I feel uninclined to communicate with Elizabeth.

JOHN: It makes you feel uninclined to communicate with Elizabeth?

LARRY: I'd say it makes it harder.

JOHN: When it's harder, what do you notice yourself doing?

[I am asking effects questions in order to understand how one experience invites another which, in turn, invites another, and so on. My questions, however, are understood by Larry as questions about Elizabeth
and the situation between them.]

LARRY: It's just one more thing that I can't talk to her about, because I
feel like she avoids talking about it. She won't look at the realities
with me. I would like her to share it with me, to feel like she was
more of a partner.

JOHN: So you prefer to have the two of you in it together, but your
experience is that the two of you can't talk about it. So what does
that get you to do? Do you try to avoid talking about it, or what do
you do?

LARRY: I try to avoid talking about it; I avoid bringing it up. Or if I do, I
get no response.

JOHN: And when Elizabeth doesn't speak of it, what do you do?

LARRY: I just wait.

[I now understand how the experience of feeling alone and responsible
invites Larry to "avoid" and "wait." I am interested in how these experiences create other unwanted experiences or if they create unhelpful
ways of experiencing Elizabeth, the relationship, and Larry himself.]

JOHN: Does this encourage you to see the relationship in certain ways?

LARRY: Yes, that I'm alone.

JOHN: So feeling alone is a lot of what this does to you? And when
you're feeling alone, do you notice yourself thinking about or seeing
Elizabeth in certain ways?

LARRY: Yes, the way I see Elizabeth around money is something that she
just puts out of her mind.

JOHN: And how do you make sense of that? I mean, what do you imagine are the reasons that she would do that?

LARRY: She has a problem with numbers, and she comes from a background where she didn't deal with this. Someone would be responsible, but she's never had to deal with harsh realities.

JOHN: What gets you to think that she's wanting to put it out of her head?

LARRY: I think it's obvious most of the time. I should also say that it has been better lately. I used to distrust her, but she has been more responsible in the last few years.

[This is an example of a moment in which potential definitions of what is "true" reflect the invisible operation of power. Characterizations of women (as "responsible" or "irresponsible") by men reproduce in the moment power relationships that establish the man in a hierarchically superior position. Because we understand intimacy as a shared negotiation of meaning between persons (Weingarten, 1991), we try in one way or another to question or challenge such uses of power.]

JOHN: "More responsible"? Can you help me understand what you mean?

LARRY: The degree that she's had problems (with money) and the degree that she's been willing to deal with money have been greater than in the past. She's been making an effort to be more responsible.

JOHN: I'm not sure what you mean by "responsible."

LARRY: The way she's been handling money individually. She's tried to be more responsible about it.

JOHN: Let me restate this to I make sure I understand. In spite of this history, you notice Elizabeth dealing with money more and more in a way that you are comfortable with?

LARRY: Yes.

> Vicki: John, I want to ask you a bit more about what you're thinking here. I'm imagining that you might think it would help Larry understand that his ideas about money and Elizabeth don't have to do with settled certainties but more with what fits for him.
>
> John: I was thinking that I needed to stay close to Larry's experience without imposing my ideas on him about how men's culture operates (at the expense of Elizabeth and their relationship). To challenge Larry's statements directly could easily be interpreted as if I am making attributions about Larry as a person (e.g., "controlling," "condescending," etc.) rather than about the effects of men's culture in

which we all participate. I understood that Larry's view of responsibility—which reflects the dominant and accepted view most of us believe—might be having negative effects on Elizabeth, the relationship, and on Larry. Although I felt uncomfortable not exploring how this accepted view affected Elizabeth and the relationship, I was more interested in making visible (for all of us) the effects of Larry's experience on him—to "deconstruct" it, in the jargon of narrative therapy (i.e., to make the assumptions visible as reflections of male culture), and that might not be consistent with other values he might hold.

John: Okay. So let me restate my understanding to make sure I'm getting this. (*I summarize the conversation and then say:*) Am I getting it right?

LARRY: Well, Elizabeth has become more responsible, but we still can't talk about things at all. We have an inability to talk about money. That's no better.

JOHN: Does this create *distance*?

Vicki: Coming back to what Jeff and I were noticing above, here you seem to be continuing to work at what we call "constructing a problem." You called this problem distance with Elizabeth, and you are doing the same here. Are you are thinking about the problem as something "between" them, and would you comment on that?

John: I was wondering if the experience of distance reflected a shared experience of the problem. I'm not sure I think of a shared experience as "between" them in the sense of a behavioral pattern. But I am thinking of distance as the effect of a pattern produced by the reciprocal invitations we discussed above. This distance is a shared experience that then invites certain kinds of understanding in each of them that further promotes reciprocal invitations to interpret and behave in ways that promote distance. I know this sounds confusing, but I do believe this reflects how the "inside" of a problem works.

LARRY: Yes, our inability to talk about money creates distance between us.

JOHN: What happens when you try to talk about money, and it doesn't work?

LARRY: We've made only a few real attempts to talk about it. I've actually been fairly happy when we have talked about it. Most recently, about two months ago we sat down and talked about a budget and communicated with each other about it, and it was better. And then we just stopped talking about it again.

[Talk continues about communication about money working better.]

> *Vicki:* Will you say why you followed with how things worked better, rather than more about the problem?
>
> *John:* As you know and have asked this question to illustrate, this is an initial attempt to explore experiences that exist outside the effects of problems, or at least to notice them as something we might want to come back to at some later point. My interest in these experiences is determined by the members of the couple. When they notice how these experiences might illuminate things they haven't ever thought about, I am more likely to pursue them. When there is a sense that they want to talk more about their experience of the problem, then it is best to leave these and follow their lead in further exploring their experience of the problem.

JOHN: *(to Larry)* When it was working better what were you noticing?

LARRY: Elizabeth was opening up about it and willing to talk.

JOHN: *(to Elizabeth)* Was that your experience also?

ELIZABETH: Yes.

JOHN: Wow, that takes a lot of courage to open up to something like that. My own experience is that to open up about something you don't feel so good about is to open yourself up for criticism, and I think that's not easy.

ELIZABETH: Yes, I think it did, and Larry was good about it. He was helpful and more understanding. At the same time, I wish he would open up more so we could both talk about it. I don't think he really says much about how he's dealing or not dealing with it, and I can't really say anything.

JOHN: What did you notice about Larry when it (i.e., the communication) was working?

ELIZABETH: He was paying attention. I see Larry checking out when things are difficult. He just withdraws.

JOHN: And do you see it this way, Larry?

LARRY: Well, it is true that I withdraw when I feel frustrated and when things are difficult.

JOHN: And is this money situation one of the things that makes you feel this way?

LARRY: Yes.

JOHN: Okay, let me summarize my understanding again to make sure I've got it right. Certain things are difficult to talk about that create trouble between the two of you, money being the most difficult. And the way it works is that the trouble about this creates distance; that this distance gets Larry to withdraw rather than bring things up, to kind of "check out," as Elizabeth says. And the distance puts Elizabeth in the position of not being able to bring things up, of putting the relationship on the "back burner" out of concern, that if she does bring it up, she will say the wrong thing. In spite of the ways this trouble has created distance, there have been some periods when the two of you have found ways to talk. Elizabeth, in spite of this, has found a way over the past few years to open up about how dealing with money is difficult. And Elizabeth, you noticed that Larry is more present at these times, right? (*She nods affirmatively.*) I think it is time to bring in the reflecting team and see what they have to say. Is that all right?

[I am summarizing here to make certain I am understanding the effects of the problem and the instances in which Larry and Elizabeth have found ways to avoid it. My use of language also reflects my understanding of problems. I am using externalizing descriptions here not as a technique, but because I understand problems to affect people in these ways.]

LARRY: Yes.

ELIZABETH: Yes.

We want to make certain we are understanding each person's experiences in the way that the member of the couple who is explaining it does. To do this, we constantly and explicitly check out our understanding by voicing our thinking and asking if it is accurate. It is also useful to look for opportunities to notice the effects of gender constructions on the identities of each partner. Problems can be thought of as "colonizing" culturally dominant ways of being a person. So we all know that men must be "strong," even when problems are making them feel inadequate and requiring that they pretend this is not the case. Similarly, the culture requires over-responsibility in women, so that when problems take over, they make women feel badly for not being able to do the (impossible) job of making everyone feel okay. As we mentioned above, dominant cultural notions of problems have "individualizing" effects: They convince people that these experiences reflect something negative about them as opposed to being cultural "truths." An important opportunity to challenge problems—to separate the person from the problem—occurs when the role of cultural beliefs in problems is made visible. This occurred for Larry and Elizabeth in response to a comment from Jeff as a member of the reflecting team.

JEFF: [Reflecting team comment:] I was interested myself in this whole issue of men feeling responsible for finances. I know in my house, we have fairly equal incomes and equal division of responsibilities, but when push comes to shove, I worry about the money, and my partner worries about the kids and managing the house. I know the effect on me if finances go badly would be to recruit me into a lot of feelings of personal inadequacy, so I was wondering how Larry was able to put that aside enough, and, instead of "checking out," how he was able to "check in" the way that Elizabeth mentioned, despite—at least as I am imagining it—having to fight *feelings of inadequacy*? I also wondered if Elizabeth understood that this might be some of the issue for Larry. If she did understand that, what difference that would make?

Later, when I (John) return to the room with Larry and Elizabeth, the following ensues.

JOHN: Were there particular things they mentioned that you found yourself thinking about?

LARRY: The thing about the *feelings of inadequacy*. I do wonder if Elizabeth understands that's part of the pressure I feel.

JOHN: When you find yourself feeling alone, does that make it hard to make those feelings visible to Elizabeth, or do you find a way to do that?

LARRY: Yes, it's hard to do that.

JOHN: Have there been times that you have made those feelings visible to Elizabeth?

LARRY: I don't think so.

JOHN: Do you have any ideas about how that might be helpful if Elizabeth did understand?

LARRY: I haven't really imagined her ever understanding.

JOHN: But these are the feelings that operate on you. Would you be surprised to learn that I don't know a man, including myself, that these feelings do not operate on?

[The problem is restraining Larry from noticing how *feelings of inadequacy* affect him and get him to see Elizabeth in a way that supports the problem. Bringing in my experience is intended to create greater separation between Larry and the problem.]

LARRY: Uh, no, it doesn't.

JOHN: So, that's your experience also?

LARRY: Yes.

JOHN: And when you remember that most men have these kinds of feelings, does that make a difference in how you feel about yourself?

LARRY: Well, when I remember that it makes me feel better, but that doesn't help me out with Elizabeth.

JOHN: So let me make sure I am understanding this correctly. The financial situation makes *feelings of inadequacy* appear, and these make you feel awkward and stop you from explaining what you're thinking and feeling to Elizabeth.

LARRY: Right. It's awkward.

JOHN: And is it the awkwardness that stops you from expressing this to Elizabeth?

LARRY: Yes, I guess it is.

JOHN: So these *feelings of inadequacy* that we men carry around with ourselves have stopped you from explaining this to Elizabeth?

LARRY: Yes, I guess they have.

JOHN: And they tell you to withdraw instead?

LARRY: Well, I don't know if they tell me to, but I do withdraw when I'm feeling these ways.

JOHN: And these *feelings of inadequacy* convince you that she is not going to understand you?

LARRY: Yes.

JOHN: (*to Elizabeth*) Was there anything said that you found yourself interested in?

ELIZABETH: Yeah. It's the thing that Jeff said, and I guess you are also saying it. I've never understood that's how Larry feels. I guess it's kind of obvious, and if I thought about it, I've always known that it was going on. But I've never heard Larry acknowledge it.

JOHN: How is it helpful for you to know about that?

ELIZABETH: Well, it changes what I think is going on with him. I mean, I know what he's going through is really hard, but it seems like hearing this makes me feel like we're more in it together. But I don't know what to say when I know he's feeling this way. If I try to say something supportive, he takes it that I'm criticizing him and withdraws.

JOHN: Yeah, we men are like that. I know that when my wife tells me something that makes me uncomfortable, the first thing I feel is criticized. I have to fight that, I'm guessing the same way Larry fights to "check in" when he does. (*to Larry*) Is that right, do you have to fight those feelings to stay present?

LARRY: Yes, I do and sometimes I'm successful, and sometimes the criticism feels like too much.

JOHN: I wonder if the *feelings of inadequacy* use Elizabeth's fears or emotional upsets as "evidence" that they're the "truth" about you. I know it can work this way—although I'd like to say it doesn't— when my wife is upset about things.

LARRY: Yes, they certainly do (*laughing*).

Vicki: Jeff, at first I had a concern about your reflecting team response in that it seemed to reproduce the need for women to "understand" men, as John talks about throughout this chapter. I see that you were talking first about Larry's "checking-in" instead of "checking-out," but I would want him to take responsibility for that, primarily. Elizabeth's understanding is, of course, helpful, but I think it might be a mistake to make Larry's "checking-in" dependent on that. I don't think that's what you meant, but my concern is that the question might have that effect. I see, from Larry's reaction, that what you said was helpful to him, and in the second session, Elizabeth comments on how these ideas were helpful to her, but you couldn't have known that at the time.

Jeff: My intention was *not* to link the two. I was wondering if Larry did take the responsibility to "check in" and make his experience more visible to Elizabeth, what effect would it have for her to know that *feelings of inadequacy* were affecting his response.

Vicki: Also John, I would like you to comment on your reason for the attention to Larry's experience, letting him know (and Elizabeth know) that you can appreciate his experience, as yours is similar. I wonder how it is for Elizabeth to have a male therapist and a male colleague on the reflecting team appreciate her husband's experience without a concomitant appreciation of her experience. Might this make it even more "necessary" for her to "understand" her husband and, thus, again replicate the cultural imperative for women? I do know from the next session that these comments had good effects, but since we don't know that beforehand, I am concerned about her continuing to feel "responsible."

John: It was my thinking that locating these *feelings of inadequacy* in the larger culture and thus challenging the "truth" of them would allow Elizabeth to feel less responsible. She would feel less pressured to make Larry feel okay about things that were not really true about him anyway. When these feelings that all men struggle with are understood as inevitable effects of how we are taught to measure ourselves, they lose much of their power for both the man and woman.

The session ends shortly, and we set a meeting time in 2 weeks. Unfortunately, holidays and a flu epidemic interfere, and we do not meet again for 6 weeks.

Jeff: John, a good piece of the work with this couple involved helping the man notice aspects of his own experience that are shaped by cultural specifications and then making this visible to his wife.

John: My experience as a man is that we are led to believe that we are supposed to be competent, effective, and always loved by the people that are important to us. I think our performance of masculinity prevents us from acknowledging experiences that do not fit these specifications. In other words, when we have effects we do not intend, it is difficult to acknowledge them, because the effect on us is to "feel inadequate." As men we have been recruited into notions of "truth" and "objectivity," into "rightness" as a thing we might have, and this makes it easier to insist that what we intend is how others should feel. As Hare-Mustin and Marecek (1994) have explained, we men are usually baffled when women express that these particular ways of "doing" masculinity, so to speak, disqualify women and ignore their experience. We do not tend to notice how our male ways of making sense get us to do this. So, the embedded nature of power within male–female relationships interferes with interactions that create the sense of shared experience and understanding we experience as "intimacy" (Weingarten, 1991). Less noticed, but also important, is how the embeddedness of power within men's ways of being requires us to ignore how we make sense of experiences that do not fit how we are supposed to be as men.

Vicki: Can you say more about some of the effects for women of this?

John: The particular ways power is embedded within and shapes relationship patterns profoundly influence how people experience and define problems. When one person, most often the man in heterosexual couples, knowingly, or more often unknowingly, possesses greater influence over the definition of "truth" (i.e., what is thought to be more "objective" or "rational"), then the other person's "truth," the woman's, is likely to remain invisible or be viewed as less worthy of consideration. This is one of the ways power operates "through" meaning between men and women in their relationships.

Miller (1976) made this point years ago about women's psychology—it tends to be invisible to men, whereas women, who are often in a less powerful position relative to men, are required to understand the experience of men. And when women's experience *is* noticed by men, we may experience it as a strange and foreign culture that academic anthropologists study, but it is a subject that we may or may not think about. My understanding is that for women who notice, it is like the experience of any group of persons who are less privileged, they swim inside it all the time. It is the air that surrounds them.

When the cultural specifications of masculinity and femininity support a relationship in which the woman's experience is invisible to the man (and the woman knows this), there is often anger, distance, and a sense that he is unable or unwilling to understand. In other instances, in which neither of them notice that the woman's experience is invisible—her experience and understanding are viewed by both of them as subordinate and less valid than his—then one is more likely to witness individual expressions of distress that many people think of as "symptoms" of individual psychological problems, such as depression and anxiety.

Vicki: Just a comment here, John. One of the most useful ways of thinking about depression—both for me and also for my clients—is to consider it as an effect of some experience of oppression. I think this thinking picks up an appreciation of the effects of power differentials in people's lives quite well.

Phase 3: Finding and Exploring Preferred Experiences of Self and Relationship Separate from the Influence of the Problem

In the course of exploring the effects of problems, narrative therapists inevitably notice subjective experiences and intentions or behaviors and events, in the present or past, in which the problem has not had the effects one might predict. This again is sometimes strange and foreign (and, hence, invisible) to therapists who have been skillfully trained to notice problems and "pathology." This invisibility also occurs when problems have been successful in making the therapist feel as hopeless as the members of the couple. However, one of the joys of postmodern reality is that experiences always exist outside the problem-saturated descriptions of us. Problems may not allow us to make sense of these other experiences without help from persons who are outside their influence, but these experiences are always there in the present, past, and usually both. As the therapist explores the effects of problems, she or he makes a list (mental or real) of potential experiences of this kind.

With Larry and Elizabeth, there were a number of moments that might be useful for future meetings. There was Larry's personal preference that they be partners in decision making. There was Larry's experience that *feelings of inadequacy* were not the "truth" about him. There was their shared understanding that there had been periods in which they felt like partners in dealing with money. There was Elizabeth's willingness to open up in the face of Larry's and her own feelings about the ways she managed money. There was acknowledgment that Elizabeth sometimes experienced Larry as "checking in" rather than "checking out." There was Elizabeth's internal resistance to finding herself blaming Larry for things. There were Elizabeth's empathic reactions to the *feelings of inadequacy* that were influencing Larry as a man. And there was Larry's witnessing of Elizabeth's empathic reaction toward him and these feelings.

Phase 4: Separating from the Influence of Gender Practices in Favor of Preferred Re-Remembered Experiences of Self and Relationship

This first meeting also opened a bit of space between Larry's experience of his identity as "inadequate" in favor of the idea that as a man, *feelings of inadequacy* were inevitable in the face of the economic pressures he faced. As it turned out, this "externalization" of the personal "truth" about him and noticing of his willingness to "check in" the relationship were the first steps toward Larry reconnecting with preferred experiences of himself and preferred ways of being in the relationship. Similarly, Elizabeth's connection to her willingness to open up and speak her mind reminded her of a preferred experience of herself that was to become an important part of the work. This could not be known in the first meeting, only guessed at as a possibility based on the understanding of how people tend to make preferred experiences of self more a part of their relationship when they notice the constructive effects of doing so in the present and in the past. When they resurrect or sometimes construct for the first time preferred narrative histories of themselves and their relationship rather than the identities and the histories promoted by problems, they come to feel more like themselves and more like the person they've wanted to be.

In this first meeting, the separation of the problem (*feelings of inadequacy*) from Larry's identity was only beginning. However, the conversation with Larry exemplifies how "externalizing" may take a variety of forms and focuses and may include the separation of the problem from the identities of each member of the couple, from each person's view of the relationship, and/or from each person's view of the other. With some couples and with some problems, there already exists enough separation of the problem from preferred ways of experiencing self, each other, and the relationship. In these instances, the work to "reauthor" proceeds concurrently with the construction of the problem.

> *Vicki:* John and Jeff, I'm wondering if anyone is noticing here that much of the interview time is spent with Larry and is focused on his experience and how the problem affects him, particularly looking at what was co-constructed as *feelings of inadequacy.* I believe that this is appropriate, given what I find most helpful in work with couples, which is to help the male member of the couple notice the effects of power in the relationship. However, I also suspect that therapists from other ways of thinking might question this practice. Could you comment on this?

> *John:* It is true that there is much more focus on Larry and not much interaction is encouraged between (members of) the couple. The reasons for this are first for Elizabeth to be in a reflexive position so that she can think about what is occurring but not have to initially respond. This lessens the chance of Larry feeling attacked while it also encourages him to explore how his experience of the problem affects what he thinks, feels, and does. Secondly, it allows me to engage Larry, as I think you imply, in ways that invite him to become more aware of and willing to counter, when appropriate, the effects that his participation in men's culture have on him, Elizabeth, and their relationship.

> *Jeff:* Because men are put in a position of greater power by the culture (i.e., they experience greater entitlement and are given by both men and women greater privilege and authority), the effects of their responses are more pronounced. For example, their often-used withdrawal response can shut off the interactional process completely. Once they begin to move, to leave certain habits behind, there can be a more mutual conversation by the couple, one that allows them to leave problems behind together.

Phase 5: Exploring the Performance of Preferred Identity and Relationships in the Past, Present, and Future by Co-Constructing a Coherent Narrative Truth about Them

A few minutes into the second meeting . . .

JOHN: So I was thinking about our meeting and wondering if there was anything that stayed with you or that might have been helpful or unhelpful in dealing with the trouble and the distance it puts between the two of you?

LARRY: Nothing specific that I can remember.

ELIZABETH: I can think of some things. I noticed a big difference . . .

LARRY: Well, I noticed the difference, but as far as what we talked about, I can't think of anything in particular that explained the difference.

ELIZABETH: For me, I felt like some things did help that happened here. It helped me to understand Larry better when he was talking and when you were talking. When you guys were talking, it made me understand things that Larry's been trying to say but that he's been having a hard time saying. So when you guys were talking, it helped me to understand. Hearing Larry talk and hearing you talk together about these things helped me a lot. Sometimes I think I know where he's coming from, and that's not always where he is coming from. I appreciate that he's willing to be here. It's not easy for Larry to be here. I realize that I'm lucky in that way, that a lot of women have to give the man an ultimatum, and I don't have to do that with Larry.

JOHN: And the conversation that you are remembering, that was helpful, was . . . ?

ELIZABETH: The talk about shutting down, walking away, and feeling inadequate. That helped me to remember that it's not me doing that to him. Sometimes I feel like I'm the one making him feel inadequate or that he's shutting down, because I've said something rather than that's just something he does that I'm not responsible for. That was really helpful for me.

> *Vicki:* I would not have predicted Elizabeth's response here, nor how helpful it was for her to separate from an experience of *responsibility* for Larry, once she could appreciate his *feelings of inadequacy*. The way I would make sense of it, and I wonder if this is also how you, John and Jeff, think about it, is that once she could locate Larry's experience in the realm of how the culture produces for men *inadequacy feelings* around certain concerns, like money and not being able to talk about it, she could see that it was not about her being somehow deficient or about him being somehow deficient. She could then see that a *responsibility* for his feelings or for the lack of communication was unnecessary, and was, in fact, also a culturally produced phenomenon for women that she did not have to respond to.

> *Jeff:* That's my theory as well. When one situates the problem in the culture, the effect is often to shift blame away from the person, her or

his partner, and the relationship. I think it was important, however, to explicitly address the *responsibility* issue for Elizabeth as a similar social construction.

John: I agree completely with what you both are saying. To raise the *responsibility* issue as a similar social construction for Elizabeth, I think, is especially and equally important to helping Larry separate a bit from *feelings of inadequacy.*

JOHN: So that's been helpful for making you less responsible for things that we men all struggle with?

ELIZABETH: (*Laughs.*) Yeah, and that helps give me a much better perspective.

JOHN: Was that helpful for the way you were feeling or thinking about yourself?

ELIZABETH: Yes, I guess it was. I have been feeling better about myself.

JOHN: If my colleague Vicki Dickerson were here, I think she might raise the question at this moment about these *feelings of responsibility* that you had for Larry's experience and the ways these feelings made you feel about yourself. I have the idea that she might be asking whether you thought these are some of the things that women are required to feel that don't always help them out. Vicki is quite sensitive to the ways the culture requires women to feel about themselves and what it makes you feel you are supposed to do for us men. I am wondering whether you think you are alone in feeling responsible for what is going on with Larry emotionally, or do you think this might be a bit like the *feelings of inadequacy* all we men are required to feel?

ELIZABETH: No, I guess it isn't me, but I sure feel it a lot.

JOHN: What would you call this experience that women are made to feel?

ELIZABETH: It's that I should be giving more. I'm the one who should be overseeing feelings. So when he's feeling badly, I feel responsible, as if I did it to him.

JOHN: I know that Vicki sometimes views this as a kind of *over-responsibility* that is unfair and unhelpful. Is that like your experience?

ELIZABETH: Yes.

Vicki: I appreciate being brought into the room here through your comment, John. I find that it is helpful for men to appreciate that other men share their experience. Men can then perhaps more easily invite other men toward accountability for their actions. So likewise, I think it is helpful for women to have their experience appreciated by other women. When I am working with men, I often call upon my knowledge of men's experience through my association with my male colleagues, such as both you, John, and Jeff.

John: Yes, and I wanted to locate these experiences of feeling emotionally responsible and not being able to say the "right" thing within an understanding of the "cultural" as opposed to something about Elizabeth as a person (i.e., her individual psychology) or as a reflection of their relationship. So we talked about what other women clients, and women on the reflecting team, said about feeling emotionally responsible (e.g., "I have to remind myself that it's not true") and finding the "right" thing to say (e.g., "it's impossible"). Then we went back to her statement that she had been feeling better about herself to explore its significance.

Phase 6: Reauthoring Practices—
Relating Preferred Experiences
to Preferred Narratives

From here the work moves into what we call "reauthoring." To do this we explore moments in the couple's relationship and in their personal histories in which preferred experiences of "presence" (a term Larry liked better than "checking-in") and being a "partner" (for Elizabeth) occur. If these experiences had not been meaningful, then it would have been necessary to extend the conversation about the effects of men's *feelings of inadequacy* and women's sense of *overresponsibility*. But these moments reconnected each of them to their shared history as a couple. It helped them to "re-remember" (White, 1996) things that were important about themselves, each other, and the relationship.

JOHN: So (*turning to Larry*) *feelings of inadequacy* and (*turning to Elizabeth*) *overresponsibility* have been interfering in your relationship. But you [Elizabeth] said sometimes you've been feeling that it's not you?

ELIZABETH: Yes, the two times I thought about it I didn't feel defensive . . . and I didn't feel angry. And things have been better in general.

JOHN: During these two times, you were feeling better about yourself?

ELIZABETH: Yes, I could understand that Larry was struggling and let him know I understood [it was hard]. So we've been communicating better.

JOHN: Did this cause problems for the distance?

[This is intended to enhance the *shared experience* of success against the problem.]

ELIZABETH: (*laughing*) Yes, you could say that.

LARRY: (*also laughing*) I would agree.

JOHN: (*to Elizabeth*) In the moments when you felt better about your-self—can you tell me a bit more about that?

[I am exploring Elizabeth's experiences in order to understand how they may reflect important histories and aspects of their identities.]

ELIZABETH: Well, maybe because I wasn't defensive, he was more like he used to be, really listening to me.

JOHN: And how did that affect you.?

ELIZABETH: Well, it was *really* great (*smiling*). That's what gave *distance* the trouble.

JOHN: Was that like the earlier times in the relationship that we talked about a bit in the last meeting, the time before kids?

ELIZABETH: Yes, it was.

JOHN: Remembering back then, did you feel less over-responsible then and more like a partner—if that makes sense?

ELIZABETH: Yes, it makes sense, but I'm not sure.

JOHN: I'm asking about this because I'm wondering where this sense of yourself as a "partner" comes from. I'd like to explain why I'm wondering about it, if it's okay. It has been my experience that these kinds of habits, these ways of being, don't come out of nothing. So I'm guessing this way of being a partner has been with you for a while.

ELIZABETH: Well, I think it's a way I've always wanted us to be in the marriage.

JOHN: Thinking back to other times in your life, who would be least surprised that this sense of partnership is important to you and that you have been making it a part of your marriage?

[This is a question intended to bring forth persons in one's history who were witnesses to a preferred story. This is the basis for a future development of a "membered" community.]

ELIZABETH: That's easy. My mom. She wouldn't be surprised. She talked a lot about being a partner with my dad. How important it was.

JOHN: Is she still alive?

ELIZABETH: No, she died 5 years ago.

Elizabeth went on to remember incidents in which she had witnessed her parents as "partners." This led to the recollections of how she and Larry had gotten together. Our conversation ended with her reconnection to the ways Larry had played the key role of a partner—in the child rearing, in projects they had done together on the house, in their shared interests. As Elizabeth mentioned these, she commented on the times she experienced respect and the sense of shared decision making. Larry seemed moved as he listened to this. I then turned to Larry to explore his steps against *feelings of inadequacy* and its friend *distance*.

JOHN: So you noticed a difference between the two of you also? What was your experience?

LARRY: Things have been better, and I've been feeling better, too.

JOHN: When you were aware of that, what was going on?

LARRY: Elizabeth has been different, and I thought about what you and Jeff said, that the *feelings of inadequacy* are there for everybody. It's not true [that I'm inadequate]. I've always known that's true, but I've never really thought about it in terms of feeling badly about myself.

JOHN: And that's helped give *distance* a run for it?

LARRY: (*again laughing*) Sometimes.

JOHN: Are you surprised that Elizabeth is seeing you differently at these times?

LARRY: Not really. I think I have been different.

JOHN: It makes for you being different in the relationship. Is this something that used to be much more a part of the relationship?

[Here I begin to bring the history of the preferred developments into the room. Preferred developments always have a history, albeit often trivialized or ignored in the face of the effects of the problem.]

LARRY: Yes, things used to be like this a lot more.

JOHN: If you think back to that time, was that before the kids?

LARRY: Yes.

JOHN: Right after you were married?

LARRY: Yes.

JOHN: If back then, you could have looked into the future and seen the last few weeks, would either you or Elizabeth been surprised that the two of you have been giving distance a run for it?

[This question invites Larry to connect his experience of himself in the past with his recent experience. Questions of this kind help to put a person in touch with how the present reflects something of her or his identity over time.]

LARRY: No, not at all.

JOHN: So it speaks to something that was true of you back then?

LARRY: Yes. I've always felt, or I used to feel, that we wanted to understand each other. She made the effort to understand me, and I think I was good at being present for her.

ELIZABETH: That's definitely true. It was one of the things that attracted me to Larry. I felt respected, and we were real partners.

Reauthoring processes reconnect persons to historical moments in order to place preferred experiences ("presence" and being a "partner") into a meaningful (alternative) story about themselves, each other, and the relationship. The experience of being "inside" these remembered moments and events is the experience of being inside the story of oneself, and the "thickening" of these alternative stories is the act of making sense of (and "reauthoring") one's identity and the "identity" of the relationship. For Larry and Elizabeth, these experiences reconnected them to the early stages of their relationship.

JOHN: (*to Larry*) This respect and partnership [that Elizabeth just mentioned], is that something you remember as well?

LARRY: Yes, I do. It's always been there to some extent—except when things are bad.

JOHN: I guess I'm wondering how to understand where this comes from. Does it reflect shared values of some kind?

[I ask this because experiences of self and relationship that are preferred often reflect very personal and closely held values. Linking preferred experiences to values helps to links these to each person's experience of identity.]

LARRY: I can't say I've ever thought about it, but I suppose it's true.

Sometimes the shared relief of separating from problematic patterns, like *distance,* enable people to reconnect spontaneously to these preferred histories. More often, questions that connect the present to the past and to the future are important. Over time and with continued pursuit of these experiences, the past, present, and (imagined) future, preferred alternatives can be experienced more of the time as the dominant frame in which people view themselves and the relationship. The details of the ways these histories are explored, the kinds of questions asked and the focuses pursued, are outlined in detail elsewhere (cf. Freedman & Combs, 1996; White, 1993b, 1995; Zimmerman & Dickerson, 1996).

This reauthoring process is helped also by extending the influence of the preferred stories of each other and the relationship. This includes the use of reflecting teams (Freedman & Combs, 1996; White, 1995; Zimmerman & Dickerson, 1996) and "communities of concern" (Madigan, 1997; Madigan & Epston, 1995). Each of these is intended to enlarge the community of those who recognize the preferred developments in the relationship. In the instance of Larry and Elizabeth, this involved conversations with their two children about the changes they were noticing in their parents and in the relationship. One incident in particular occurred when their adolescent daughter made a disparaging comment about her father. According to Elizabeth's account, Larry stood his ground and yet surprised his daughter. He calmly sat down and explained to her what he had been learning about himself and the ways his withdrawal had previously placed her mother in a difficult position. He explained that they were working on it together and that it was now different between them. Elizabeth heard the interchange and spoke up for Larry by agreeing that things were changing. Evidently, this stunned their adolescent daughter, who had been used to tension between her parents and silence from her dad. She later told her mom she could see what they were talking about.

Like every couple fighting problems, Larry and Elizabeth could be drawn temporarily back into the influence of (for Larry) *feelings of inadequacy* and (for Elizabeth) *feelings of helplessness* and *over-responsibility.* In any case it is important to acknowledge the pain and difficulties that these problems created for them and then to focus on areas in which they had extended the breadth of the preferred ways of relating to each other.

RELEVANT LITERATURE

For those interested in learning more about narrative therapy, we offer the following suggestions. Narrative couple therapy reflects ideas from cultural anthropology, poststructural philosophy, and literary criticism that White and Epston (1990; Epston, 1993; Epston & White, 1992; White, 1991, 1993a, 1993b, 1995) introduced into family therapy. Paré (1996) provides a useful map that discusses the importance of these ideas for narrative therapy, locates how narrative therapy is related to and distinct from other family therapy approaches, and discusses how these distinctions reflect the evolution and current status of family therapy ideas as a whole. Zimmerman and Dickerson's (1994) paper on the narrative metaphor is useful for understanding how some of the ideas that characterize narrative thinking evolved out of other family therapy ideas and illustrates the use of the narrative metaphor in their thinking and practices.

For comprehensive descriptions of narrative therapy as a whole, two new books are available. Zimmerman and Dickerson (1996), in *If Problems Talked: Narrative Therapy in Action,* write in a way to bring the reader closer to the *experience* of narrative therapy. The book includes detailed descriptions of the process of therapy. One chapter is devoted specifically to working with couples. Freedman and Combs (1996), in *Narrative Therapy: The Social Construction of Preferred Reality,* include an excellent summary of the thinking that organizes the work, outline the process of therapy in detail, and provide detailed examples of therapeutic conversations.

Of course, the writings of White and Epston, as cited above, describe numerous aspects of the thinking and work. White's (1993a) description of how the concept of "deconstruction" is translated into clinical work is especially helpful for understanding the thinking that organizes the interviewing of couples about problems in a respectful and helpful way.

Weingarten's (1991, 1992) discussions of the implications of social constructionist thinking describe completely different views of persons and relationships reflected by practices of narrative therapy. Weingarten (1991) distinguishes social constructionist from more commonly held beliefs about the "self," relationships, and intimacy and discusses the implications of adhering to one as opposed to the other set of ideas. In a follow-up article, Weingarten (1992) describes how this social constructionist understanding of persons, relationships, and intimacy translates into the process of therapy.

There are also a number of papers that describe the process of narrative work with couples. Epston (1993) outlines a procedure for interviewing couples that helps them escape the influences of problems and reestablish preferred views of each other and preferred ways of relating to each other. Neal (1998) describes the process of "externalizing" through a focus on engaging men into the process of separating themselves from cultural notions about masculinity that promote and support the operation of problems. Two papers by Zimmerman and Dickerson (1993a, 1993b) outline how, from a narrative perspective, problems are understood to affect couples and describe ways to intervene in these effects. The chapter on couples in Zimmerman and Dickerson (1996) also provides a detailed description of the process of therapy and includes a thorough discussion of the ideas that influence the thinking of the therapist and how this relates to the kinds of questions asked and not asked.

CONCLUSION

John: In ending this chapter, I am thinking we might each emphasize what we hope readers take with them. For me, there are two things. First, in working with couples, it is important to pursue each person's personal experience to make sense of how the cultural operates within their understanding of themselves and of their relationship. Proceeding in this way helps address the influence of gender and power in relationships with respect for women *and* men. Second, by emphasizing the work with a man in this chapter, I hoped to show how therapists can challenge the effects of masculinity without demeaning the character or intentions of men. Thinking and speaking of problems as distinct from and operating upon persons facilitate this experience with clients. If we had more space, I would have wanted to emphasize the importance of the narrative metaphor for making sense of experience. But this has been done in other places (e.g., White & Epston, 1990). What about for the two of you?

Vicki: I am interested in people noticing how their work may or may not replicate the cultural requirements of men and women, and hopefully see from this chapter some ways to challenge those requirements. It is important to me, as a therapist, to respect the experiences of both members of a couple, really wanting to help people experience themselves in their more preferred ways.

Jeff: For me, what I would want to emphasize is just how different this work is from work that evaluates (based on past or personality), pathologizes, or instructs. And how exciting it is when couples reclaim their relationship in a way that reflects their preferences and intentions.

NOTES

1. In focusing on gender and power, we are not suggesting that gender is always the distinction that matters with couples. It is our experience that, when working with heterosexual and same-sex couples, it is useful to assume that gender involved in one way or another. However, this is not always the case,

and sometimes the couple does not experience the operation of power that supports problems as linked to gender. In any case, the operation of power within problems is assumed by the therapist who finds the domain of experience (i.e., by asking questions and showing interest in the client's experience) in which this occurs rather than imposing his or her ideas about what "really" is.

2. Vicki attended later interviews. The rationale for this has to do with the structure of the training program—in which there are always ytwo of us teaching—rather than with the organization of the therapy.

REFERENCES

Epston, D. (1993). Internalizing discourses versus externalizing discourses. In S. Gilligan & R. Price (Eds.), *Therapeutic conversations* (pp. 161–177). New York: Norton.

Epston, D., & White, M. (1992). *Experience, contradiction, narrative, and imagination: Selected papers of David Epston and Michael White, 1989–1991.* Adelaide, South Australia: Dulwich Centre Publications.

Freedman, J., & Combs, G. (1996). *Narrative therapy: The social construction of preferred realities.* New York: Norton.

Gilligan, C. (1990). Joining the resistance: Psychology, politics, girls, and women. *Michigan Quarterly Review, 29,* 501–536.

Hare-Mustin, R., & Marecek, J. (1994). Feminism and postmodernism: Dilemmas and points of resistance. *Dulwich Centre Newsletter, 4,* 13–19.

Janowsky, Z. M., Dickerson, V. C., & Zimmerman, J. L. (1995). Through Susan's eyes: Reflections on a reflecting team experience. In S. Friedman (Ed.), *The reflecting team in action: Collaborative practice in family therapy* (pp. 167–183). New York: Guilford Press.

Madigan, S. (1997). Re-considering memory: Re-remembering lost identities back toward re-membered selves. In C. Smith & D. Nylund (Eds.), *Narrative therapies with children and adolescents* (pp. 338–355). New York: Guilford Press.

Madigan, S., & Epston, D. (1995). From "spy-chiatric gaze" to communities of concern: From professional monologue to dialogue. In S. Friedman (Ed.), *The reflecting team in action: Collaborative practice in family theray* (pp. 257–276). New York: Guilford Press.

Miller, J. (1976). *Toward a new psychology of women.* Boston: Beacon Press.

Neal, J. H. (1996). Narrative therapy training and supervision. *Journal of Systemic Therapies, 15,* 63–78.

Neal, J. H. (1998). Narrative ideas and practices in couples therapy: Separating men from the unhelpful performance of masculinity.[Online]. Available on the World Wide Web, http://www.jhneal.com/prof/nctm.pdf. (Available for reading or downloading as pdf file).

Paré, D. A. (1996). Culture and meaning: Expanding the metaphorical repertoire of family therapy. *Family Process, 34,* 1–20.

Singh, A. (1996). *Narrative reflecting teams: Clients' experiences.* Unpublished doctoral dissertation. California School of Professional Psychology, Alameda, CA.

Weingarten, K. (1991). The discourses of intimacy: Adding a social constructionist and feminist view. *Family Process, 30,* 285–305.

Weingarten, K. (1992). A consideration of intimate and non-intimate interactions in therapy. *Family Process, 31,* 45–59.

White, M. (1993a). Deconstruction and therapy. In S. Gilligan & R. Price (Eds.), *Therapeutic conversations* (pp. 22–61). New York: Norton.

White, M. (1993b). Commentary: The histories of the present. In S. Gilligan & R. Price (Eds.), *Therapeutic conversations* (pp. 121–135). New York: Norton.

White, M. (1995). *Re-authoring lives: Interviews and essays.* Adelaide, South Australia: Dulwich Centre Publications.

White, M. (1996, October). *Narrative therapy renewed.* Presentation at Bay Area Family Therapy Training Associates, Cupertino, CA.

White, M., &. Epston., D. (1990). *Narrative means to therapeutic ends.* New York: Norton.

Zimmerman, J. L., & Dickerson, V. C. (1993a). Bringing forth the restraining influence of pattern and relationship discourse in couple's therapy. In S. Gilligan & R. Price (Eds.), *Therapeutic conversations* (pp. 197–214). New York: Norton.

Zimmerman, J. L., & Dickerson, V. C. (1993b). Separating couples from restraining patterns and the relationship discourse that supports them. *Journal of Marital and Family Therapy, 19,* 403–413.

Zimmerman, J. L., & Dickerson, V. C. (1994). Using a narrative metaphor: Implications for theory and clinical practice. *Family Process, 33,* 233–246.

Zimmerman, J. L., & Dickerson, V. C. (1996). *If problems talked: Narrative therapy in action.* New York: Guilford Press.

15

◄O►

SHORT-TERM
COUPLE THERAPY

The Present and the Future

JAMES M. DONOVAN

Powerfully built, 36-year-old Frank and his slender, vivacious 34-year-old wife, Janine, enter the office and offer their recurring conflict, their "fight," to you the therapist. Janine speaks first, animated and immediately accusatory. Frank, while polite and a good earner, offers her and the children no emotional involvement. He doesn't assume any responsibility for child care, or share his feelings with her, or empathize with her daily anxiety over their two children, a 5-year-old daughter and 7-year-old son. Their overtly peaceful family seems an emotional wasteland to her. Janine's social work experience may have attuned her to emotional issues, but it has also increased her fears that off-kilter family life can irremediably damage a child's self-esteem. As the parentified oldest daughter of an alcoholic father, Janine knows all about overfunctioning. She feels convinced that her passive husband pushes her toward the kind of behavior that was so damaging to her growing up: compulsive caretaking, expressing the feelings for everyone in the family, recognizing her own needs but putting them last.

Frank, a successful attorney, prizes independence and achievement above all. He's bewildered by the ferocity of Janine's complaints, and he can't find sympathy in himself for her "dependent," "self-doubting obsessions." If he allowed himself such feelings at his office, he would be lost. He's angry that she freely gives reign to her fears and to her seemingly endless criticisms of him. He's begun to withdraw more and more into his study. When Janine pursues him in his lair, he is at first peremptory but now more often explodes in resentment. "Exactly whose income and self-discipline provides your comfortable surroundings and pays for your expensive personal psychotherapy for that matter?"

Each partner brings his or her own complicated past to the office. Janine's alcoholic father, demanded her support but gave little of his own and rarely praised her for her high grades and hard work in the family. He wanted so much from her, but what she gave never seemed enough. Janine's mother, burdened with her husband's drinking and the pressure of raising a family almost alone, needed Janine's help but had no energy or heart left over to worry about her daughter's interests. Frank's family, free of overt psychopathology, apparently raised him and his two brothers to grow up as independent agents with high self-confidence. The family was competitive and focused; failure was not a possibility in this high-achieving home. Frank felt he could only share his successes but not his doubts with his parents. He could never remember seeing either parent or his brothers cry. Frank told himself that this was unimportant, not what his family was about, but he also realized that he would have no idea of what to do if one of his family did break into tears. Needless to say, he feels equally unprepared to deal with Janine's stormy outbursts.

What a challenge for any therapist to grapple with these complicated family histories, adult personality styles, and characteristic, intense grievances. Each partner brings his or her own quota of rage and pain. Both feel blamed, helpless, angry, and demoralized. You, the therapist, can easily empathize with both husband and wife but to do so would inevitably risk alienating the diametrically opposed partner. Beginning to treat this couple seems a daunting task indeed, but our 24 authors have promised that they can meet the challenge.

Now readers, this is your final exam. What is your first move with this couple? If you called Susan Johnson, Michael Nichols and Salvador Minuchin, or Daniel Wile what would they advise? How would James Donovan translate their suggestions?

Begin with the principles of brief treatment. First scratch through the details of the presenting complaint to find the focus. Behind the details of that complaint lies the specific recurring conflict, what I call "the fight," and it is here that most of our authors focus. Carefully describe the repetitive action gone wrong. Susan Johnson counsels you to begin looking right away for the "soft" affects, the hurt and the longing, that underlie Janine's accusations and Frank's stonewalling. Michael

Nichols and Salvador Minuchin guide you to check for diffuse boundaries, possibly between Janine and one or more of her children, which freeze the conflict in place. If you're enmeshed with your child, how free are you to be involved with your spouse? Daniel Wile observes that both partners are entitled to their anger and their hurt. Begin to write a script for them to help them express these injuries.

Joseph Eron and Thomas Lund caution you to search immediately under the bubbling antagonism for each person's preferred view, to wonder with them how an effective, caring man comes to act like a cold and unsympathetic husband. How does a supportive, emotionally attuned woman come to act so bitingly critical toward a man whom she loves? We need to lead each partner back to his or her preferred adult identity. Frank sees himself as an independent problem solver. Help him define the problem he needs to solve with Janine. Janine wishes to be an empathic, team player. How can she begin to understand Frank's withdrawal and ally with him rather than berate him? Steven Friedman and Eve Lipchik urge us as therapists to look for the positive in what is already going on. Grasp it and don't let it go.

How can I or you, the therapist, respond to the heat of the anger and the hurt? How to confront the emotional intensity? Jim Donovan and Phyllis Cohen respond "Great, emotional intensity is our friend." Follow those feelings back to their source into the families of origin. Help the patient see where those emotions came from and support the individual in confronting the original, unresolved family problem. John Neal and his colleagues will guide you in relating these powerful feelings to gender role conflicts in the society at large. Frank is silent and strong like the thrice-divorced John Wayne. Janine must over-function for everyone as a prototypical 1990s, "soccer Mom." Of course the strongest feelings become involved in these basic, dominant cultural conversations. Explain this gently to each partner. Richard Vogel will help you ponder whose separation or survivor guilt may be provoking these affective storms. Frank can't betray his taciturn, powerful, idealized father and descend into "mushiness." In his mind this might kill the old man or at least Frank's internalized image of him.

Simon Budman, a 20-year veteran of working with limited mental health insurance benefits, advises you to plan your treatment carefully, with frequent meetings at the beginning, more space between sessions in the second half of the year—follow-up after January when the new benefits kick in. Daniel Wile worries less about planning. For him couple therapy is like bowling lessons, some sessions now, some later, look for cumulative results. Your couple will be a little more competent at script writing after each meeting.

Okay, reader, you learned to search for that focus and then practice your trade with the principles of brief treatment evenly held in your hand: maintaining flexibility, building the alliance, responding to emotional intensity, actively planning the treatment. You've learned much of what you need to pass your exam with distinction.

My advice to learn and practice these guidelines to time-effective treatment seems worthwhile enough, but these chapters have even more truths to divulge. Perhaps new meaning can be discovered not in the authors explicit suggestions about core techniques but in the meta-message, the paradigm shift. We can track what our writers do, but how do they think about what they do? What, probably preconscious, assumptions guided them as they worked out their models?

PARADIGM SHIFT 1: PAST, PRESENT, FUTURE

Only two of our panel, James Donovan and Phyllis Cohen, speak much about the past, and they bring it as rapidly as possible to bear on the couple's present fight. Michael Nichols and Salvador Minuchin, Steven Friedman and Eve Lipchik, James Keim, Andrew Christensen and Neil Jacobson and their colleagues, and particularly Daniel Wile, stay stubbornly in the present. How can we increase acceptance now? What positive experiences can we emphasize today? What strategic exercise fits the issues of the present visit? Rarely do any of this coterie delve into personal history. This paradigm shift, though subtle, carries great significance for the immediacy and the brevity of the treatment.

Many of our writers aren't satisfied with the present focus, however; they're interested in the future as well. Joseph Eron and Thomas Lund wouldn't care much about how Frank's ferocious temper developed. They would want to know how, according to his preferred view, will he modulate it when Janine, in tears, next bursts into his study? Erika Lawrence, Kathleen Eldridge, Andrew Christensen, and Neil Jacobson would role play with Frank and Janine picturing the next time she dissolves into self-doubt and desperately grabs for Frank's support.

PARADIGM SHIFT 2:
IN HERE VERSUS OUT THERE

The psychoanalytic paradigm focuses on the transference neurosis. What happens in the office between patient and therapist must be worked through to heal the patient. Our writers would not pass muster at any traditional psychoanalytic institute. James Donovan coaches his couples to develop "tools" to mitigate their fight at home. Daniel Wile teaches his couples to "write" and "perform" scripts to practice away from the office. Simon Budman gives homework assignments. Erica Lawrence, Kathleen Eldridge, Andrew Christensen, and Neil Jacobson prescribe behavioral exchange and problem-solving techniques to be carried out at home. The location of the action changes from here to out there, rendering the treatment more time effective.

PARADIGM SHIFT 3: THE REFRAME

Shift 1 encompasses an alteration in tense, from past to present to future. Shift 2 involves a change in location from here to there, but, as we'll see in a moment, Shift 3 implies a profound change in meaning. Behind the principles of brief therapy, lies the reframe, the art of time-managed couple work. The distressing behavior *doesn't mean what the couple is so convinced it means.* Daniel Wile encourages partners to own their anger. Of course they're jealous. Of course they feel slighted and exploited. These feelings represent simply the facts of everyday married life. Susan Johnson might demonstrate to her couples that Janine's rage doesn't mean that she despises Frank but, rather, that she's always felt emotionally abandoned, and there it just happened again. John Neal observes that of course Frank feels inadequate when he cannot buoy Janine's self-image. American men are supposed to solve everyone's problems practically and efficiently. James Donovan explains that Janine's feelings of aloneness and desertion make perfect psychological if not actual sense, given her unreliable father and preoccupied mother. Richard Vogel reframes Janine's affective storm as an expression of alliance with her downtrodden mother who could never stand up for herself.

All the paradigm shifts, but particularly the reframe, lead us closer to the core of short-term couple psychotherapy. They all point the couple before, after, behind, or above the bitter, utterly preoccupying fight that snares them. There must be a new look, and it must be an emotional one. Joseph Eron and Thomas Lund's couples must reconnect in their guts with their life-long preferred view. Daniel Wile's couples need to emotionally embrace their entitlement to anger and jealousy. Phyllis Cohen's and James Donovan's couples need to feel their emotional connection to the troubled past. Without the paradigm shifts, so different in detail from model to model, but so similar in effect, there would be no short-term couple therapy. The meetings would simply fall flat, rehashing more of the same. In treatments that do not work, the paradigm change is not embraced by the couple, and the therapy travels around in a circle to no productive end. The reframe for couple therapy represents, then, the analog of emotional insight for individual treatment. In the reframe, we discover the essence of brief couple work, no effective reframe, no effective treatment.

WHITHER COUPLE THERAPY?

Although all our authors hold certain common assumptions that we have just struggled to understand, their approaches also seem to spread across a wide conceptual and technical spectrum. If this be the current state of brief couple therapy, where in the world is this enterprise headed?

Susan Johnson (1991) has lamented that since the field lacks a unifying theory of intimacy, and thus of couple dysfunction, consistent progress in developing and studying treatment models has endured developmental delay. Ironically, she then beautifully explicates Bowlby's attachment theory and illustrates its relevance to her system of emotionally focused therapy.

Our authors have described the broadest choices in theoretical outlook from psychodynamic (Cohen and Donovan) to structural (Nichols and Minuchin) to social learning (Lawrence, Eldridge, Christensen, and Jacobson) to solution-focused (Friedman and Lipchik) to narrative (Neal, Zimmerman, and Dickerson). Given this panoply of approaches it appears that Susan Johnson is right. We don't have a unified theory of couple treatment, and there isn't one in sight.

In what direction, then, should we look for the next progress? Although the word "integrated" may now be a bit overused, new developments in our field will be solidly integrative ones. The term is not overused when referring to models that have a clear conceptual focus and combine two or perhaps three important elements from different approaches, all of which the writer really understands. Simon Budman solidly grasps Prochaska's stages of change model and his own systemic approach so he can artfully combine the two.

Our theorists have already begun to combine one model with another, with exciting results. In this book we see examples of solid, creative, integrative approaches. Andrew Christensen and Neil Jacobson, the integrative behaviorists, have performed true to their name—radically altering their social exchange thinking by combining it with something akin to Daniel Wile's acceptance approach to fashion their integrative behavioral couple therapy system. Joseph Eron and Thomas Lund have deftly melded strategic, narrative, and solution-focused work. Steven Friedman and Eve Lipchik have effected the same combination less explicitly. Phyllis Cohen presents a cross-fertilization of systemic and dynamic approaches, and her mentor Gerson (1996) is hard at work on the same project. Who will be next?

Richard Vogel emphasizes the need to master unconscious separation and survivor guilt. This orientation could easily be folded into any dynamic model such as Johnson's, Donovan's, or Cohen's. Simon Budman's systemic-dynamic approach, so broad in scope and pragmatically oriented, could easily encompass narrative or solution-focused methods within it. In other words, the arc of distinct approaches is compacting toward the center. More and more models will be used to augment one another, and most of the new systems we will see probably will be combinations of their forebearers.

I think we will also encounter greater testing of well-established approaches. Neil Jacobson's original behavioral model has been the most rigorously studied couple treatment ever. Some 30 projects have examined it both in the United States and abroad. Johnson and colleagues have begun to systematically study emotionally focused treatment as well. These two camps are so enthusiastic about process and outcome research that they will certainly contribute many further reports evaluating at least their two major models. This scholarly activity may be contagious as other authors catch the spirit and begin testing their approaches as well. Susan Johnson and the Christensen–Jacobson group have also already built upon their research findings to publish treatment manuals for their respective approaches. However, because the narrative and solution-focused people remain staunchly "anti-normative" and "anti-linear," we may never see them submit their systems to "scientific" review or manualization. Yet courageous outside researchers might venture into this territory.

Although graduate educational programs remain notoriously slow to teach the methods forced upon the practicing clinician by the real world, in the future we will encounter, to our surprise perhaps, courses on couple therapy becoming a major part of doctoral and internship training. The needs of the public will simply exert too much pressure in this direction to be denied.

Couple therapy is here to stay. In 50 years, we will see many more well-known, well-studied and appropriately applied models of time-effective couple work. This statement could not have been responsibly made perhaps even 10 years ago. Widespread clinical practice, cross-fertilization of models, evaluation research, publication of treatment manuals, inclusion in graduate training—it looks like the beginning of a consolidation phase to me. This book hopefully contributes to the dawning of that phase, first by presenting the spectrum of models currently available and second by supplying perspective on the commonalities and points of contrast between those models. The bullet train of couple treatment is picking up speed. We've enjoyed our role as guide for this section of the trip, and we hope you have enjoyed the tour as well.

REFERENCES

Gerson, M. J. (1996). *The embedded self*. Hillsdale, NJ: Analytic Press.
Johnson, S. M. (1991). Marital therapy: Issues and challenges. *Journal of Psychiatric Neuroscience, 16,* 176–181.

INDEX